ULTRASOUND
SCANNING

ULTRASOUND SCANNING

PRINCIPLES AND PROTOCOLS

SECOND EDITION

Betty Bates Tempkin, BA, RT(R), RDMS

Ultrasound Consultant
Formerly Clinical Director of the Diagnostic Medical Sonography Program,
Hillsborough Community College, Tampa, Florida

W.B. SAUNDERS COMPANY
A Harcourt Health Sciences Company
Philadelphia ■ London ■ New York ■ St. Louis ■ Sydney ■ Toronto

W.B. SAUNDERS COMPANY
A Harcourt Health Sciences Company

The Curtis Center
Independence Square West
Philadelphia, Pennsylvania 19106

Library of Congress Cataloging-in-Publication Data

Tempkin, Betty Bates.
    Ultrasound scanning: principles and protocols / B.B. Tempkin.—
2nd ed.
      p.   cm.
    Includes index.
    ISBN 0–7216–6879–8
    1. Diagnosis, Ultrasonic.   I. Title.
    [DNLM: 1. Ultrasonography—methods. 2. Ultrasonography—
standards. 3. Clinical Protocols—standards. WN 208 T283u 1999]
RC78.7.U4T46 1999
616.07′543—dc21
DNLM/DLC   97-44164

Ultrasound Scanning: Principles and Protocols   ISBN 0–7216–6879–8

Printed in the United States of America

Last digit is the print number: 9   8   7   6   5   4   3

To Max

Contributors

Kristen Dykstra-Downey, AAS, RT(R), RDMS
Staff Sonographer
Women's Hospital
St. Petersburg, Florida
Formerly Director of the Diagnostic Medical
Sonography Program
Hillsborough Community College
Tampa, Florida

Neonatal Brain Scanning Protocol

Felicia M. Jones, AS, BS, RVT, RDMS
Director, Ultrasound Program
Tidewater Community College
Virginia Beach, Virginia

Breast Scanning Protocol

Wayne C. Leonhardt, BA, RT(R), RVT, RDMS
Faculty
Foothill College School of Ultrasound
Los Altos, California
Staff Sonographer, Technical Director, and
Continuing Education Director
Summit Medical Center
Oakland, California

*Scrotum Scanning Protocol; Thyroid and Parathyroid
Glands Scanning Protocols*

Maureen E. McDonald, BS, RDMS, RDCS
Staff Echocardiographer and Adult Echocardiography
Instructor and Lecturer
Thomas Jefferson University Hospital
Philadelphia, Pennsylvania

Adult Echocardiography Scanning Protocol;
Pediatric Echocardiography Scanning Protocol

Marsha M. Neumyer, BS, RVT
Assistant Professor of General and Vascular Surgery and
Director of the Vascular Studies Section
The Milton S. Hershey Medical Center
Pennsylvania State University College of Medicine
Hershey, Pennsylvania

Abdominal Doppler and Color Flow;
Cerebrovascular Duplex Scanning Protocol;
Peripheral Arterial and Venous Duplex Scanning Protocols

G. William Shepherd, PhD, RVT, RDMS
Clinical Instructor
Ultrasound Research and Educational Institute
Thomas Jefferson University
Philadelphia, Pennsylvania

Obstetrical Scanning Protocol

B. B. Tempkin, BA, RT(R), RDMS
Ultrasound Consultant
Formerly Clinical Director of the Diagnostic Medical
Sonography Program
Hillsborough Community College
Tampa, Florida

Scanning Planes and Scanning Methods; Pathology
Scanning Protocol; Abdominal Aorta Scanning Protocol;
Inferior Vena Cava Scanning Protocol; Liver Scanning
Protocol; Gallbladder and Biliary Tract Scanning Protocol;
Pancreas Scanning Protocol; Renal Scanning Protocol;
Spleen Scanning Protocol; Scanning Protocols for Full and
Limited Studies of the Abdomen; Female Pelvis Scanning
Protocol; Obstetrical Scanning Protocol; Male Pelvis
Scanning Protocol; Scrotum Scanning Protocol; Thyroid
and Parathyroid Glands Scanning Protocols; Breast
Scanning Protocol

Deborah D. Werneburg, MBA, BS, RDMS
Manager of Managed Care and Finance
Family Health Alliance
Columbus, Ohio
Formerly Technical Coordinator
Ultrasound Research & Educational Institute
Thomas Jefferson University
Philadelphia, Pennsylvania

Female Pelvis Scanning Protocol

Preface

Ultrasound Scanning Principles and Protocols came about as a result of my teaching, and practical scanning experience.

During my seventeen years as a sonographer—most of which I have spent as a clinical director and teaching in scanning labs as well as the hospital setting—I realized that sonographers needed a basic approach to the performance of scans, a pattern as well as a benchmark for their work. My purpose in writing this text is to provide a step-by-step method for scanning and image documentation for physician diagnostic interpretation. I hope this "how to" scanning approach takes the struggle out of scanning and ensures thoroughness and accuracy. Scanning principles and specific instructions on how to scan and document images is provided to improve the quality of sonographic studies and establish standardization.

The structure of this text should make it easy to read, simple to follow, and practical to use. The text begins with an introduction that includes topics such as the purpose and general use of the text, scanning standards to adopt, and criteria for professionalism and clinical skills. Requisites for handling ultrasound equipment, film labeling, image technique, and film-case presentation are also discussed. The text proceeds with technical parameters that include scanning planes and their anatomical interpretations and scanning methods. Prior to the protocol chapters a universal method for scanning and documenting pathologies is provided. Next, the protocol chapters proffer scanning protocols for the major blood vessels and organs of the abdomen, the male and female pelvic organs, and obstetrics. Protocols for the scrotum, thyroid gland, breast, and neonatal brain are also included.

The protocol chapters conclude with protocols for vascular and cardiac studies. Applicable protocols are patterned after the American Institute of Ultrasound in Medicine's scanning guidelines which, along with an abbreviation glossary are included in the appendices of the text.

The scanning protocol chapters selectively address organ, vasculature, or fetal location, as well as, anatomy, physiology, sonographic appearance, and normal variations. In addition, patient preparation, position, and breathing techniques are discussed. Steps are specified for transducer placement, surveys, and required images. Other features to assist the reader are illustrations for anatomy, patient positions, the placement, position, and direction to move the transducer, and, illustrations of every ultrasound image.

What's new. This edition exclusively includes updates for the universal pathology protocol, and several of the abdominal protocols. A new abdominal chapter has been added to provide protocols for full and limited studies. Also, some authors who contributed to *Ultrasonography An Introduction To Normal Structure and Functional Anatomy, Curry and Tempkin, WB Saunders, 1995,* also contributed to this edition with chapter updates on the female pelvis, obstetrics, the scrotum, the thyroid and parathyroid glands. The vascular protocols chapter has been completely revised by a new contributor, and for the first time, scanning protocols for echocardiography have been added. Further, for this edition, the illustrations accompanying each ultrasound image have been "colored" to match the gray scale of the image thus making anatomical interpretations easier. Moreover, image quality has been significantly improved through digital reproduction. The updates, revision, new chapters, and improved illustrations and images make this edition up-to-date and comprehensive.

Since the scanning methods represent our personal scanning and teaching experiences, most chapters highlight the methods that we have found to work best. However, scanning is dependent on the individual performing it, thus finding one's personal approaches to solving imaging problems is not only expected but unavoidable. Therefore, in addition to our personal way of doing things, we discuss some alternatives and encourage you to explore other approaches.

The text reflects the assumption that the reader has thorough knowledge of gross and sectional anatomy. An in-depth course in normal anatomy and sectional anatomy are key prerequisites for comprehending scanning techniques. As an overview, gross anatomy and reference illustrations are at the beginning of most protocol chapters.

The sonographer's role in medicine is unique from those of other allied health professionals specializing in imaging modalities because sonographic image quality is directly proportional to the skill of the operator. That single reason is enough to support the fact that scanning skills must equal the level of importance attached to a sonographer's knowledge of physics, physiology, pathology, and anatomy. Currently, practical considerations prevent the American Registry of Diagnostic Medical Sonography from evaluating scanning ability. Therefore, feedback from sonography educators and sonologists and comparison of films to established guidelines and scanning protocols is vital to mastering the art of ultrasound scanning. When performed at the highest level, the collective factors that define "sonographer" become an integral part of patient evaluation. It is my hope that this text directly contributes to the achievement of excellence in the daily practice of ultrasound.

B.B. Tempkin, BA, RT(R), RDMS

Acknowledgments

It is with much pleasure that I have the opportunity to thank Jim Bowie, MD, Carol Mittelstaedt, MD, Magdalena Pogonowska, MD, Bert Newmark, MD, and Marie Mandelstamm, MD, for being instrumental in my sonography career.

Many thanks to the contributing authors. I had no idea my publishing experiences would introduce me to so many dedicated, charming, and talented individuals.

I greatly appreciate the efforts of the people whose help I could not have done without: the many that volunteered to be scanned, those that contributed images, and Kay Johnson with Dupont Film.

A special acknowledgment to the American Institute of Ultrasound in Medicine and Kathleen M. Wilson, Director of Publications for agreeing to include the AIUM's guidelines in the text. This collaboration has greatly benefitted the reader and ultimately the ultrasound community.

I am grateful to the late Earle Pitts for his artistic coordination of the first edition. For this edition, my highest regards go to Marsha Jessup for her artistic direction, expertise, and astuteness. Many thanks to Marsha and her media department staff at the Robert Wood Johnson Medical School for their exceptional artistic renderings.

Tremendous thanks to my original editor, Lisa Biello and the coordinated efforts of Helaine Barron and the excellent staff at WB Saunders.

And finally, I am much obliged to my dear parents for their support and interest and to David whose enthusiasm and unique style are perpetually stimulating!

B.B.T.

Contents

General Principles

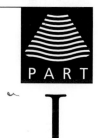

Overview

PURPOSE

The purpose of this text is to:

- Provide scanning criteria and standardization of image documentation for physician interpretation.
- Provide instructional information on how to scan.
- Clarify the anatomical directions and interpretations of ultrasound scanning planes.
- Provide step-by-step, "how-to" instructions for surveys.
- Provide examples of image documentation for sonographic studies.
- Provide applicable scanning protocols that are patterned after the American Institute of Ultrasound in Medicine's suggested guidelines (provided in the appendix).

GENERAL USE

How to use this text:

- Follow scanning protocols as you would a recipe. Specific survey steps and examples of the images to document are provided.
- Know gross anatomy. Structures are accurately identified on ultrasound images by their location, not their sonographic appearance since it may be altered by pathology or other factors. An in-depth course in gross and sectional anatomy should be a prerequisite to this text. Only as a reference, most chapters include brief sections on anatomy and physiology.
- Refer to the universal scanning protocol for documenting pathology. An abnormality does not need to be diagnosed to accurately document it for physician interpretation.
- Study the illustrations that accompany the steps of each survey. Become familiar with different patient positions and with the location, position, and direction to move the transducer. Practice on yourself (with the machine off) or

1

on scanning dummies to become comfortable with the subtle manipulations of the transducer.

- Familiarize yourself with the sonographic appearance of body structures and the terms used to describe them:

  (a) **Gray Scale:** display mode in which echo intensity is recorded as degrees of brightness or shades of gray.

  (b) **Echogenic:** capable of producing echoes. Correlate with the terms hyperechoic, hypoechoic, and anechoic which refer to the quantity of echoes produced.

  (c) **Anechoic:** an echo-free appearance on a sonographic image. The normal urine-filled urinary bladder and the normal bile-filled gallbladder are described as having anechoic lumens on sonographic images. The sound waves pass through anechoic structures because there is not enough density to attenuate or stop the beam.

  (d) **Hyperechoic:** descriptive term used to describe echoes that are brighter than normal or brighter than adjacent structures. In some cases, normal kidney parenchyma may be hyperechoic compared to the normal liver.

  (e) **Hypoechoic** and **Echopenic:** descriptive terms used to describe echoes that are not as bright as normal or less bright than adjacent structures. In some cases, the normal pancreas may be described as hypoechoic compared to the normal liver.

  (f) **Isoechoic** and **Isosonic:** descriptive terms used to describe structures with the same relative echo density. In some cases, the liver and pancreas may be described as isosonic.

  (g) **Heterogeneous:** refers to an uneven echo pattern or reflections of varying echodensities. The sonographic appearance of normal kidneys is heterogeneous because of the variation in density between the renal parenchyma and the renal sinus.

  (h) **Homogeneous:** refers to an even echo pattern or reflections that are relative and uniform in composition. The sonographic appearance of normal renal parenchyma, the normal liver, the normal urine-filled bladder, and uterine myometrium can be described as homogeneous with ranges in echogenicity. The normal liver, for example, may be described as homogeneous and moderately echogenic.

- Note that in the scanning protocol chapters, the bold-faced words under the headings Patient Position, Transducer, and Breathing Technique are the preferred option.

STANDARDS

Guidelines to follow:

- Perform thorough, methodical surveys of structures in at least two scanning planes prior to image documentation. The survey is the most important element of an ultrasound study. It is a time of evaluation and determination.
- Use surveys to:
  (a) determine the best technique to optimally image a structure.
  (b) determine the best patient position and breathing technique to ultimately give the best representation of a structure.
  (c) rule out pathology.
  (d) rule out normal variants.
- Operator-dependent, real-time scanning makes it impractical to take ultrasound images every one or two centimeters through a structure. Therefore, fewer representative images are given to the physician for diagnostic interpretation. The images are a small representation of the whole; a small sample that must accurately represent the determinations made during the survey.
- Documented areas of interest must be represented in at least two scanning planes. Single plane representation of a structure is not enough confirmation.
- Documented areas of interest must be imaged in a logical sequence. Follow imaging protocol examples.
- Use up-to-date, calibrated, ultrasound machinery.
- **Never give patients a diagnosis. Only physicians can give a legal diagnostic impression.**
- Always practice professional and courteous behavior with patients. Put them at ease and make them as comfortable as possible.

PROFESSIONALISM

Standards to set:

- Introduce yourself to patients.
- Practice courteous and respectful interaction with patients and staff.
- Remember that the patient is paying for your service.
- Conversations with patients should be proper and professional.
- Dress appropriately and wear an identification badge.
- **Unless you are a physician, do not give a diagnosis.**

CLINICAL SKILLS

Criteria to follow:

- Briefly explain the examination to the patient.
- Instruct the patient in a slow, clear, and appropriate manner.
- Make sure you have the correct patient. Check identification bracelets (or patient numbers) against patient charts.
- When required, assist the patient in dressing in a gown.
- Assist the patient with any medical equipment attached to him or her.
- Assist the patient onto the examination table. Drape the patient properly for the exam and make sure he or she is as comfortable as possible.
- Handle medical equipment attached to the patient and ultrasound equipment in a safe manner.
- Be familiar with sterile procedures.
- Be familiar with procedures to assist physicians with special studies.

EQUIPMENT

Criteria for proper use of ultrasound machinery:

- Begin with a transducer best suited to the structure(s) of interest.
- Attach and detach transducers with ease.
- Use a coupling agent such as gel to remove the air between the transducer and the surface of the patient's skin.
- Be familiar with key controls to expedite the study and produce interpretable images.
- Ready films and/or tapes for exposure. Make sure labeling is up-to-date and accurate.

FILM LABELING

The following information **must** be included on films and/or tapes:

- Patient's name
- Patient's identification number
- Date and time
- Scanning site (name of hospital or private office)
- Name or initials of the person scanning

N O T E : Endocavital studies should be witnessed by another health professional and his or her name or initials should be labeled on the film or tape.

- Transducer megahertz
- Area of interest: general area and specific area
  example: Aorta is the general area and the proximal aorta is the specific area
- Patient position
- Scanning plane

N O T E : Film labeling should be confined to the margins surrounding the image. Never label over the image unless you take the very same image again without any labels. Labels could cover important diagnostic information for the interpreting physician.

TECHNIQUE

The following criteria should be optimal:

- Select the correct transducer megahertz for the area of interest.
- Adjust the field size to best view the area of interest.
- Focus near- and far-gain settings to enhance visualization of the area of interest.
- Set contrast to delineate structures well from one another.
- Adjust gain settings so borders are well defined.
- Power settings should be low. Compensate with adjusted TGC (time-gain compensation) slope.
- Avoid areas of fade-out whenever possible. Try increasing or adjusting the TGC slope or switch to a more powerful transducer.
- **Document accurate images for diagnostic interpretation.**

FILM CASE PRESENTATION

The appropriate method of presenting films to the radiologist/sonologist is to:

- State the exam and reason for it.
- Present patient history.
- Present patient lab data and other known correlative data such as reports and films from other imaging modalities.
- Present the films in a logical sequence (follow the sequence in which the images were documented).
- Be able to discuss and justify techniques and procedures used.
- Be able to discuss related anatomy and any abnormal findings.

N O T E : Never give or put in writing a clinical impression that includes a diagnosis unless you are a physician.
Abnormal findings should be described according to location, size, and composition.

Scanning Planes and Scanning Methods

PU

The purpose of this chapter is to:

- Explain the way ultrasound uses body or scanning planes to image the body.
- Define scanning planes and show how they divide the body.
- Define the anatomic areas of each scanning plane.
- Provide scanning techniques and methods.
- Define patient positions.
- Provide surface landmarks used as scanning references.

STANDARDS

Criteria to follow when scanning:

- Know the two-dimensional anatomic areas appreciated on each scanning plane.
- Use proper scanning methods.
- Be familiar with the surface landmarks used as scanning references.
- Follow the survey steps and take the required images recommended in the scanning protocol chapters.

SCANNING PLANES

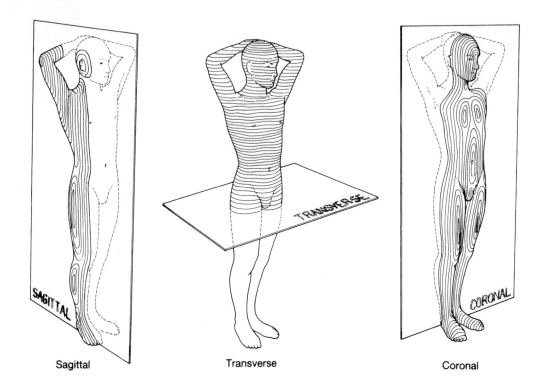

Sagittal   Transverse   Coronal

- Scanning planes include sagittal planes, transverse planes, and coronal planes.
  - (a) Sagittal Planes: divide the body into unequal right and left sections.
  - (b) Transverse Planes: divide the body into unequal superior and inferior sections.
  - (c) Coronal Planes: divide the body into unequal anterior and posterior sections.
- Scanning planes are used to establish the direction that the ultrasound beam enters the body and the anatomic portion of anatomy being visualized from that particular direction.
- Scanning planes are two dimensional.

SAGITTAL SCANNING PLANE

Anatomic areas seen on a sagittal scan:

- Anterior or posterior approach:
  - (a) Anterior   (c) Superior
  - (b) Posterior   (d) Inferior

N O T E : Right and left lateral are *not* seen on a sagittal scan; therefore, the transducer must be moved to either the right or left of a sagittal plane to visualize adjacent anatomy.

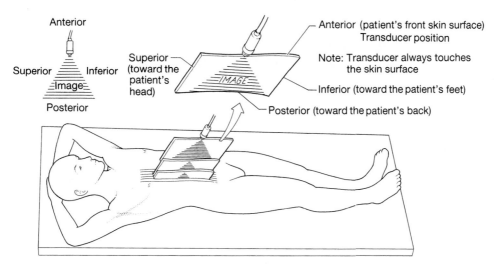

Sagittal scan from an anterior approach.

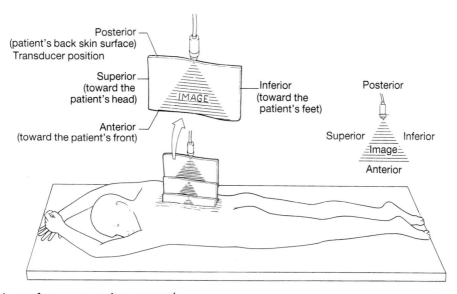

Sagittal scan from a posterior approach.

TRANSVERSE SCANNING PLANE

Anatomic areas seen on a transverse scan:

- Anterior or posterior approach:
    - (a) Anterior
    - (b) Posterior
    - (c) Right Lateral
    - (d) Left Lateral
- Right or left lateral approach:
    - (a) Lateral (right or left)
    - (b) Medial
    - (c) Anterior
    - (d) Posterior

N O T E :   Superior and inferior are *not* seen on a transverse scan; therefore, the transducer must be moved either superiorly or inferiorly from a transverse plane to visualize adjacent anatomy.

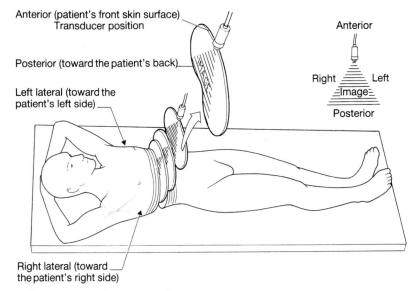

Transverse scan from an anterior approach.

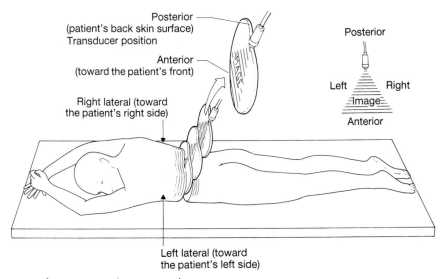

Transverse scan from a posterior approach.

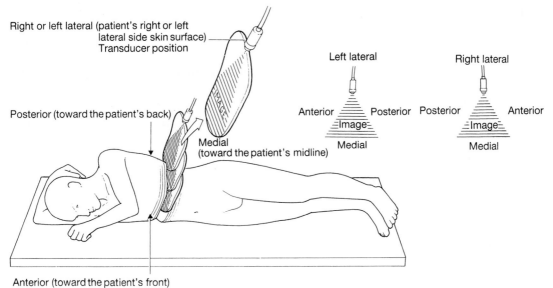

Transverse scan from a lateral approach.

CORONAL SCANNING PLANE

Anatomic areas seen on a coronal scan:

- Right or left lateral approach:
    - (a) Lateral (right or left)
    - (b) Medial
    - (c) Superior
    - (d) Inferior

N O T E :   Anterior and posterior are *not* seen on a coronal scan; therefore, the transducer must be moved either anteriorly or posteriorly from a coronal plane to visualize adjacent anatomy.

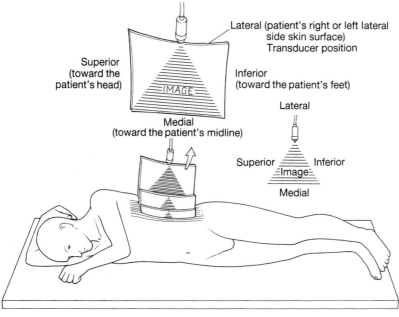

Coronal scan from a lateral approach.

SCANNING METHODS

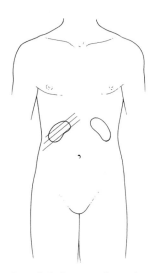

Criteria to follow when scanning:

- Always use a scanning couplant, such as scanning gel, to reduce the air between the transducer and surface of the skin.
- Scan according to the lie of the organ. Scanning plane may therefore be oblique.
- To better evaluate a structure, slightly rock-and-slide the transducer while scanning.

By slightly rotating the transducer, oblique sagittal planes are used to visualize the lie or longitudinal views of the kidney.

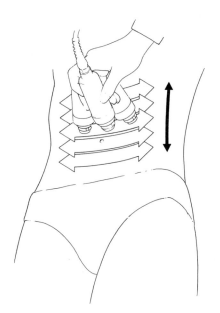

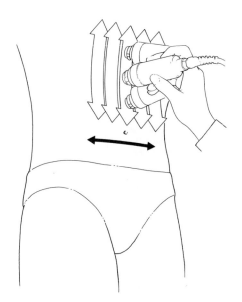

While scanning in a sagittal plane, slightly rock the transducer right and left while slowly sliding the transducer superiorly and inferiorly.

While scanning in a transverse plane, slightly rock the transducer superiorly and inferiorly while slowly sliding the transducer laterally.

• Different transducer positions are used according to the area of interest being evaluated.

    (a) Perpendicular: the transducer is straight up and down to the scanning surface.

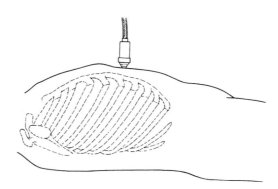

    (b) Angled: the transducer is angled superiorly, inferiorly, or right and left laterally at varying degrees.

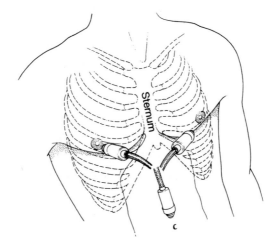

(c) Subcostal: the transducer is angled superiorly just beneath the inferior costal margin.

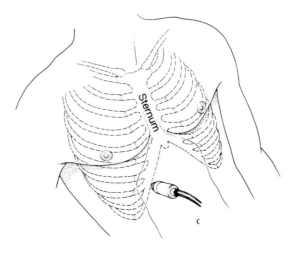

(d) Intercostal: the transducer is positioned between the
ribs; it can be perpendicular, angled, or subcostal.

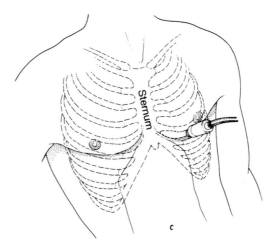

(e) Rotated: the transducer is rotated varying degrees to
oblique the scanning plane.

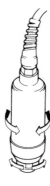

- To accurately measure structures, find the long axis or longest length. The long axis of a structure can be seen in any scanning plane depending on how that structure lies in the body. For example:
  (a) The abdominal aorta lies superior to inferior in the body; therefore, its long axis can be viewed from a sagital or coronal plane approach:

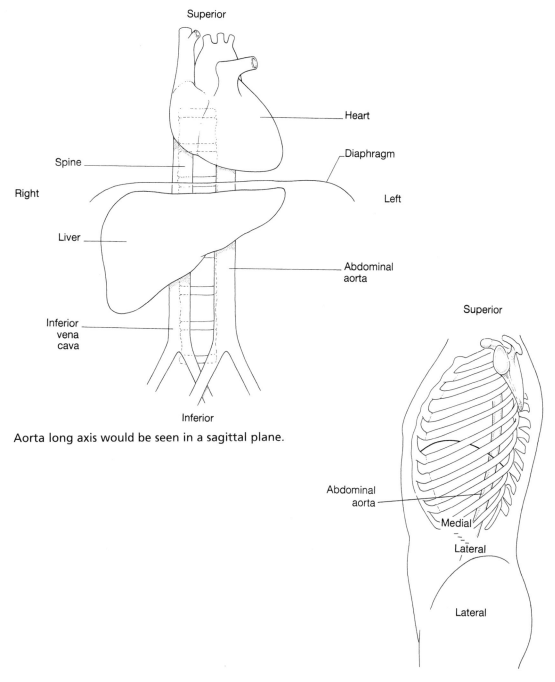

Aorta long axis would be seen in a sagittal plane.

Aorta long axis would be seen in a coronal plane.

(b) The gallbladder lie is variable in the body. The gallbladder can lie superior to inferior or laterally.

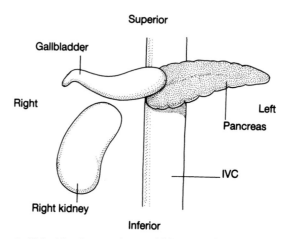

Gallbladder long axis would be seen in a transverse plane.

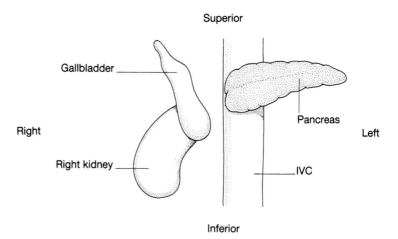

Gallbladder long axis would be seen in a sagittal plane.

Superior

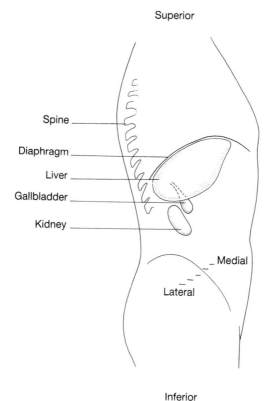

Inferior

Gallbladder long axis would be seen in a coronal plane.

- Different patient positions are used depending on the area of interest being evaluated.
  (a) Supine: the patient lies on his or her back.
  (b) Prone: the patient lies on his or her front.
  (c) Sitting: erect or semi-erect.
  (d) Right lateral decubitus (RLD): the patient lies on his or her right side with the left arm up over the head.
  (e) Left lateral decubitus (LLD): the patient lies on his or her left side with the right arm up over the head.
  (f) Right posterior oblique (RPO): The patient lies on his or her back with the right side of the body elevated at a 45-degree angle.
  (g) Left posterior oblique (LPO): the patient lies on his or her back with the left side of the body elevated at a 45-degree angle.

N O T E :   The best patient position should be determined during the survey of a structure and should not be changed while taking images of that structure. Occasionally patient position must be changed during imaging because of gas obliteration, etc. If this occurs then the required images must be retaken from the beginning of the series.

• Use the following surface landmarks as references when scanning.

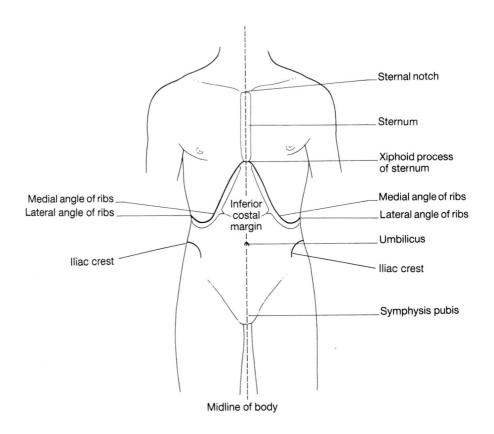

Pathology Scanning Protocol

CHAPTER

2

The purpose of this chapter is to:

- Provide a universal scanning protocol for evaluating and documenting pathology no matter the type.
- Provide the criteria to accurately describe the sonographic findings of a structure without giving a diagnosis.
- Support the legal premise that only physicians can give a diagnostic interpretation of a study.
- Support the fact that sonographers must possess the knowledge about pathologies, how they interact with different body systems, and their typical sonographic presentations.

STANDARDS

Criteria to follow when scanning and documenting abnormal findings:

- Abnormalities must be surveyed in at least two scanning planes *following* the survey of the area(s) of interest. This is not to say that the abnormality is not evaluated as the area of interest is evaluated, but it ensures that a total evaluation is made of a structure, not just its abnormal part.
- Image documentation must be in at least two scanning planes. Single-plane representation of an abnormality is not enough confirmation.
- Image documentation must include volume measurements of the abnormality.
- Image documentation must include views of the abnormality with high- and low-gain settings in at least two scanning planes.
- Abnormal findings should be described according to location, size, and composition.
- **Only physicians can give a legal diagnostic impression.**

19

DESCRIBING PATHOLOGY

Criteria for describing the sonographic findings of an abnormal structure:

- Location
  - (a) Described by the organ or structure that the abnormality is located in or originates from.

    example: ...the mass lies within the tail of the pancreas, just anterior to the left kidney, slightly indenting the abdominal aorta...

  - (b) Described by structures immediately adjacent to the abnormality.

    example: ...the mass is superior to the iliac arteries, inferior to the superior mesenteric artery, and posterior to the splenic vein and a portion of the body of the pancreas....

- Size
  - (a) Measurements of the abnormality must be taken in at least two scanning planes to obtain a volume measurement.
  - (b) Depending on the scanning approach (the direction the sound beam enters the body), measurements are described as:
    - (1) anterior to posterior, posterior to anterior, front to back, back to front, or thickness.
    - (2) lateral to lateral, lateral to medial, side to side, or width.
    - (3) superior to inferior, longitudinal, or length.
    - (4) long axis (longest length).

    example: ...its superior to inferior measurement is 4 cm, it measures 3 cm anterior to posterior, and it is 3 cm wide...

- Composition

Although a sonographic image cannot definitively distinguish between malignant and benign masses, it can determine the composition of an abnormality. Because most pathologies—benign or malignant—have specific sonographic compositions, a high percentage of correct diagnoses are made prior to biopsies or surgery. It is standard in sonography to confirm the composition of an abnormality by providing the interpreting physician with images of the abnormality at high- and low-gain technical settings. This technical range should demonstrate any variations in echodensities. Pathology has the following classic sonographic presentations:

(a) Solid masses:
   (1) Can appear isosonic to the organ parenchyma that it is part of, distinguishable only by its walls.
   (2) Can exhibit homogeneous, hyperechoic, hypoechoic, echopenic, or anechoic echo textures.
   (3) Can exhibit heterogeneous echo texture when it is composed of varying echodensities.
   (4) Other considerations that effect the degree of echogenicity of solid or soft tissue masses are vascular, interstitial, and collagen components, and the presence of any degeneration.
   (5) If calculi are present, they can be identified by posterior shadowing occurring from increased attenuation of the sound beam.
   (6) In some cases, walls are poorly defined and irregular.
(b) Cystic masses:
   (1) Appear anechoic with posterior through transmission or increased echo amplitude (acoustic enhancement artifact).
   (2) In most cases, walls are well defined and smooth.
   (3) In some cases, septations may be present.
(c) Complex masses:
   (1) Comprises cystic and solid portions; it is echogenic and anechoic.
   (2) Wall appearance is variable. Walls can appear poorly or well defined, and irregular or smooth.

REQUIRED IMAGES

N O T E :   The required images of pathology should always follow the images documenting the normal structures of the study.

1. Longitudinal image of the abnormality with *measurement from the most superior to most inferior margin.*

   L A B E L E D :   "ORGAN" or "SITE LOCATION" and "SCANNING PLANE"

N O T E :   In cases where the origin of an abnormality cannot be determined, adjacent structures must be noted for a site location. Look for echogenic interfaces where fat separates adjacent structures.

2. Same image and labeling as number 1, without measurement calipers.

N O T E :   Use the very same "frozen" image, just remove the measurement calipers because they could possibly obscure diagnostic information for the interpreting physician.

3. Transverse image with *measurements from the most anterior to most posterior margin and from the most lateral to lateral or lateral to medial margin.*

L A B E L E D :   "ORGAN" or "SITE LOCATION" and "SCAN-NING PLANE"

4. Same image and labeling as number 3, without measurement calipers.

5. Longitudinal image with high gain technique.

L A B E L E D :   "ORGAN" or "SITE LOCATION," "SCAN-NING PLANE," "HIGH GAIN"

6. Transverse image with high gain technique.

L A B E L E D :   "ORGAN" or "SITE LOCATION," "SCAN-NING PLANE," "HIGH GAIN"

7. Longitudinal image with low gain technique.

L A B E L E D :   "ORGAN" or "SITE LOCATION," "SCAN-NING PLANE," "LOW GAIN"

8. Transverse image with low gain technique.

L A B E L E D :   "ORGAN" or "SITE LOCATION," "SCAN-NING PLANE," "LOW GAIN"

N O T E :   Depending on the size and complexity, additional images may be necessary to document the extent of the pathology. These extra views must also be confirmed in at least two scanning planes.

Abdominal Scanning Protocols

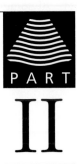

PART

II

Overview

STANDARDS

- No single-organ examinations whenever possible.
- Protocols provide specific survey steps with "how-to" illustrations.
- Protocols provide image specifications.
- Patient care and safety are always a priority.
- Use good clinical skills and always practice professional behavior.
- **Only physicians can give a legal diagnostic impression.**
- **Only physicians can give a diagnosis.**

SURVEY

- The area(s) of interest in the abdomen are completely evaluated in at least two scanning planes.
- Surveys are used to set correct imaging techniques, to rule out pathologies, and to recognize any normal variants.
- Surveys provided for the abdomen are per organ or structure. Combined, they comprise a complete abdominal survey. Typically, full abdominal surveys begin with the aorta, followed by the inferior vena cava and the liver, and then the rest of the abdominal organs and associated structures. Only if they are well visualized, survey the aorta along the

left lobe of the liver and the inferior vena cava with the right lobe, followed by the rest of the abdominal organs and associated structures.

- If an abnormality is identified, it is surveyed in at least two scanning planes *following* the completed survey of the abdominal organ(s) or structures of interest. Refer to Chapter 2 for specifics on how to survey pathology.
- Images are not taken during a survey.

IMAGE DOCUMENTATION

- Images are taken following the completed survey.
- As with the survey, documented areas of interest must be represented in at least two scanning planes. Single-plane representation is not enough confirmation.
- Documented areas of interest must be done in a logical sequence. Follow imaging protocol examples.
- After an abnormality is identified and surveyed, it must be documented in at least two scanning planes *following* the completed survey and completed images of the abdominal organs and related structures even if the abnormality is demonstrated on the standard set of required images. Refer to Chapter 2 for specifics on how to document pathology.

OTHER CONSIDERATIONS

- Patient comfort and the amount of transducer pressure on the skin is an important consideration. Experiment using different amounts of transducer pressure on the skin surface. More often than not, beginning sonographers can usually apply more pressure than they realize and in turn improve image quality. However, always make sure the patient is comfortable.
- Echo textures of abdominal organ parenchyma should be homogeneous with ranges in echogenicity. Note that parenchymal patterns change with disease processes.
- Normal sonographic patterns in the abdomen:
  (a) Organ parenchyma, muscles, and tissues: homogeneous echo textures.
  (b) Fluid-filled structures such as blood vessels, ducts, gallbladder, and urinary bladder: anechoic lumens with hyperechoic walls.

(c) Gastrointestinal tract: presentation varies depending on content. Walls are usually hypoechoic to surrounding structures. Lumens can present as highly reflective areas filled with gas or air, or have a heterogeneous appearance from a combination of fluid and gas or air, or as a fluid-filled, homogeneous, anechoic presentation (in this case, walls are hyperechoic to the fluid).

(d) Bone: highly reflective echoes, hyperechoic to adjacent structures.

(e) Fat: highly reflective echoes, hyperechoic to adjacent structures.

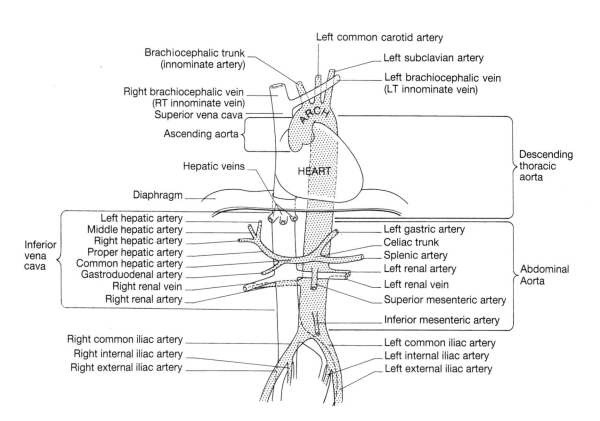

Location and anatomy of the aorta

Abdominal Aorta Scanning Protocol

LOCATION

- The abdominal aorta originates at the left ventricle.
- Ascends posterior to the pulmonary artery.
- Arches to the left.
- Descends (thoracic aorta) posterior to the diaphragm into the retroperitoneum of the abdominal cavity (abdominal aorta).
- Descends anterior to the spine to the left of the inferior vena cava.
- Bifurcates into the common iliac arteries anterior to the body of the fourth lumbar vertebra.

ANATOMY

- Consists of three muscle layers:
  - (a) Intima (innermost).
  - (b) Media (middle layer).
  - (c) Adventitia (outer).
- Largest artery in the body.
- Branches:
  - (a) Celiac trunk (branches into the left gastric artery, hepatic artery, and splenic artery).
  - (b) Superior mesenteric artery (SMA).
  - (c) Inferior mesenteric artery (IMA).
  - (d) Renal arteries.
- Size is normal up to 3 cm in diameter gradually tapering toward the bifurcation.
- Can be very tortuous.

PHYSIOLOGY

- Supplies the organs, bones, and connective structures of the body with oxygen and nutrient-rich blood.

SONOGRAPHIC APPEARANCE

- Echogenic muscular walls.
- Anechoic, echo-free lumen.

PATIENT PREP

- Fasting for at least 8 hours.
- If the patient has eaten, still attempt the examination.

PATIENT POSITION

- **Supine, right lateral decubitus.**
- Left lateral decubitus, left posterior oblique, right posterior oblique, or sitting semierect to erect as needed.

N O T E :   Different patient positions should be used whenever the suggested position does not give the desired results.

TRANSDUCER

- **3.0 MHz or 3.5 MHz.**
- 5.0 MHz for thin patients.

BREATHING TECHNIQUE

- **Normal respiration.**
- Deep, held respiration.

N O T E :   Different breathing techniques should be used whenever the suggested breathing technique does not give the desired results.

AORTA SURVEY

N O T E :   While surveying the aorta, evaluate the periaortic regions for adenopathy.

☰ LONGITUDINAL SURVEY

Sagittal Plane • Anterior Approach

1. Begin with the transducer perpendicular, at the midline of the body, just inferior to the xiphoid process of the sternum.

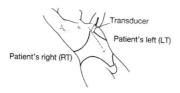

2. Move or angle the transducer to the patient's right and identify the distal IVC posterior to the liver.

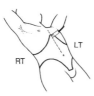

3. Move or angle the transducer to the patient's left and identify the proximal aorta posterior to the liver.

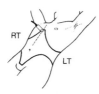

4. While viewing the proximal aorta, slowly move inferiorly, using a rock-and-slide motion. Slightly rock right to left to scan through each side of the aorta while sliding inferiorly. It may be necessary to rotate the transducer at varying degrees (to oblique the scanning plane according to the lie of the aorta) to visualize the long axis of the aorta. Note and evaluate the anterior branches: celiac, SMA.

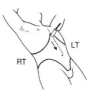

5. Continue rocking and sliding the transducer inferiorly through the middle and distal aorta to the bifurcation (usually at or just beyond the level of the umbilicus).

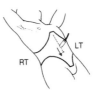

N O T E :   The aorta is posterior to the diaphragm. The IVC passes through the diaphragm.

N O T E : The longitudinal of the bifurcation can be difficult to visualize in the sagittal plane. Visualization can be easier from the coronal plane.

Sagittal Plane • Anterior Approach

- Patient **supine,** left posterior oblique, right posterior oblique, or sitting semi-erect to erect.
- From the lateral aspects of the most distal aorta, angle the transducer back toward the aorta and slightly move inferiorly until the bifurcation and common iliac arteries are seen.

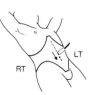

Coronal Plane • Left Lateral Approach

- Patient **right lateral decubitus,** supine, sitting semierect to erect, or left lateral decubitus.
- Begin with the transducer perpendicular, midcoronal plane, just superior to the iliac crest.

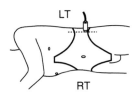

- Use the inferior pole of the left kidney as a landmark and look for the bifurcation medial and inferior.
- It may be necessary to rotate the transducer at varying degrees to visualize the long axis of the bifurcation and common iliac arteries.

N O T E : To avoid moving the patient, survey of the bifurcation in the decubitus position can be done after the transverse survey.

N O T E : While longitudinal evaluation of the proximal and middle aorta is generally easier from the sagittal plane approach, the coronal plane approach can be used. Move the transducer superiorly from the level of the bifurcation or scan intercostally, looking for the aorta medially. Label any images that follow accordingly.

≡ TRANSVERSE SURVEY

Transverse Plane • Anterior Approach

1. Begin with the transducer perpendicular, at the midline of the body, just inferior to the xiphoid process of the sternum.

2. Angle the transducer superiorly until the heart is seen. Slowly, straightening the transducer to perpendicular, look for the aorta just to the left of midline. The aorta will appear round or oval-shaped. Alternatively, in the sagittal plane locate the longitudinal of the proximal aorta, then rotate the transducer 90 degrees into the transverse plane.

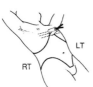

3. While viewing the proximal aorta, slowly move inferiorly, using a rock-and-slide motion. Slightly rock superiorly to inferiorly while sliding inferiorly. This way you should never lose sight of the aorta. Note and evaluate the anterior branches: celiac, SMA.

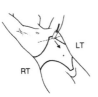

4. Continue rocking and sliding the transducer inferiorly through the middle and distal aorta to the bifurcation. Note and evaluate the lateral branches: renal arteries.

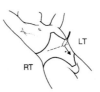

5. At the level of the bifurcation, evaluate the common iliac arteries by scanning through them inferiorly until you lose sight of them.

REQUIRED IMAGES

≡ LONGITUDINAL IMAGES

Sagittal Plane • Anterior Approach

1. Longitudinal image of the proximal aorta. (Inferior to the diaphragm and superior to the celiac trunk).

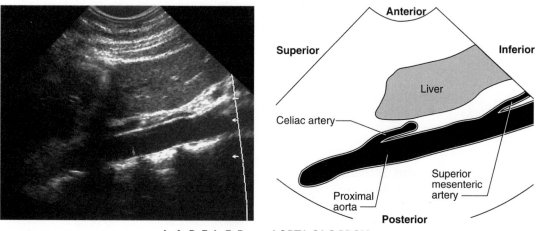

L A B E L E D :   AORTA SAG PROX

2. Longitudinal image of the middle aorta. (Inferior to the celiac trunk and along the length of the SMA).

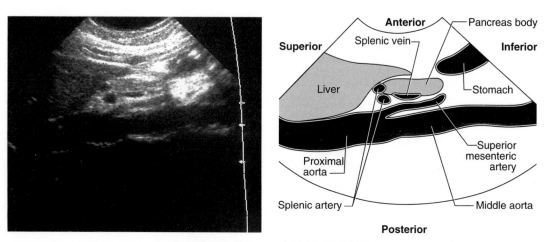

L A B E L E D :   AORTA SAG MID

3. Longitudinal image of the distal aorta. (Inferior to the SMA and superior to the bifurcation).

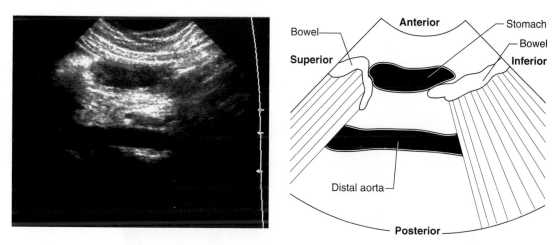

L A B E L E D :   AORTA SAG DISTAL

4. Longitudinal image of the aorta bifurcation. (Common iliac arteries).

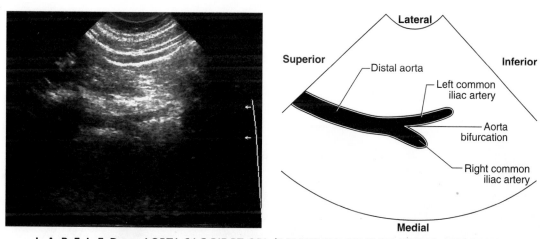

L A B E L E D :   AORTA SAG BIF RT OBL (DEPENDING ON THE LATERAL ASPECT YOU ANGLE THE TRANDUCER FROM) OR AORTA LT OR RT COR BIF

N O T E :   To avoid moving the patient, longitudinal images of the bifurcation in the decubitus position can be taken after the transverse images. Although the coronal plane approach can be used with the patient supine, the decubitus position is generally easier and can be helpful if the patient has obscuring bowel gas anteriorly.

≡ TRANSVERSE IMAGES

Transverse Plane • Anterior Approach

5. Transverse image of the proximal aorta with *anterior to posterior measurement (calipers outside wall to outside wall).* (Inferior to the diaphragm and superior to the celiac trunk).

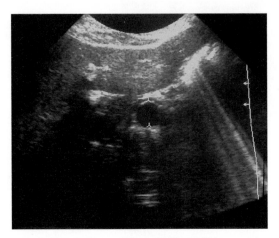

L A B E L E D :   AORTA TRV PROX

6. Same image as number 5 without calipers.

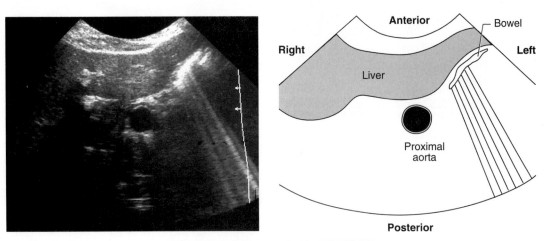

L A B E L E D :   AORTA TRV PROX

7. Transverse image of the middle aorta with *anterior to posterior measurement (calipers outside wall to outside wall).* (Inferior to the celiac trunk, *at the level of the renal arteries,* and along the length of the SMA).

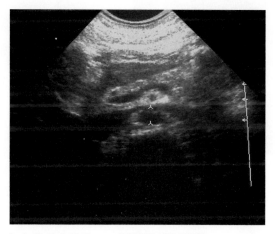

L A B E L E D :   AORTA TRV MID

8. Same image as number 7 without calipers.

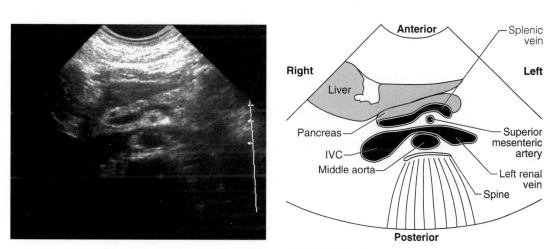

L A B E L E D :   AORTA TRV MID

N O T E :   If the renal arteries are not represented on the previous images, an additional image(s) of the renal arteries should be taken here and labeled accordingly.

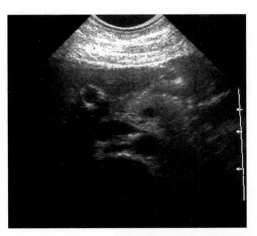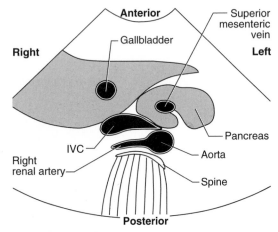

L A B E L E D :   RT RENAL ART TRV

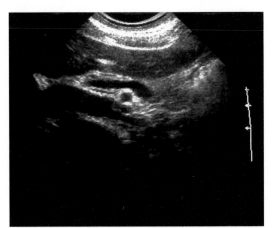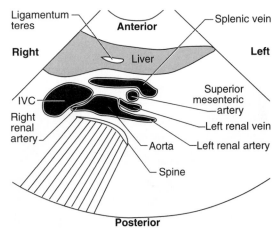

L A B E L E D :   LT RENAL ART TRV

9. Transverse image of the distal aorta with *anterior to posterior measurement (calipers outside wall to outside wall)*. (Inferior to the SMA and superior to the bifurcation).

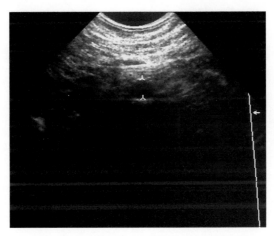

L A B E L E D : AORTA TRV DISTAL

10. Same image as number 9 without calipers.

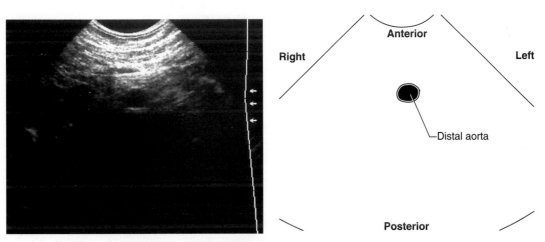

L A B E L E D : AORTA TRV DISTAL

11. Transverse image of the bifurcation. (Common iliac arteries).

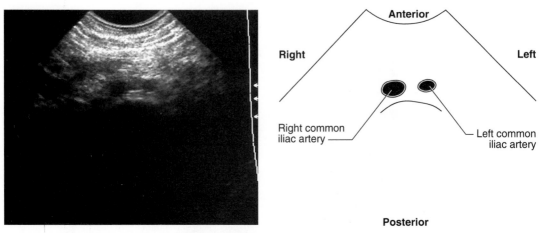

L A B E L E D :   AORTA TRV BIF

REQUIRED IMAGES WHEN THE ABDOMINAL AORTA IS NOT THE PRIMARY AREA OF INTEREST

1. Longitudinal image of the proximal and middle aorta.

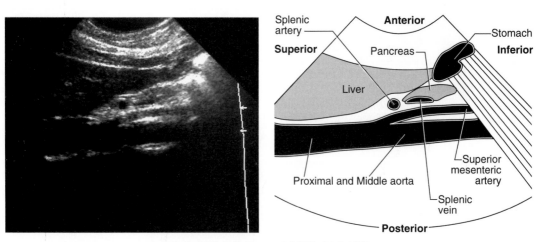

L A B E L E D :   AORTA SAG MID

2. Transverse image of the middle aorta at the level of the renal arteries.

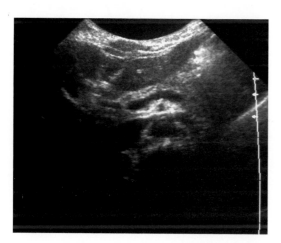 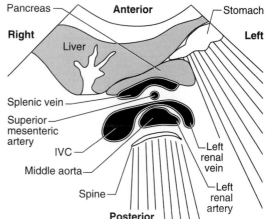

L A B E L E D :   AORTA TRV MID

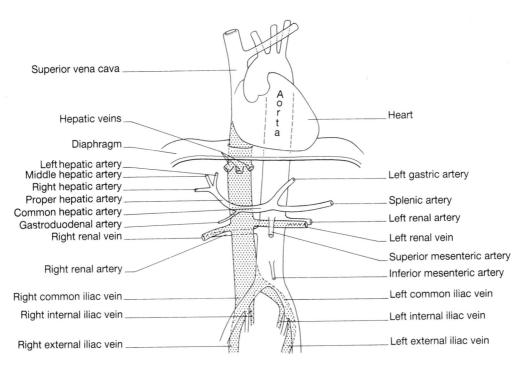

Superior vena cava

Hepatic veins

Diaphragm

Left hepatic artery
Middle hepatic artery
Right hepatic artery
Proper hepatic artery
Common hepatic artery
Gastroduodenal artery
Right renal vein

Right renal artery

Right common iliac vein

Right internal iliac vein

Right external iliac vein

Aorta

Heart

Left gastric artery

Splenic artery

Left renal artery

Left renal vein

Superior mesenteric artery

Inferior mesenteric artery

Left common iliac vein

Left internal iliac vein

Left external iliac vein

Location and anatomy of the inferior vena cava

Inferior Vena Cava Scanning Protocol

LOCATION

- The inferior vena cava originates at the junction of the two common iliac veins anterior to the body of the fifth lumbar vertebra.
- Ascends the retroperitoneum of the abdominal cavity and passes through the diaphragm to enter the right atrium.
- Ascends anterior to the spine to the right of the aorta.
- Passes through a deep fossa on the posterior surface of the liver between the caudate lobe and bare area.

ANATOMY

- Consists of three muscle layers:
  - (a) Intima (innermost).
  - (b) Media (middle layer).
  - (c) Adventitia (outer).
- Size is variable and normal up to 4 cm.
- Tributaries:
  - (a) Hepatic veins.
  - (b) Renal veins.
  - (c) Common iliac veins.
  - (d) Right adrenal vein.
  - (e) Right ovarian vein or testicular vein.
  - (f) Inferior phrenic vein.
  - (g) Four lumbar veins.
  - (h) Medial sacral vein.
- Can be very tortuous.

PHYSIOLOGY

- Returns deoxygenated blood from the tissues to the heart for oxygenation and recirculation.

SONOGRAPHIC APPEARANCE

- Echogenic muscular walls.
- Anechoic, echo-free lumen.

PATIENT PREP

- Fasting for at least 8 hours.
- If the patient has eaten, still attempt the examination.

PATIENT POSITION

- **Supine, left lateral decubitus.**
- Right lateral decubitus, left posterior oblique, right posterior oblique, or sitting semierect to erect as needed.

N O T E :   Different patient positions should be used whenever the suggested position does not give the desired results.

TRANSDUCER

- **3.0 MHz** or **3.5 MHz.**
- 5.0 MHz for thin patients.

BREATHING TECHNIQUE

- **Normal respiration** or deep, held respiration.

N O T E :   The diameter of the IVC varies depending on the level of respiration. Normal veins increase with held respiration or the Valsalva maneuver.

N O T E :   Different breathing techniques should be used whenever the suggested breathing technique does not give the desired results.

INFERIOR VENA CAVA SURVEY

N O T E :   While surveying the IVC, evaluate the surrounding soft tissue areas for adenopathy.

☰ LONGITUDINAL SURVEY

Sagittal Plane • Anterior Approach

1. Begin with the transducer perpendicular, at the midline of the body, just inferior to the xiphoid process of the sternum.

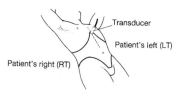

2. Move or angle the transducer to the patient's left and identify the proximal aorta posterior to the liver.

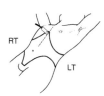

3. Move or angle the transducer to the patient's right and identify the distal IVC posterior to the liver.

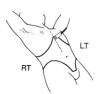

N O T E :   The IVC passes through the diaphragm. The aorta passes posterior to the diaphragm.

4. While viewing the distal IVC, slowly move inferiorly, using a rock-and-slide motion. Slightly rock right to left to scan through each side of the IVC while sliding inferiorly. It may be necessary to rotate the transducer at varying degrees (to oblique the scanning plane according to the lie of the IVC) to visualize the long axis of the IVC. Note and evaluate the anterior tributaries: hepatic veins.

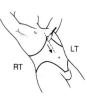

5. Continue rocking and sliding the transducer inferiorly through the middle and proximal IVC to the bifurcation (usually at or just beyond the level of the umbilicus).

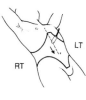

N O T E :   The longitudinal of the bifurcation can be difficult to visualize in the sagittal plane. Visualization can be easier from the coronal plane.

Sagittal Plane • Anterior Approach

- Patient **supine,** left posterior oblique, right posterior oblique, or sitting semierect to erect.
- From the lateral aspects of the most proximal IVC, angle the transducer back toward the IVC and slightly move inferiorly until the bifurcation and common iliac veins are seen.

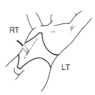

Coronal Plane • Right Lateral Approach

- Patient **left lateral decubitus,** supine, or sitting semierect to erect.
- Begin with the transducer perpendicular, midcoronal plane, just superior to the iliac crest.

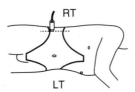

- Use the inferior pole of the right kidney as a landmark and look for the bifurcation medial and inferior.
- It may be necessary to rotate the transducer at varying degrees to visualize the

long axis of the bifurcation and common iliac veins.

N O T E :   To avoid moving the patient, survey of the bifurcation in the left lateral decubitus position can be done after the transverse survey.

N O T E :   Although longitudinal evaluation of the distal and middle IVC is generally easier from the sagittal plane approach, the right coronal plane approach can be used. Move the transducer superiorly from the level of the bifurcation or scan intercostally, looking for the IVC medially. Label any images that follow accordingly.

≡ TRANSVERSE SURVEY

Transverse Plane • Anterior Approach

1. Begin with the transducer perpendicular, at the midline of the body, just inferior to the xiphoid process of the sternum.

2. Angle the transducer superiorly until the heart is seen. Slowly, straightening the transducer to perpendicular, look for the IVC just to the right of midline. The IVC will appear oval or almond-shaped. Alternatively, in the sagittal plane, locate the longitudinal of the distal IVC, then rotate the transducer 90 degrees into the transverse plane.

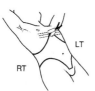

3. While viewing the distal IVC, slowly move inferiorly using a rock-and-slide motion. Slightly rock superiorly to inferiorly while sliding inferiorly. This way you should never lose sight of the IVC. Note and evaluate the anterior tributaries: hepatic veins.

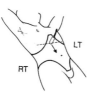

4. Continue rocking and sliding the transducer inferiorly through the middle and proximal IVC to the bifurcation. Note and evaluate the lateral tributaries: renal veins.

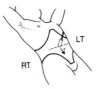

5. At the level of the bifurcation, evaluate the iliac veins by scanning through them inferiorly until you lose sight of them.

REQUIRED IMAGES

≡ LONGITUDINAL IMAGES

Sagittal Plane • Anterior Approach

1. Longitudinal image of the distal IVC to include the diaphragm and hepatic vein(s).

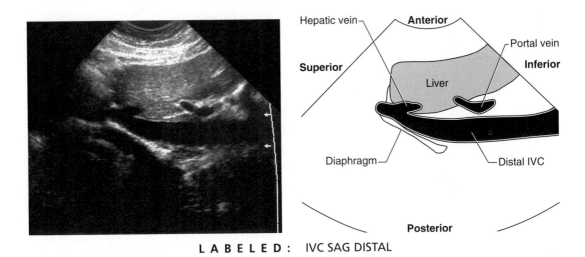

L A B E L E D : IVC SAG DISTAL

2. Longitudinal image of the middle IVC at the level of the head of the pancreas.

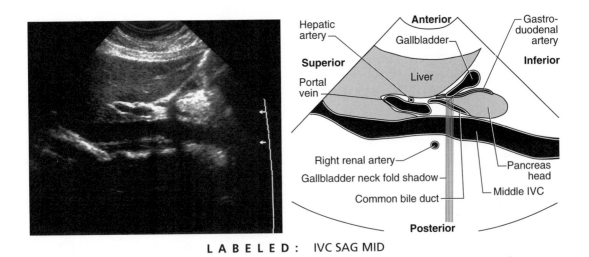

L A B E L E D : IVC SAG MID

3. Longitudinal image of the proximal IVC.

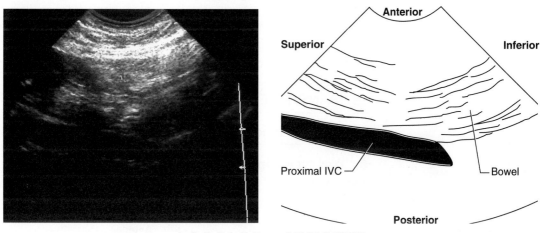

L A B E L E D :   IVC SAG PROX

4. Longitudinal image of the IVC bifurcation. (Common iliac veins).

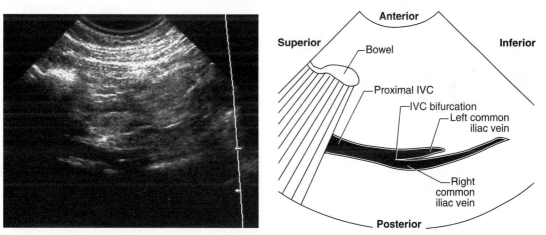

L A B E L E D :   IVC SAG BIF RT OR LT OBL (DEPENDING ON THE LATERAL ASPECT YOU ANGLE THE TRANSDUCER FROM) OR IVC RT COR BIF

N O T E :   To avoid moving the patient, longitudinal images of the bifurcation in the left lateral decubitus position can be taken after the transverse images. Although the coronal plane approach can be used with the patient supine, the left lateral decubitus position is generally easier and can be helpful if the patient has obscuring bowel gas anteriorly.

≡ TRANSVERSE IMAGES

Transverse Plane • Anterior Approach

5. Transverse image of the distal IVC to include the hepatic veins.

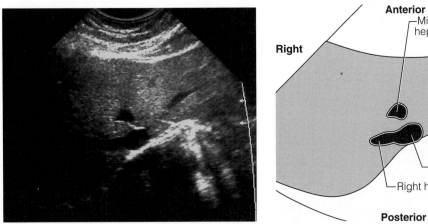
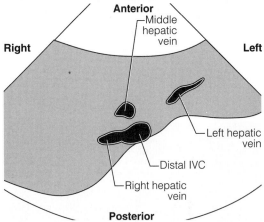

L A B E L E D :   IVC TRV DISTAL

6. Transverse image of the middle IVC at the level of the renal veins.

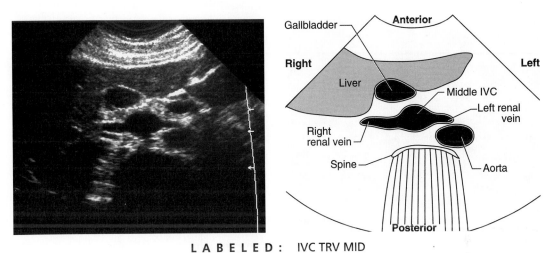

LABELED: IVC TRV MID

7. Transverse image of the proximal IVC.

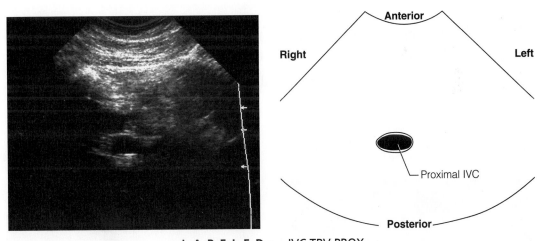

LABELED: IVC TRV PROX

8. Transverse image of the IVC bifurcation. (Common iliac veins).

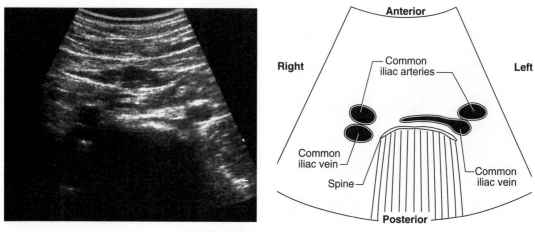

L A B E L E D :   IVC TRV BIF

N O T E :   Measurements of the IVC are not required unless indicated by pathology.

REQUIRED IMAGES WHEN THE IVC IS NOT THE PRIMARY AREA OF INTEREST

1. Longitudinal image of the distal and middle IVC.

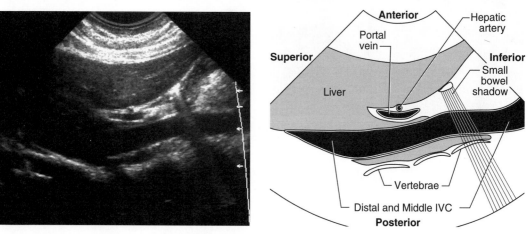

L A B E L E D :   IVC SAG DISTAL

2. Transverse image of the distal IVC to include the hepatic veins.

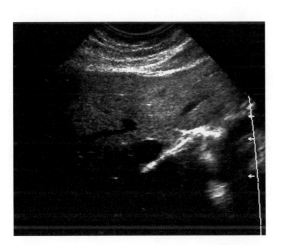 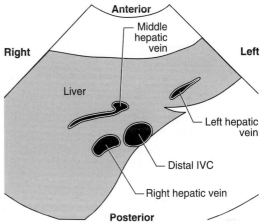

L A B E L E D :   IVC TRV DISTAL

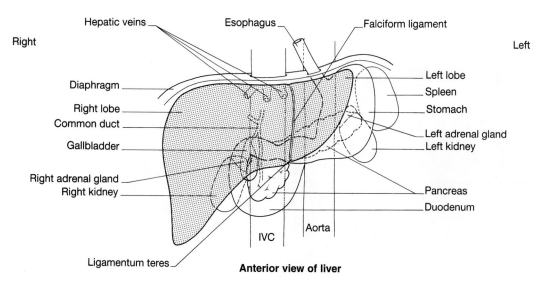

Anterior view of liver

Right

Left

Hepatic veins

Esophagus

Falciform ligament

Diaphragm

Right lobe

Common duct

Gallbladder

Right adrenal gland
Right kidney

Ligamentum teres

Left lobe

Spleen

Stomach

Left adrenal gland
Left kidney

Pancreas

Duodenum

IVC

Aorta

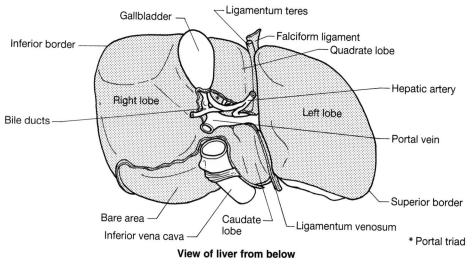

View of liver from below

Gallbladder

Ligamentum teres

Inferior border

Falciform ligament

Quadrate lobe

Right lobe

Hepatic artery

Bile ducts

Left lobe

Portal vein

Superior border

Bare area

Caudate lobe

Ligamentum venosum

Inferior vena cava

* Portal triad

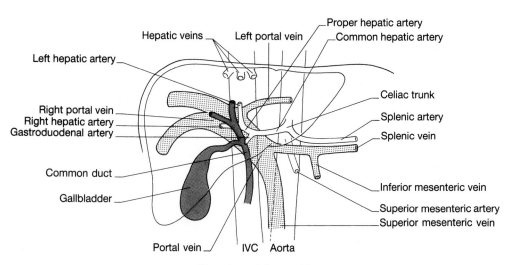

Vessels and ducts of liver

Hepatic veins

Left portal vein

Proper hepatic artery

Common hepatic artery

Left hepatic artery

Right portal vein
Right hepatic artery
Gastroduodenal artery

Celiac trunk

Splenic artery

Splenic vein

Common duct

Gallbladder

Inferior mesenteric vein

Superior mesenteric artery
Superior mesenteric vein

Portal vein

IVC

Aorta

Liver Scanning Protocol

CHAPTER

5

LOCATION

- The liver occupies the right side of the upper abdomen and often extends beyond the midline of the body to the left side. Generally, it lies between the level of the nipples to the level of the eighth or ninth rib.
- Intraperitoneal except for a bare area that encompasses most of the liver's posterior surface. Additional interruptions of the peritoneum at the liver include the gallbladder fossa, porta hepatis, falciform ligament attachment, and portions around the inferior vena cava.
- Most anterior visceral organ of the peritoneal cavity. The left lobe and majority of the right lobe are surrounded by the rib cage. The remaining portion of the right lobe is usually in contact with the abdominal wall.
- Superior, posterior, and anterior liver surfaces abut the diaphragm.
- Left lobe lies in the left hypochondriac and epigastric regions. It is bounded in front by the rib cage and abdominal wall and posteriorly it rests on the stomach.
- Right lobe occupies the right hypochondrium. It is bounded in front by the rib cage and abdominal wall and posteriorly it rests on the gallbladder, head of the pancreas, right adrenal gland, and right kidney (primarily the superior pole).
- Caudate lobe located on the posterior surface of the liver. Lies posterior to the porta hepatis between the fissure for the ligamentum venosum and the inferior vena cava.

ANATOMY

- Largest internal organ.
- Size and shape are variable. Viewed anteriorly has a basic wedge shape, tapering toward the left side. Right lobe significantly larger than left lobe.

- Encased by Glisson's capsule, a thick, fibrous, connective tissue layer that contains nerves, blood vessels, and lymphatic vessels. In turn, encased liver largely covered by the peritoneum.
- Divided into lobes according to anatomy and into segments according to function.

A. **Liver Lobes:** Using the traditional anatomic system, the liver is divided based on the sonographic identification of specific anatomic landmarks.

(a) **Left Lobe:** Anatomically separated from the right lobe by the falciform ligament on its superior surface. Divided from the caudate lobe by the fissure for the ligamentum venosum and on its inferior (visceral) surface from the quadrate lobe by the fissure for the ligamentum teres.

(b) **Right Lobe:** Anatomically separated from the left lobe by the falciform ligament on its superior (diaphragmatic) surface and by the left intersegmental fissure on its inferior surface. Riedel's lobe, a normal anatomic variant, is a projection of the right lobe that can extend as far as the iliac crest.

(c) **Caudate Lobe:** Anatomically separated from the left lobe by the fissure for the ligamentum venosum. Boundaries are the inferior vena cava on the right, its margin on the left, which forms the hepatic boundary of the superior recess of the lesser sac, and the porta hepatis anteriorly.

(d) **Quadrate Lobe:** Distinguished sonographically and physiologically as the medial portion of the left lobe. The porta hepatis borders posteriorly, the margin of the liver anteriorly, the gallbladder fossa right laterally, and on the left, the fissure for the ligamentum teres.

B. **Liver Segments:** Liver segments are based on hepatic function. Segments are determined according to blood supply and biliary drainage. Segmental liver anatomy is clinically significant for localizing potentially resectable liver lesions.

(a) **Two Main Functional Divisions:** Right and Left. Middle hepatic veins located in the main lobar fissure delineate the liver into intrahepatic (functional), right and left lobes.

(b) **Right Functional Lobe:** Is everything to the right of the plane through the gallbladder fossa and inferior vena cava (analogous to the anatomic right lobe).

Two Divisions: Anterior Segment and Posterior Segment.

The right hepatic vein located in the right intersegmental fissure delineates the anterior and posterior segments. These segments are also separated by the right portal vein that passes centrally within them.

(c) **Left Functional Lobe:** Is everything to the left of the plane through the gallbladder fossa and inferior vena cava (analogous to the anatomic left lobe, caudate lobe, and quadrate lobe).

Two Divisions: Medial Segment and Lateral Segment. The medial segment is analogous to the traditional quadrate lobe. The lateral segment is analogous to the anatomic left lobe. The ascending portion of the left portal vein (in the left intersegmental fissure) delineates the medial and lateral segments. These segments are also separated by the left hepatic vein (in the left intersegmental fissure) superiorly and the ligamentum teres inferiorly.

(d) **Caudate Lobe:** The portion of the liver lying posterior to the porta hepatis, between the fissure for the ligamentum venosum and the inferior vena cava (analogous to the caudate lobe).

No Divisions.

It distinctly receives hepatic arterial and portal venous blood from both the right and left systems that otherwise individually supply respective right and left lobes. The left portal vein separates the caudate lobe from the medial segment of the left lobe. The left portal vein runs anterior to the caudate and posterior to the medial segment. The fissure for the ligamentum venosum runs along the left anterior margin of the caudate separating it from medial and lateral segments of the functional left lobe.

- **Liver Surfaces:**
  (a) **Posterior Surface:**
  (1) caudate lobe.
  (2) bare area.
  (3) deeply indented area centrally where it lies on the spine.
  (4) fossae for the inferior vena cava and ligamentum venosum.
  (5) attachment to the diaphragm by loose connective tissue.
  (6) most of this surface is not covered by peritoneum.

  (b) **Anterior Surface:**
  (1) lies inside the peritoneum immediately posterior to the xiphoid process of the sternum.
  (2) is part of the diaphragmatic surface until it loses contact on the left at the 7th or 8th costal cartilage and on the right anywhere from the 6th to 10th costal cartilage.
  (3) is accentuated by a deep notch. The ligamentum teres ascends from the umbilicus to the umbilical notch of the anterior surface.

  (c) **Superior Surface:**
  (1) is intraperitoneal.

(2) is a convex diaphragmatic, smooth surface, separated from the pleura, lungs, pericardium, and heart by the dome of the diaphragm.

(d) **Inferior Surface:**

(1) is covered by peritoneum except at the porta hepatis and site of the gallbladder attachment.

(2) is a concave visceral surface acccentuated by fossae and indentations from organs that rest against its surface.

(3) of the left lobe is deeply indented by the anterior surface of the stomach.

(4) of the right lobe is accentuated by the hepatic flexure of the colon, right kidney and adrenal gland, and the duodenum where it lies adjacent to the gallbladder neck.

(5) anterior mid portion is the quadrate lobe (medial left lobe) bound by the falciform ligament on the left.

(6) posterior mid portion of the inferior surface is the caudate lobe. The posterior portion of the caudate forms a part of the anterior boundary of the lesser sac.

- **Liver Ligaments:** Ligaments attach the liver to the diaphragm, stomach, anterior abdominal wall, and retroperitoneum.

(a) **Falciform Ligament:**

Parietal peritoneal, anteroposterior fold that attaches the bare area of the liver to the right rectus muscle of the anterior abdominal wall. It extends from the diaphragm to the umbilicus, running along the liver's anterior surface. It is continuous with the ligamentum teres which is contained within its layers. On the liver's superior (diaphragmatic) surface, it is described as the anatomical divider of the right and left lobes and along with the ligamentum teres, functionally designates the boundary of the left lobe's medial and lateral segments.

(b) **Ligamentum Teres:**

Fibrous, round ligament formed by the obliterated left umbilical vein. Arises from the umbilicus and courses within the falciform ligament to the umbilical notch on the anterior surface of the liver. Coursing along the inferior (visceral) surface it continues as the ligamentum venosum (obliterated ductus venosus) running posteriorly to the inferior vena cava.

(c) **Coronary Ligament:**

Parietal peritoneal, bifold layer that attaches the liver's posterior surface to the diaphragm. Anterior and posterior layers are continuous anteriorly with the falciform ligament and laterally with the triangular ligaments.

(d) **Right and Left Triangular Ligaments:**

Formed by continuations of the coronary ligament. Triangular extensions on the right from the far right border of the bare area to the diaphragm and on the left from the superior surface of the left lobe to just anterior of the esophageal opening in the diaphragm.

(e) **Gastrohepatic Ligament:**

Visceral peritoneal, bifold layer also known as the lesser omentum. From the undersurface of the liver it is continuous with the ligamentum venosum. Ascending, it attaches the undersurface with the lesser curvature of the stomach and the first portion of the duodenum.

(f) **Hepatoduodenal Ligament:**

Portion of the lesser omentum that is located on the right free edge of the gastrohepatic ligament. Extends to the duodenum and right hepatic flexure and forms the ventral portion of the foramen of Winslow or the epiploic foramen. Surrounds the portal triad immediately adjacent to the porta hepatis.

- **Liver Fissures:**

(a) **Main Lobar Fissure:**

Runs obliquely between the neck of the gallbladder and right portal vein. Contains the middle hepatic vein and separates the right and left hepatic lobes. Its course is short and variable.

(b) **Left Intersegmental Fissure:**

Subdivides the right lobe into anterior and posterior portions.

(c) **Fissure for the Ligamentum Venosum:**

Contains the gastrohepatic ligament and separates the left lobe and caudate lobe.

(d) **Fissure for the Ligamentum Teres:**

Forms the left boundary of the quadrate or medial portion of the left lobe.

- **Liver Vessels and Ducts:**

(a) **Hepatic Veins:**

The right, middle, and left hepatic veins drain the blood from the liver and dump it into the inferior vena cava.

(b) **Hepatic Arteries:**

Supply the liver with oxygenated blood from the aorta. The celiac axis branch of the aorta divides into the splenic, left gastric, and common hepatic arteries.

(1) The common hepatic artery runs directly toward the right side of the body, anterior to the portal vein and left of the common bile duct. Here, it divides into the gastroduodenal artery and the ascending proper hepatic artery.

(2) The proper hepatic artery divides into two main branches, the right and left hepatic arteries which supply the right and left segmental lobes respectively.

(3) The middle hepatic artery generally arises from the left hepatic artery.

(4) The cystic artery arises from the right hepatic artery.

(c) **Portal Vein:**

The main portal vein enters the liver at the porta hepatis, posterior to the hepatic artery and common bile duct. It then divides into the right and left branches. These branches become intrasegmental veins that branch into medial and lateral portions of the left lobe and anterior and posterior portions of the right lobe.

(d) **Portal Venous System:**

Supplies the greatest percentage of total blood flow to the liver. Formed by the confluence of three tributaries: the splenic vein, superior mesenteric vein, and inferior mesenteric vein. This system carries blood from the spleen and bowel to the liver.

(e) **Bile Ducts:**

Transport bile, a fluid made in the liver, to the gallbladder where it is stored. When bile is needed to aid digestion of fat, the bile ducts carry it into the duodenum.

(f) **Portal Triad:**

Refers to the hepatic artery, bile duct, and portal vein at the level of the porta hepatis. When there is a question of dilated bile ducts, a distinction between these structures is important. At the level of the porta, the portal vein is posterior to (or behind) the hepatic artery on the right and the common bile duct on the left. Passing into the liver, the bile duct referred to as the common hepatic duct at this level is immediately anterior to the right hepatic artery, which in turn, is immediately anterior to the portal vein. The right and left main portal vein branches are located immediately posterior to the right and left hepatic ducts.

PHYSIOLOGY

- Vascular Functions:

  For the storage and filtration of blood. Expands to act as a blood reservoir in times of excess blood volume and supplies extra blood in times of diminished blood volume. Kupffer cells that line hepatic sinuses cleanse the blood of up to all but approximately 1% of bacteria found in portal blood from the intestine.

- Metabolic Functions:

  Synthesizes many substances sent to other areas of the body and performs a vast number of other metabolic functions. Functions include protein, fat, and carbohydrate metabolisms. Storage of glycogen, vitamins, and iron. Forms most of the substances utilized in blood coagulation. Excretes drugs, hormones, and other substances into bile and ultimately the feces.

- Secretory and Excretory Bile Functions:
  Produces and releases bile through the biliary tract into the small bowel where it is used for the digestion of fat.

SONOGRAPHIC APPEARANCE

- Homogeneous, mid-gray (medium-level echoes) lobes.
- Normal parenchyma may be described as hyperechoic to normal renal parenchyma.
- Normal parenchyma may be described as hypoechoic to normal pancreas parenchyma.
- Blood vessels and bile ducts have anechoic lumens surrounded by hyperechoic walls.
- Portal and hepatic veins are seen as anechoic tubular structures branching throughout the lobes. For differentiation, follow branches toward the porta hepatis or IVC, respectively.

N O T E : Major portal vein branches are surrounded by highly reflective or echogenic fibrofatty tissues. Smaller portal vein branches may lack these surrounding echoes. Hyperechoic walls can also be seen surrounding the larger hepatic vein tributaries. Because of this variability these features *are not* a reliable distinction between these two vessel systems.

- Highly reflective or very echogenic ligaments and fissures.

NORMAL VARIANTS

- Reidel's lobe:
  Inferior extension of the right lobe.
- Absence of left lobe:
  Very rare. Results from occlusion of the left hepatic vein due to abnormal extension of neonatal spasm of the ligamentum venosum.
- Many variations in size and shape.

PATIENT PREP

- Fasting for 8 to 12 hours, because the gallbladder, biliary tract, and pancreas will be evaluated. This guarantees normal gallbladder and biliary tract dilatation and reduces the stomach and bowel gas anterior to the pancreas.
- If the patient has eaten, still do the liver exam.

N O T E : Liver evaluation is not usually limited by bowel gas, since the bowel tract is anatomically inferior to the liver.

PATIENT POSITION

- **Supine.**
- Left posterior oblique, left lateral decubitus, sitting semi-erect to erect or prone as needed.

N O T E : Different patient positions should be used whenever the suggested position does not give the desired results.

TRANSDUCER

- **3.0 MHz or 3.5 MHz.**
- 5.0 MHz for very thin patient.

N O T E : It may be necessary to use 5.0 MHz for a patient's left lobe and 3.0 or 3.5 MHz on the right lobe.

BREATHING TECHNIQUE

- **Deep, held inspiration.**

N O T E : Different breathing techniques should be used whenever the suggested breathing technique does not give the desired results.

LIVER SURVEY

≡ LONGITUDINAL SURVEY

Sagittal Plane • Anterior Approach

1. Begin with the transducer perpendicular, at the midline of the body, just inferior to the xiphoid process of the sternum.

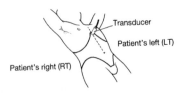

This is the general area of the left lobe.

Note the ligamentum venosum, caudate lobe, and aorta or IVC.

N O T E : Depending on liver shape and patient respiration, varying degrees of subcostal and inferior angles may have to be used when scanning the liver longitudinally to completely survey the superior and inferior liver margins. In some cases intercostal scanning will be necessary.

2. While viewing the left lobe, use subcostal angles and move the transducer to the patient's left, lateral and inferior along the costal margin until you are beyond the left lobe. Note the aorta.

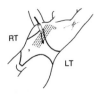

3. Return to midline just inferior to the xiphoid process.

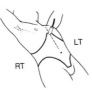

4. To evaluate the right lobe, use subcostal angles and move the transducer to the patient's right, lateral and inferior along the costal margin until you are beyond the right lateral, inferior lobe.

Note the IVC, hepatic veins, portal vein, portal triad, porta hepatis, main lobar fissure, bile ducts, gallbladder, right kidney, and perinephric space.

5. Move the transducer back onto the right lateral inferior lobe. Place the transducer at the most lateral edge of the right costal margin and use a very sharp subcostal angle to view the right lateral superior lobe. Move or angle the transducer right lateral and sweep through and beyond the right lateral superior lobe.

Note the dome of the right lobe and adjacent pleural space.

N O T E : The longitudinal of the right lateral superior lobe can be difficult to visualize from a sagittal plane subcostal angle. Sagittal plane intercostal scanning or right coronal plane subcostal or intercostal scanning can be used.

Sagittal Plane • Anterior Intercostal Approach

- Patient **supine,** left posterior oblique or sitting semierect to erect.
- Begin with the transducer perpendicular in an intercostal space immediately anterior to the right lateral superior lobe.

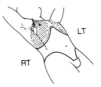

- Suspended respiration should make the area more viewable.
- Move the transducer to adjacent intercostal spaces to evaluate the entire right lateral superior lobe.
- Angling the transducer within the intercostal spaces and using different breathing techniques can aid evaluation.
- Note the dome of the right lobe and adjacent pleural space.

Coronal Plane • Right Lateral Subcostal Approach

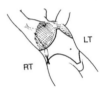

- Patient **supine,** left posterior oblique, left lateral decubitus, sitting semierect to erect.
- Begin with the transducer angled subcostally, midcoronal plane. Varying degrees of subcostal angles and deep, held respiration should make the right lateral superior lobe viewable.

- Note the dome of the right lobe and adjacent pleural space.

Coronal Plane • Right Lateral Intercostal Approach

- Patient **supine,** left posterior oblique, left lateral decubitus, sitting semierect to erect.
- Begin with the transducer perpendicular, midcoronal plane, just inferior to the costal margin. Move superiorly into the first intercostal space.

cent intercostal spaces until you scan through and beyond the right lateral superior lobe.

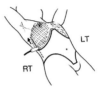

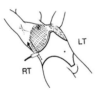

- Using suspended or deep, held respiration, move superiorly through the adjacent intercostal spaces until you scan

- Angling the transducer within the intercostal spaces and using different breathing techniques can aid evaluation.
- Note the dome of the right lobe and adjacent pleural space.

≡ TRANSVERSE SURVEY

Transverse Plane • Anterior Approach

1. Begin with the transducer perpendicular, at the midline of the body, just inferior to the xiphoid process of the sternum. This is the general area of the left lobe.

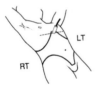

Note the ligamentum venosum, caudate lobe, hepatic vein(s), IVC, and aorta.

N O T E :   Depending on liver shape and patient respiration, varying degrees of subcostal and inferior angles may have to be used when scanning the liver transversely to completely survey the superior and inferior liver margins. In some cases intercostal scanning may be necessary.

2. While viewing the left lobe, move the transducer inferior until you scan through and beyond the left lobe. Note the portal vein and ligamentum teres.

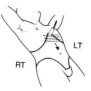

3. Depending on liver shape and size, all of the left lateral aspect of the left lobe may be seen in its entirety from midline. If not, return to midline, just inferior to the xiphoid process. Use subcostal and inferior angles and move the transducer to the patient's left, lateral and inferior along the costal margin until you are beyond the left lobe.

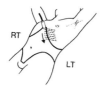

4. Return to midline, just inferior to the xiphoid process.

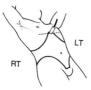

5. To evaluate the right lobe, use subcostal and inferior angles and move the transducer to the patient's right, lateral and inferior along the costal margin until you are beyond the right lateral inferior lobe.

Note the IVC, hepatic veins, portal vein, portal triad, right and left portal branches, porta hepatis, main lobar fissure, bile ducts, gallbladder, right kidney, and perinephric space.

6. Move the transducer back onto the right lateral inferior lobe. Place the transducer at the most lateral edge of the right costal margin and use a very sharp subcostal angle to view the right lateral superior lobe. Move or angle the transducer right lateral and sweep through and beyond the right lateral superior lobe. Note the dome of the right lobe and adjacent pleural space.

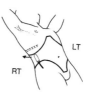

N O T E : The transverse of the right lateral superior lobe can be difficult to visualize from a transverse plane subcostal angle. Transverse plane intercostal scanning or transverse plane right lateral subcostal or right lateral intercostal scanning can be used.

Transverse plane/anterior intercostal approach

Transverse plane/right lateral subcostal approach

Transverse plane/right lateral intercostal approach

Use the same suggested scanning methods as those for the longitudinal surveys of the right lateral superior lobe.

REQUIRED IMAGES

≡ LONGITUDINAL IMAGES

Sagittal Plane • Anterior Approach

1. Longitudinal image of the left lobe to include the inferior margin and the aorta.

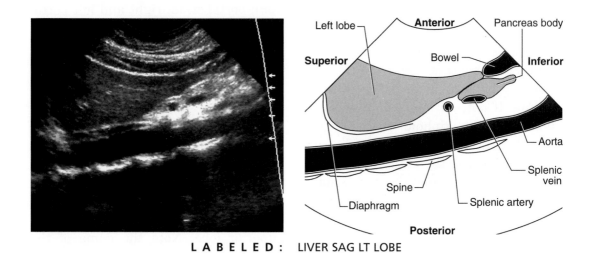

L A B E L E D :   LIVER SAG LT LOBE

2. Longitudinal image of the left lobe to include the diaphragm and caudate lobe.

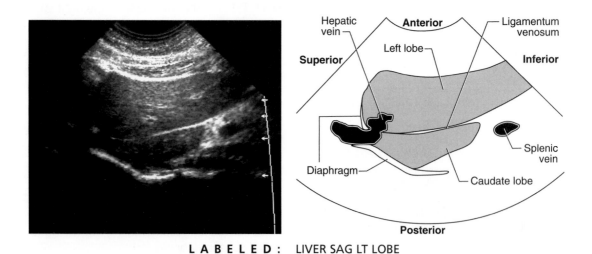

L A B E L E D :   LIVER SAG LT LOBE

3. Longitudinal image of the right lobe to include the IVC where it passes through the liver.

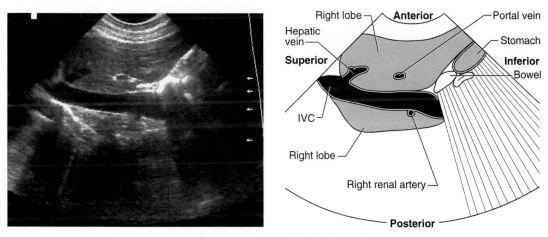

L A B E L E D :   LIVER SAG RT LOBE

4. Longitudinal image of the right lobe to include the main lobar fissure, gallbladder, and portal vein.

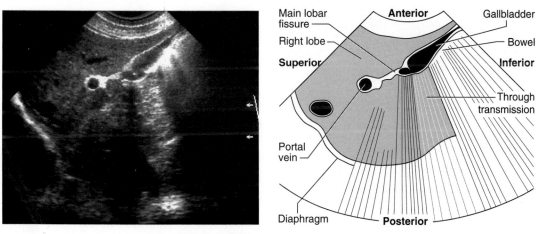

L A B E L E D :   LIVER SAG RT LOBE

5. Longitudinal image of the right lobe to include part of the right kidney for parenchyma comparison.

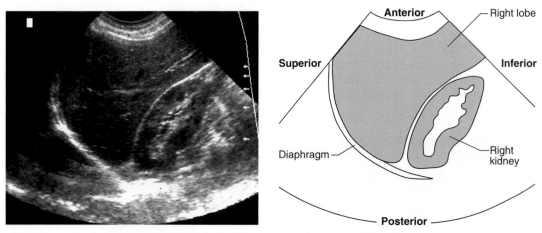

L A B E L E D :   LIVER SAG RT LOBE

6. Longitudinal image of the right lobe to include the dome and the adjacent pleural space.

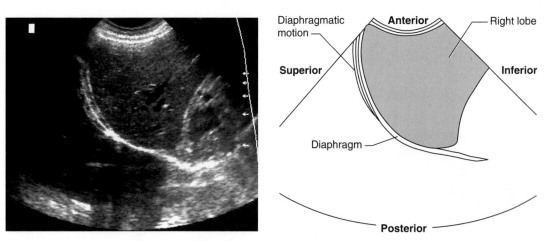

L A B E L E D :   LIVER SAG RT LOBE

☰ TRANSVERSE IMAGES

Transverse Plane • Anterior Approach

7. Transverse image of the left lobe to include its lateral margin.

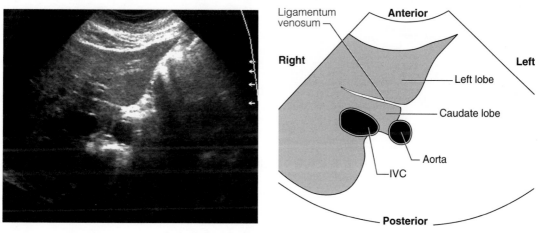

L A B E L E D :   LIVER TRV LT LOBE

8. Transverse image of the left lobe to include the ligamentum teres.

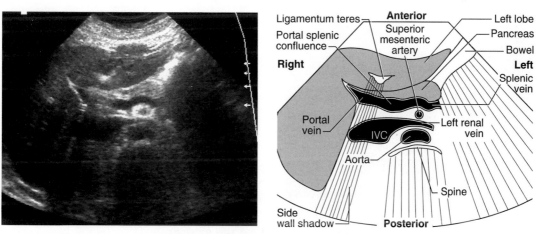

L A B E L E D :   LIVER TRV LT LOBE

N O T E :   Depending on liver size and shape, it may be possible to take a transverse image that includes the left lobe's lateral margin and the ligamentum teres. If so, label: liver trv lt lobe

9. Transverse image of the right lobe to include the hepatic veins.

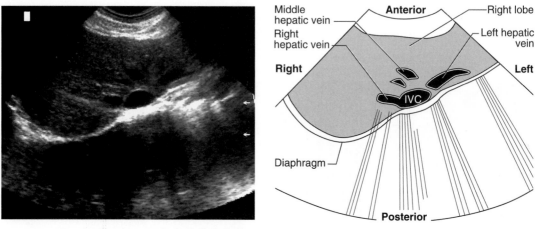

L A B E L E D :   LIVER TRV RT LOBE

10. Transverse image of the right lobe to include the right and left branches of the portal vein.

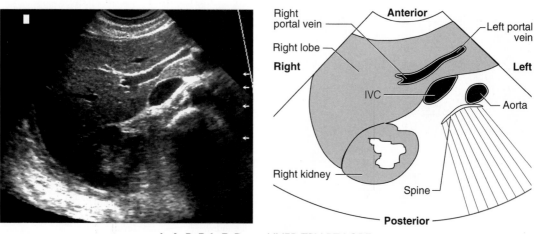

L A B E L E D :   LIVER TRV RT LOBE

11. Transverse image of the right lateral inferior lobe.

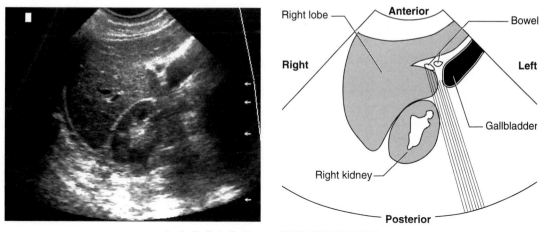

L A B E L E D :   LIVER TRV RT LOBE

12. Transverse image of the right lobe to include the dome and the adjacent pleural space.

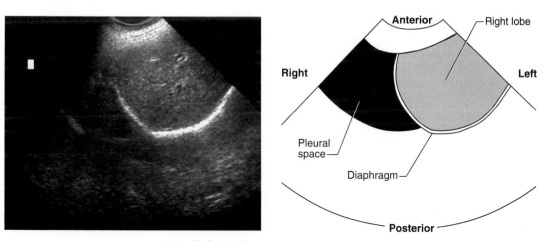

L A B E L E D :   LIVER TRV RT LOBE

N O T E :   Measurements of the liver are not required unless indicated by pathology.

REQUIRED IMAGES WHEN THE LIVER IS NOT THE PRIMARY AREA OF INTEREST

Required images of the liver are always the same, whether it is the primary area of interest of the study or not.

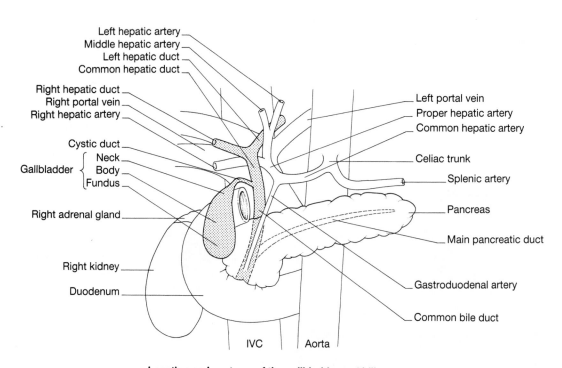

Left hepatic artery

Middle hepatic artery

Left hepatic duct

Common hepatic duct

Right hepatic duct

Right portal vein

Right hepatic artery

Cystic duct

Neck

Body

Fundus

Gallbladder

Right adrenal gland

Right kidney

Duodenum

Left portal vein

Proper hepatic artery

Common hepatic artery

Celiac trunk

Splenic artery

Pancreas

Main pancreatic duct

Gastroduodenal artery

Common bile duct

IVC

Aorta

Location and anatomy of the gallbladder and biliary tract

Gallbladder and Biliary Tract Scanning Protocol

CHAPTER 6

LOCATION

- The gallbladder is in the right upper quadrant.
- Intraperitoneal.
- Immediately posterior to the liver.
- Neck of the gallbladder is fixed in its position at the main lobar fissure.
- Body and fundus of the gallbladder are extremely variable in position.
- Fundus of the gallbladder may be anterior to the superior pole of the right kidney.
- Cystic duct is superior to the gallbladder neck.
- Common bile duct is inferior to the gallbladder. It can also be posterior to the gallbladder, depending on the lie of the gallbladder.
- Common bile duct is right lateral to the common hepatic artery.
- Common duct is anterior to the portal vein.

ANATOMY

- Right and left hepatic ducts exit from the liver at the porta hepatis and meet to form the common duct.
- The superior (proximal) portion of the common duct is referred to as the common hepatic duct, and the inferior (distal) portion as the common bile duct.
- The common hepatic duct courses inferomedially and meets with the cystic duct of the gallbladder to form the common bile duct.
- The common bile duct courses inferomedially running behind the duodenum on its way to the head of the pancreas.
- The common bile duct either passes through the pancreatic head or runs along a groove on its posterior surface to meet with the main pancreatic duct. Joined together or separately, the ducts enter the duodenum at the ampulla of Vater.

- The gallbladder is pear-shaped. Its rounded inferior portion is the fundus and its superior tapering portion is the neck. The middle portion of the gallbladder is referred to as its body.
- Normal gallbladder size is variable according to the amount of bile it is storing. Up to 3 cm wide and 7 cm to 10 cm long is normal size for the gallbladder.
- Normal common duct size is variable according to the amount of bile in it and patient age. Common duct may enlarge with age.
- Up to 4 mm is normal for the common hepatic duct near the porta hepatis.
- Up to 7 mm is normal for the common bile duct distally.

N O T E :   The common duct assumes bile storage function following loss of gallbladder function resulting from cholecystectomy or gallbladder disease. Up to 10 mm is normal for size.

- The cystic duct connects the gallbladder neck with the common duct.
- The area where the cystic duct and gallbladder neck join is tortuous and referred to as the spiral valve. This reference is to appearance only because there is no valvular action.

PHYSIOLOGY

- Accessory to the digestive system.
- Liver manufactures bile, a fat emulsifier and carrier of liver waste. Bile is stored and concentrated in the gallbladder, then travels via the bile ducts to the small intestine when needed to aid digestion.

SONOGRAPHIC APPEARANCE

- The bile-filled gallbladder is an anechoic oblong structure with echogenic walls.
- The bile-filled common duct is an anechoic tubular structure with echogenic walls.

NORMAL VARIANTS

- Shape variations:
  (a) Segmental contractions that disappear after fasting or changing patient position.
  (b) Phrygian cap is an example of where the gallbladder fundus is folded over.

- Position variations:
  (a) The gallbladder can be found throughout the abdomen because it is suspended on long mesentery.
  (b) Very rare deep fossa intrahepatic gallbladder.
- Septations:
  (a) May partially or totally divide the gallbladder.
  (b) May partially or totally divide the cystic duct, producing various degrees of double gallbladder.
- Duplication of the common duct:
  (a) Very rare. Can be partial or complete.
- The level of the junction of the cystic duct and common hepatic duct is variable.

PATIENT PREP

- Fasting for 8 to 12 hours to guarantee maximum gallbladder and biliary tract dilatation but may be scanned after 4 to 6 hours.

N O T E :   Before a gallbladder exam it is very important to determine when a patient last ate because the inability to visualize the gallbladder with ultrasound is indicative of gallbladder disease.

PATIENT POSITION

- **Supine** and **left lateral decubitus.**
- Left posterior oblique, sitting semierect to erect or prone as needed.

N O T E :   Biliary system examinations must be done in two patient positions. This allows for differentiation between pathologies. For example, gallstones and sludge move, and other considerations such as polyps and gallbladder carcinoma are stationary.

N O T E :   Different patient positions should be used whenever the suggested position does not give the desired results.

TRANSDUCER

- **3.0 MHz** or **3.5 MHz.**
- 5.0 MHz for thin patients and anterior-lying gallbladders.

BREATHING TECHNIQUE

- **Deep, held inspiration.**

N O T E :   Different breathing techniques should be used whenever the suggested breathing technique does not give the desired results.

GALLBLADDER SURVEY

N O T E :   Gallbladder and biliary tract surveys **must be done in two patient positions.** Use the following scanning methods for both positions.

☰ LONGITUDINAL SURVEY

Sagittal Plane • Anterior Approach

1. Begin with the transducer perpendicular, just inferior to the costal margin at the right medial angle of the ribs.

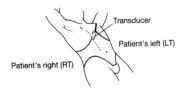

Usually this is the area of the portal vein and gallbladder neck. If the gallbladder is not seen here, find the main lobar fissure that extends from the gallbladder to the right portal vein.

N O T E :   Subcostal transducer angles can help locate the gallbladder. In some cases intercostal scanning will be necessary. Also, the gallbladder tends to lie in the area between the right medial angle of the ribs and the superior pole of the right kidney. Therefore, moving the transducer inferior and right lateral can be another way to locate the gallbladder.

2. Once the gallbladder is located, determine its longitudinal lie. This can be accomplished by rotating the transducer to oblique the scanning plane. Occasionally, no oblique is required.

N O T E :   The longitudinal of the gallbladder can lie in either the sagittal plane or transverse plane because of the variability in gallbladder position.

3. Assuming the longitudinal is seen in an oblique sagittal plane, slightly rock the transducer right to left, sweeping through both sides of the gallbladder and at the same time slide inferiorly through and beyond the fundus.

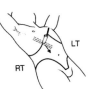

4. Rocking and sliding, move the transducer superiorly back onto the fundus and continue scanning up through the body and neck until you are beyond the gallbladder.

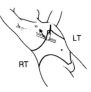

≡ TRANSVERSE SURVEY

Transverse Plane • Anterior Approach

1. Still in the sagittal scanning plane, locate the fundus of the gallbladder. Rotate the transducer 90 degrees into the transverse scanning plane and traverse the fundus. The fundus will appear round or oval.

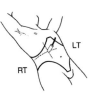

NOTE: An optional method for locating the gallbladder in the transverse plane is locating the superior pole of the right kidney first. In most cases, the fundus of the gallbladder is seen immediately anterior to the superior right pole.

2. Slightly rock the transducer superior to inferior and at the same time slide inferiorly through and beyond the fundus.

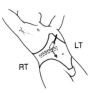

3. Continue rocking and slide the transducer superiorly back onto the fundus and continue scanning up through the body and neck until you are beyond the gallbladder.

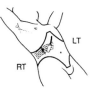

BILIARY TRACT SURVEY

☰ LONGITUDINAL SURVEY

Sagittal Plane • Anterior Approach

1. Begin by locating the neck of the gallbladder or the main lobar fissure. Note the portal vein and look for the longitudinal of the common duct anteriorly. It may be necessary to rotate the transducer at varying degrees (to oblique the scanning plane according to the lie of the duct) to visualize the long axis of the common duct. Note that the common duct usually lies at a right angle to the costal margin.

N O T E : In a sagittal oblique plane the portal vein at the level of the porta hepatis will be traversed, seen as round or oval. Inferior to this the portal vein appears longitudinal as it runs posterior and parallel to the duct.

2. *Slightly* rock the transducer right to left sweeping through both sides of the duct and at the same time *slowly* slide the transducer *slightly* superior and right lateral through and beyond the common hepatic duct.

Note that the distance you move is small.

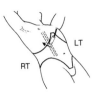

Note the traversed hepatic artery between the duct and the portal vein.

3. Move the transducer back onto the common hepatic duct and return to the level of the gallbladder neck or main lobar fissure.

4. Continue by *slightly* rocking the transducer right to left and at the same time *slowly* slide the transducer *slightly* inferior and medial through the common bile duct to the head of the pancreas.

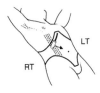

Note that the distance you move is small.

Note the traversed hepatic artery between the duct and the portal vein.

Stay at this location to begin the transverse survey.

N O T E : The common bile duct can be difficult to see when it is behind the duodenum because of bowel gas. Continue to scan through the duodenum and pick up the duct again just inferior to the duodenum or at the head of the pancreas. Giving the patient enough water to drink to fill the duodenum can aid in the evaluation of the retroduodenal portion of the common bile duct, as the water displaces the bowel gas.

☰ TRANSVERSE SURVEY

Transverse Plane • Anterior Approach

N O T E :   Because of the small size of the common duct, transverse evaluation can be difficult. Therefore, common hepatic duct (proximal) evaluation is done at the gallbladder neck and common bile duct (distal) evaluation is done at the head of the pancreas.

1. Still in the sagittal scanning plane evaluating the longitudinal of the common bile duct at the head of the pancreas, rotate the transducer 90 degrees into the transverse scanning plane and traverse the common bile duct.

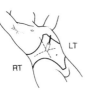

2. If you lose sight of the duct while rotating the transducer, look for the small round or oval duct in the lateral and posterior portions of the pancreatic head. Note the traversed gastroduodenal artery anterior to the duct.

3. Return to the sagittal scanning plane and locate the neck of the gallbladder and just superior to it the longitudinal common hepatic duct. Rotate the transducer 90 degrees into the transverse scanning plane and traverse the common hepatic duct.

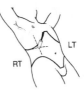

4. If you lose sight of the duct while rotating the transducer, look for the small round or oval duct anterior to the portal vein.

REQUIRED IMAGES

> **N O T E :**   Gallbladder and biliary tract pictures **must be done in two patient positions.**

First Position/Supine

☰ LONGITUDINAL GALLBLADDER IMAGES

Sagittal Plane • Anterior Approach

1. Long axis image of the gallbladder.

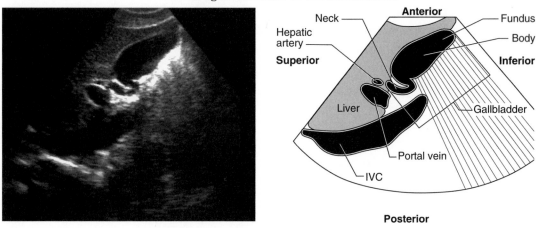

L A B E L E D :   GB SAG LONG AXIS

> **N O T E :**   In many cases gallbladder definition is sacrificed to achieve the long axis. Therefore, additional longitudinal images of the gallbladder fundus, body, and neck should be taken.

2. Longitudinal image of the gallbladder fundus and body.

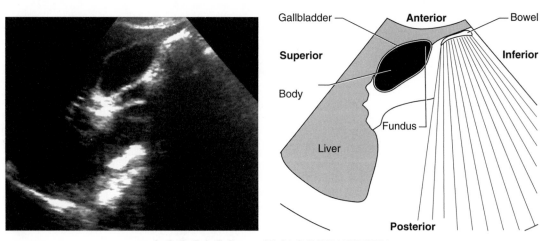

L A B E L E D :   GB SAG FUNDUS/BODY

3. Longitudinal image of the gallbladder neck.

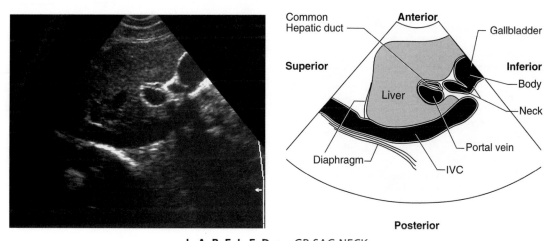

L A B E L E D :   GB SAG NECK

☰ TRANSVERSE GALLBLADDER IMAGES

Transverse Plane • Anterior Approach

4. Transverse image of the gallbladder fundus.

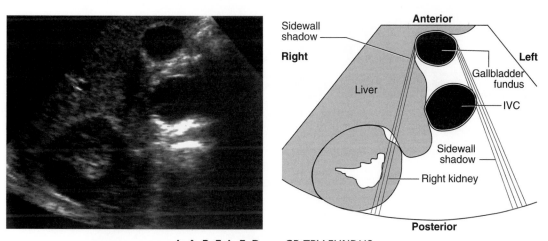

L A B E L E D :   GB TRV FUNDUS

5. Transverse image of the gallbladder body.

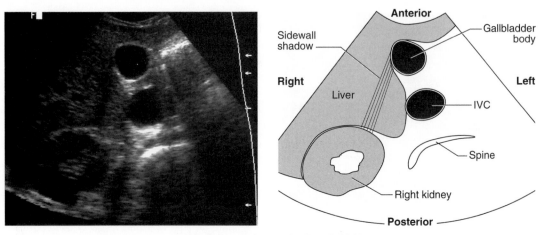

L A B E L E D :   GB TRV BODY

6. Transverse image of the gallbladder neck.

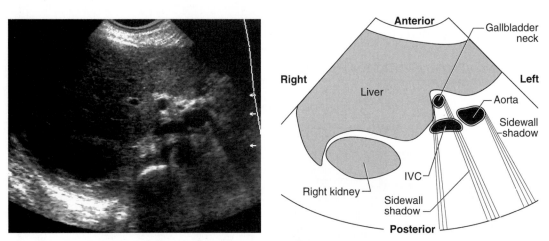

L A B E L E D :   GB TRV NECK

≡ LONGITUDINAL BILIARY TRACT IMAGES

Sagittal Plane • Anterior Approach

N O T E :   Images of the common duct may be taken in the second patient position if they were better visualized there during the survey.

N O T E :   Images of the common duct can be magnified to aid interpretation.

7. Longitudinal image of the common hepatic duct.

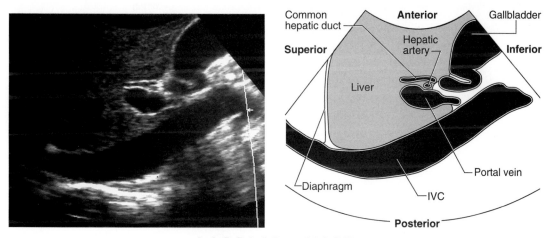

L A B E L E D :   SAG CHD

N O T E :   The longitudinal common hepatic duct image can be eliminated if the common hepatic duct was imaged with the gallbladder long axis image or longitudinal neck image.

8. Longitudinal image of the common bile duct with *anterior to posterior measurement.*

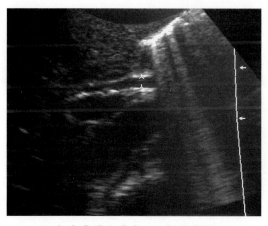

L A B E L E D :   SAG CBD

9. Same image as number 8 without calipers.

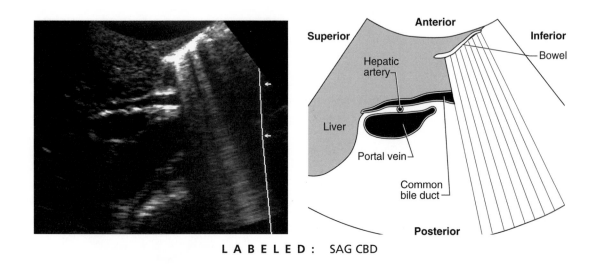

L A B E L E D :   SAG CBD

N O T E :   Measurement of the duct should be at the widest part of the lumen.

Second Position/Left Lateral Decubitus

≡ LONGITUDINAL GALLBLADDER IMAGE

Sagittal Plane • Anterior Approach

10. Long axis image of the gallbladder.

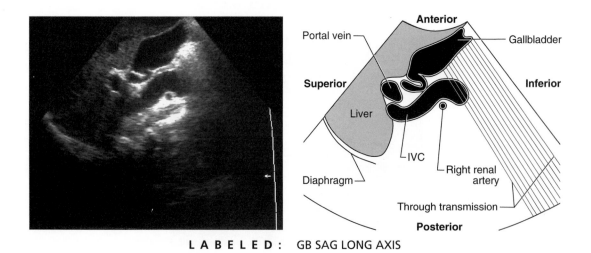

L A B E L E D :   GB SAG LONG AXIS

≡ TRANSVERSE GALLBLADDER IMAGE

Transverse Plane • Anterior Approach

11. Transverse image of the gallbladder fundus.

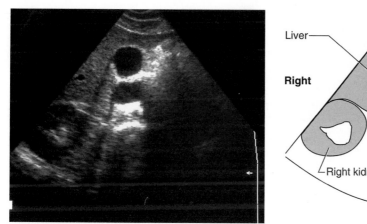 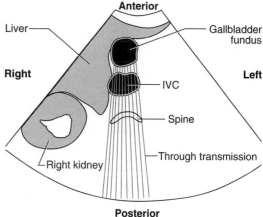

L A B E L E D :   GB TRV FUNDUS

REQUIRED IMAGES WHEN THE GALLBLADDER AND BILIARY TRACT ARE NOT THE PRIMARY AREA OF INTEREST

Single Position

≡ LONGITUDINAL GALLBLADDER IMAGE

Sagittal Plane • Anterior Approach

1. Long axis image of the gallbladder.

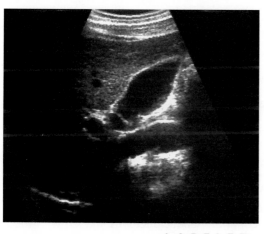 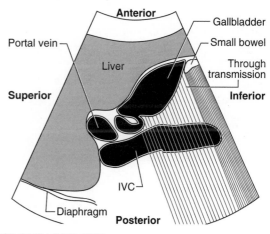

L A B E L E D :   GB SAG LONG AXIS

≡ TRANSVERSE GALLBLADDER IMAGE

Transverse Plane • Anterior Approach

2. Transverse image of the gallbladder fundus.

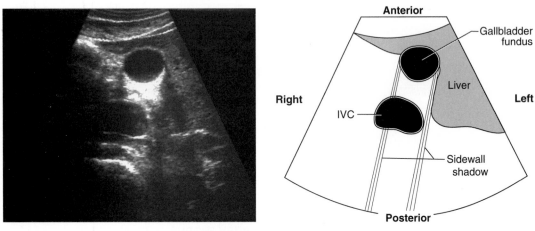

LABELED: GB TRV FUNDUS

≡ LONGITUDINAL BILIARY TRACT IMAGES

Sagittal Plane • Anterior Approach

NOTE: Images of the common duct can be magnified to aid interpretation.

3. Longitudinal image of the common hepatic duct.

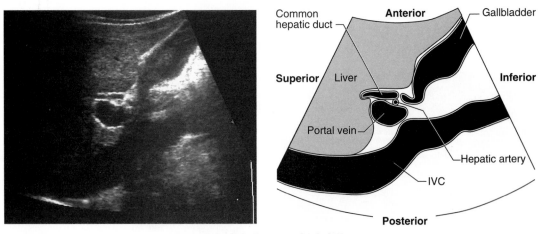

LABELED: SAG CHD

NOTE: The longitudinal common hepatic duct image can be eliminated if the common hepatic duct was imaged with the gallbladder long axis image.

4. Longitudinal image of the common bile duct with *anterior to posterior measurement*.

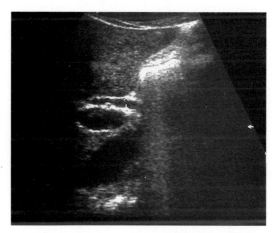

L A B E L E D :   SAG CBD

5. Same image as number 4 without calipers.

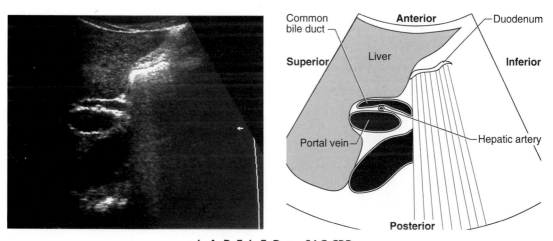

L A B E L E D :   SAG CBD

N O T E :   Measurement of the duct should be at the widest part of the lumen.

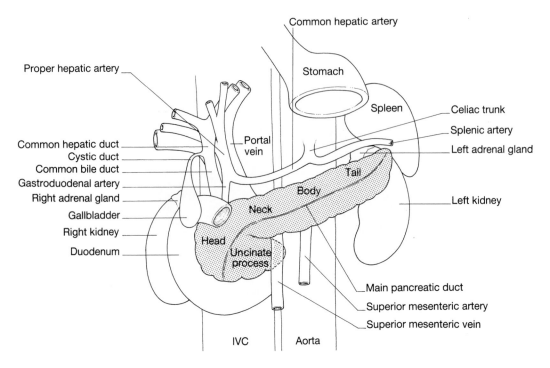

Location and anatomy of the pancreas

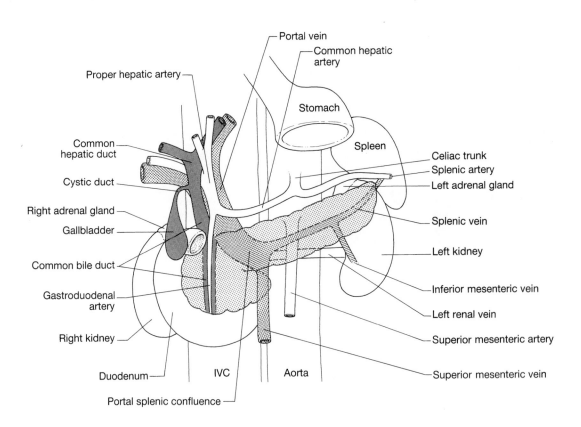

Location and anatomy of the pancreas

Pancreas Scanning Protocol

CHAPTER

7

LOCATION

- The pancreas traverses the body, extending from the hilum of the spleen to the duodenum.
- Retroperitoneal.
- Pancreas head and uncinate are anterior to the IVC.
- The uncinate is posterior to the superior mesenteric vein.
- Pancreas neck is anterior to the superior mesenteric vein.
- Pancreas body is posterior to the stomach.
- Pancreas body is anterior to the splenic vein, superior mesenteric artery, left renal vein, and aorta.
- Pancreas body and tail are inferior to the splenic artery.
- Pancreas tail is anterior to the splenic vein and left kidney.

ANATOMY

- The pancreas is 15 to 20 cm long, and though it is not actually segmented, it is described in segments.

  (a) **Head:** Lies to the right of the superior mesenteric vein against the medial curve of the duodenum and immediately anterior to the IVC.

  The gastroduodenal artery lies at the anterolateral border. The common bile duct lies at the posterolateral border.

  The anterior to posterior dimensions of the head range from 2.0 to 2.5 cm.

  (b) **Uncinate process:** The medial portion of the head that lies immediately posterior to the superior mesenteric vein. Variable in size, it can extend left lateral and lie immediately posterior to the superior mesenteric artery.

  (c) **Neck:** Lies immediately anterior to the superior mesenteric vein, and slightly superior to that level lies anterior to the formation of the portal vein.

  The anterior to posterior dimensions of the neck range from 1.0 to 2.0 cm.

(d) **Body:** Lies to the left of the neck, immediately anterior to the splenic vein, and extends left lateral toward the pancreas tail.

The anterior to posterior dimensions of the body range from 1.0 to 2.0 cm.

(e) **Tail:** Lies to the left of the pancreas body, immediately anterior to the splenic vein, and extends left lateral to the hilum of the spleen.

The anterior to posterior dimensions of the tail range from 1.0 to 2.0 cm.

- Size, shape, and lie are variable. Viewed anteriorly the pancreas can be seen head to tail, with the head appearing slightly larger.
- The pancreas decreases in size with age.
- Wirsung's duct, the main pancreatic duct, extends the length of the pancreas and enlarges toward the head up to 3 mm. It meets with the common bile duct at the pancreas head, and joined together or separately the ducts enter the duodenum.
- Santorini's duct, an accessory duct, is small and sometimes absent. It enters the duodenum separately from Wirsung's duct.

PHYSIOLOGY

- Endocrine function produces the hormone insulin to prevent diabetes mellitus.
- Exocrine function produces pancreatic enzymes that, via the pancreatic duct(s), aid digestion.

SONOGRAPHIC APPEARANCE

- Pancreas is homogeneous, midgray or medium-level echoes with even texture that is equal to or more echogenic than the normal liver.
- The pancreas becomes more echogenic with age.
- The contour of the normal pancreas should always be smooth.

N O T E :　The pancreas is not encapsulated, and therefore retroperitoneal fat may infiltrate the gland and make the contour difficult to evaluate.

- Wirsung's duct and Santorini's duct are anechoic tubular structures with echogenic walls.

NORMAL VARIANTS

- Size, shape, and lie are variable.

PATIENT PREP

- Fasting for 8 to 12 hours to reduce the stomach and bowel gas anterior to the pancreas. Also to ensure gallbladder and biliary tract dilatation for evaluation because certain pathologies of the pancreas, gallbladder, and biliary tract affect each other.
- If the patient has eaten, still do the exam. Stomach content can displace gas and act as a window for the sound beam. For this reason, 2 to 4 cups of water or noncarbonated drink can be given to the patient to aid evaluation if gas is obscuring the pancreas. This fluid technique works best if the patient is sitting erect.
- Peristalsis can cause the fluid to pass quickly through the stomach and duodenum, making evaluation of the pancreas inadequate. Peristaltic-reducing drugs such as glucagon can be given to prevent this.

PATIENT POSITION

- **Supine.**
- Sitting semierect to erect, left posterior oblique, left lateral decubitus, or prone as needed.

N O T E : Different patient positions should be used whenever the suggested position does not give the desired results.

TRANSDUCER

- **3.0 MHz or 3.5 MHz.**
- 5.0 MHz for thin patients and the anterior lying pancreas.

BREATHING TECHNIQUE

- **Deep, held inspiration.**

N O T E : Different breathing techniques should be used whenever the suggested breathing technique does not give the desired results.

PANCREAS SURVEY

N O T E :   While surveying the pancreas, evaluate the peri-pancreatic regions for adenopathy.

≡ LONGITUDINAL SURVEY

Transverse Plane • Anterior Approach

1. Begin with the transducer perpendicular, at the midline of the body, just inferior to the xiphoid process of the sternum.

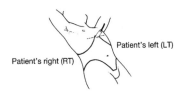

2. Slightly rock the transducer superior to inferior and slowly slide the transducer inferiorly.

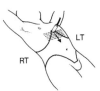

Note that the body of the pancreas lies just inferior to the traversed celiac trunk and longitudinal splenic artery and just anterior to the longitudinal splenic vein, which is immediately anterior to the traversed superior mesenteric artery.

3. Once you locate the pancreas body, it may be necessary to rotate the transducer at varying degrees (to oblique the scanning plane according to the lie of the pancreas) to visualize the longitudinal of the body. Note the anterior lying stomach between the pancreas body and liver. Look for the pancreatic duct in the center of the pancreas body.

4. Continue to scan inferiorly through the pancreas body until you are beyond it.

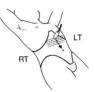

N O T E :   Angling the transducer inferiorly from the midline of the body and superior to the pancreas body may aid evaluation.

5. Move the transducer back onto the pancreas body and move the transducer left lateral onto the pancreas tail. Rotating the transducer can help visualize the longitudinal of the tail.

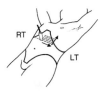

Once located, scan superiorly through the pancreas tail until you are beyond it.

6. Move the transducer back onto the tail and scan inferiorly through the pancreas tail until you are beyond it.

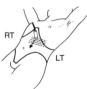

Note that the tail lies just posterior to the stomach and just anterior to the longitudinal splenic vein, which is immediately anterior to the traversed superior pole of the left kidney. Also, in most cases the pancreas tail is left lateral to the superior mesenteric artery and aorta. Look for the pancreatic duct in the center of the tail.

N O T E : Angling the transducer left lateral toward the pancreas tail from the midline of the body at the level of the pancreas body may aid evaluation. Also, using a posterior approach can aid evaluation. Look for the pancreas tail anterior to the superior pole of the left kidney.

7. Return to the pancreas body and move the transducer right lateral onto the pancreas neck. Rotating the transducer can help visualize the longitudinal of the neck. Once located, scan superiorly through the neck until you are beyond it.

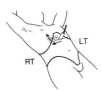

Note that the superior portion of the neck lies just anterior to the longitudinal portal splenic confluence. Look for the pancreatic duct in the center of the neck.

8. Move back onto the neck and scan slightly inferior through the neck and onto the pancreatic head.

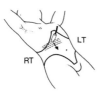

Note that the inferior portion of the neck is just anterior to the traversed superior mesenteric vein that separates the neck from the uncinate process.

N O T E : Angling the transducer right lateral toward the pancreatic neck from the midline of the body at the level of the pancreas body may aid evaluation.

9. Move back onto the neck and scan slightly right lateral and inferior onto the pancreatic head. If necessary, adjust the position of the transducer to visualize both sides of the head, then continue scanning inferiorly through the head until you are beyond it.

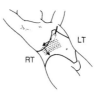

Note that the head and uncinate are just anterior to the traversed IVC. Note the traversed common bile duct at the posterior right lateral border and the traversed gastroduodenal artery at the anterior right lateral border. Note the duodenum immediately right lateral to the head. Look for the pancreatic duct in the center of the head.

N O T E : Angling the transducer right lateral toward the pancreatic head from the midline of the body at a level inferior to the pancreatic body may aid evaluation.

☰ TRANSVERSE SURVEY

Sagittal Plane • Anterior Approach

1. Begin with the transducer perpendicular and locate the distal long axis portion of the IVC where it passes through the liver. Move inferiorly along the IVC until you locate the head of the pancreas immediately anterior to it. In most cases this is at the level of the IVC where the traversed right renal artery passes posterior to it.

3. Move the transducer slightly toward the midline of the body and onto the uncinate process.

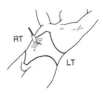

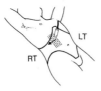

2. Once the pancreas head is located, move the transducer right lateral scanning through the head until you are beyond it. Move back onto this lateral portion of the head and note the traversed portal vein and proper hepatic artery superiorly.

Note the longitudinal superior mesenteric vein immediately anterior to the uncinate separating it from the pancreatic neck. In most cases the uncinate lies just anterior to the IVC, but it may extend left lateral and anterior to the aorta.

4. Scan left lateral through the pancreatic neck and uncinate and onto the pancreatic body. It may be helpful to rotate the transducer varying degrees to visualize the long axis of the aorta and superior mesenteric artery and look for the pancreas body anteriorly.

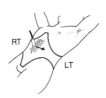

Note the longitudinal common bile duct posteriorly and the longitudinal gastroduodenal artery anteriorly. Note that the pancreatic head lies between the IVC and the liver. Look for the pancreatic duct in the center of the head.

Once the pancreas body is located, note that it lies immediately anterior to the traversed splenic vein. Note the traversed splenic artery immediately superior. Look for the pancreatic duct in the center of the body. Note the anterior and inferior lying stomach between the pancreas body and liver.

5. Scan left lateral through and beyond the pancreas body onto the pancreas tail.

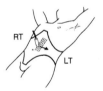

Note that the tail lies just posterior to the stomach, just inferior to the splenic artery, and just anterior to the traversed splenic vein, which is immediately anterior to the longitudinal left kidney. Also, in most cases the tail lies left lateral to the aorta. Look for the pancreatic duct in the center of the tail.

6. Continue to scan left laterally through the pancreas tail until you are beyond it.

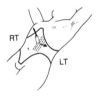

N O T E : Using a posterior approach can aid evaluation. Look for the pancreas tail anterior to the longitudinal left kidney.

REQUIRED IMAGES

☰ LONGITUDINAL IMAGES

Transverse Plane • Anterior Approach

1. Long axis image of the pancreas to include as much head, uncinate, neck, body, tail, and pancreatic duct as possible.

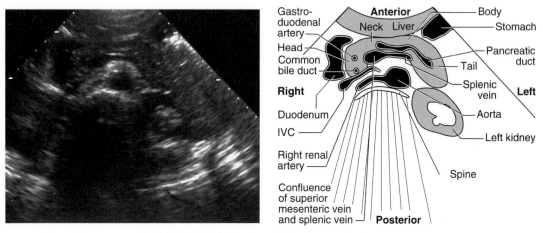

L A B E L E D :   PANCREAS TRV LONG AXIS

2. Longitudinal image of the pancreas body and neck to include the splenic vein.

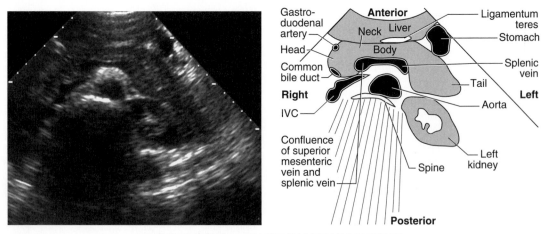

L A B E L E D :   PANCREAS TRV BODY/NECK

3. Longitudinal image of the pancreas tail.

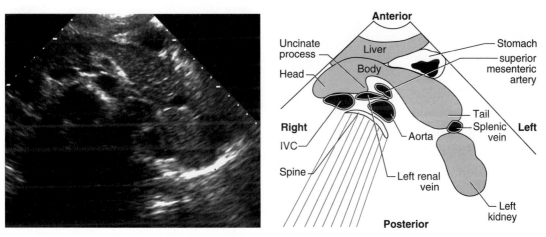

L A B E L E D : PANCREAS TRV TAIL

4. Longitudinal image of the pancreas head to include the uncinate process and common bile duct (if bile-filled).

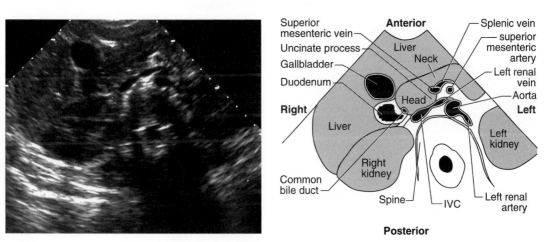

L A B E L E D : PANCREAS TRV HEAD

☰ TRANSVERSE IMAGES

Sagittal Plane • Anterior Approach

5. Transverse image of the pancreas head to include the common bile duct (if bile-filled).

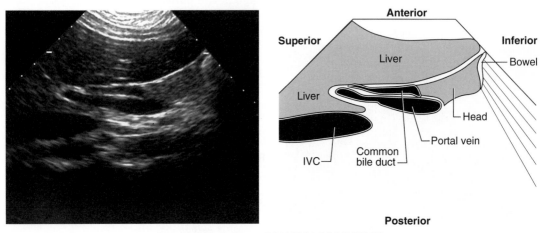

L A B E L E D :   PANCREAS SAG HEAD

6. Transverse image of the pancreas neck and uncinate process to include the superior mesenteric vein.

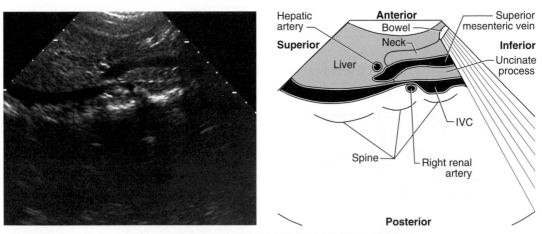

L A B E L E D :   PANCREAS SAG NECK/UNCINATE

7. Transverse image of the pancreas body to include the splenic vein.

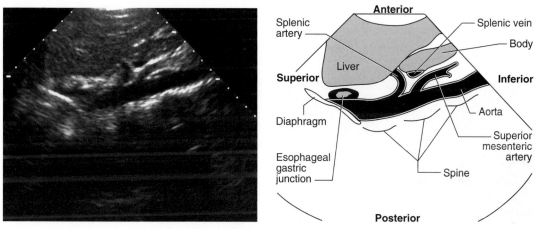

L A B E L E D :   PANCREAS SAG BODY

8. Transverse image of the pancreas tail.

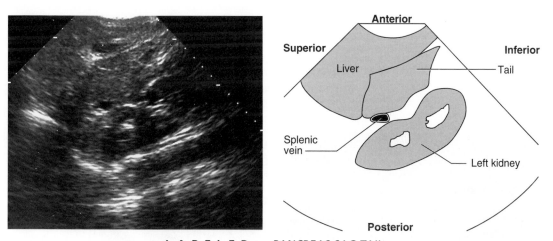

L A B E L E D :   PANCREAS SAG TAIL

N O T E :   Measurements of the normal pancreas are not required.

N O T E :   If the pancreas cannot be seen because of overlying bowel gas, and the patient cannot be given fluids and every effort has been made to image the pancreas, take the above images in the designated area and add "area" to the labeling.

REQUIRED IMAGES WHEN THE PANCREAS IS NOT THE PRIMARY AREA OF INTEREST

☰ LONGITUDINAL IMAGES

Transverse Plane • Anterior Approach

1. Long axis image of the pancreas to include as much head, uncinate, neck, body, tail, and pancreatic duct as possible.

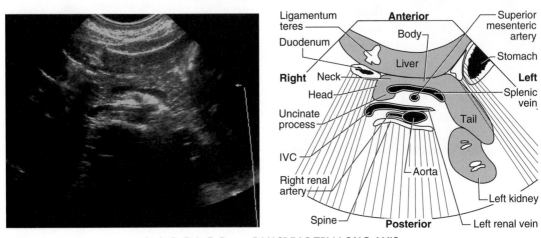

L A B E L E D :   PANCREAS TRV LONG AXIS

2. Longitudinal image of the pancreas head to include the uncinate process and common bile duct (if bile-filled).

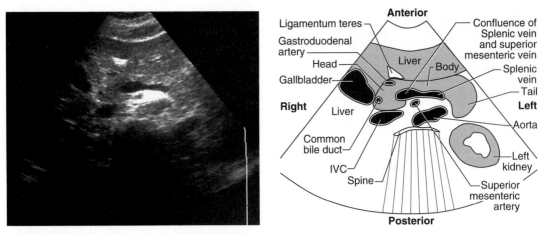

L A B E L E D :   PANCREAS TRV HEAD

≡ TRANSVERSE IMAGE

Sagittal Plane • Anterior Approach

3. Transverse image of the pancreas head to include the common bile duct (if bile-filled).

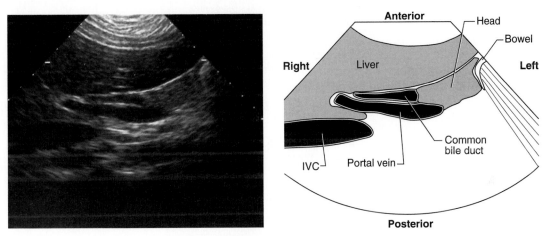

L A B E L E D :   PANCREAS SAG HEAD

N O T E :   If the pancreas cannot be seen because of overlying bowel gas and the patient cannot be given fluids and every effort has been made to image the pancreas, take the above images in the designated areas and add "area" to the labeling.

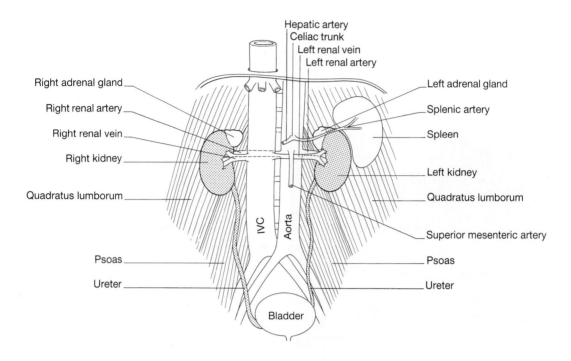

Location of the urinary system

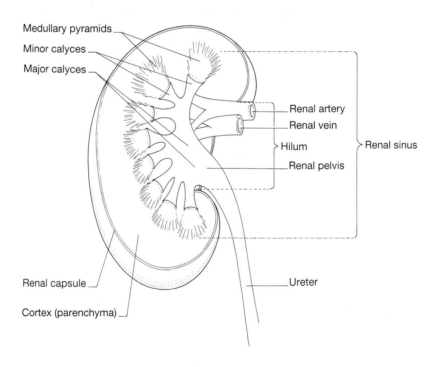

Anatomy of the kidney

Renal Scanning Protocol

LOCATION

- The kidneys lie on each side of the spine in the area between the 12th thoracic and 4th lumbar vertebrae.
- Retroperitoneal.
- The right kidney is lower than the left kidney.
- The right kidney is posteroinferior to the liver and gallbladder.
- The left kidney is inferior and medial to the spleen.
- The kidneys lie immediately anterior to the psoas and quadratus lumborum muscles.
- Located superior, anterior, and medial to each kidney is the adrenal gland.

ANATOMY

- The kidneys are covered by a fibrous "renal or true capsule."
- Fat surrounds the encapsulated kidneys in the perinephric space.
- Gerota's fascia is a fibrous sheath that encloses each kidney, perinephric fat, and adrenal gland.
- Normal adult kidneys are 9 to 12 cm long, 2.5 to 3.5 cm thick, and 4 to 5 cm wide.
- The kidneys are composed of two distinct areas:
    (a) **Sinus:**

    The entrance to the sinus is referred to as the hilum. Through it passes the renal arteries, veins, nerves, lymphatic vessels, and ureter.

    The sinus contains fat and the renal pelvis, which is formed by the expanded superior end of the ureter. The renal pelvis is a urine reservoir or collecting system that divides into the infundibula: two or three major calyces that in turn divide into 8 or 18 minor calyces. Each minor calyx is indented by the top or apex of a medullary pyramid, from which it receives urine.

    (b) **Parenchyma:**

    Surrounds the sinus.

    Outer cortex:

    Contains millions of nephrons, the microscopic func-

101

tional units of the kidney. Site of urine formation. The cortex lies between the renal capsule and the medulla. Inner medulla:

Consists of 8 to 18 renal pyramids that pass urine to the minor calyces. The bases of the pyramids form a margin with the cortex. The apices of the pyramids project into the bottom or side of the renal sinus and into the minor calyces. The pyramids are separated from each other by bands of cortical tissue referred to as the columns of Bertin, which extend inward to the renal sinus.

PHYSIOLOGY

- As part of the excretory system, kidneys function to get rid of metabolic wastes.
- Kidneys purify the blood by excreting urine (excess water, salt, toxins).

SONOGRAPHIC APPEARANCE

- Because of the fat, the renal sinus is echogenic with variable contour. Parenchyma surrounds the sinus.
- The infundibula and renal pelvis are not seen if collapsed; otherwise, they appear anechoic.
- The cortex is homogeneous, midgray or medium- to low-level echoes with even texture that is less echogenic than the normal liver or spleen. The contour of the normal cortex should appear smooth. The cortex is surrounded by the echogenic renal capsule.
- The medullary pyramids appear as triangular, round, or blunted by hypoechoic areas to the more urine-filled anechoic areas.
- Arcuate vessels can be seen at the corticomedullary junction as echogenic dots.
- The ureters are not normally seen.

NORMAL VARIANTS

- Dromedary humps:
  (a) Cortical bulge(s) on the lateral border of the kidney.
  (b) Sonographic appearance is the same as normal renal cortex.
- Hypertrophied column of Bertin:
  (a) At varying degrees of size, cortical tissue indents the renal sinus.
  (b) Sonographic appearance is the same as normal renal cortex.

- Double collecting system:
  - (a) The renal sinus is divided by a hypertrophied column of Bertin.
  - (b) Sonographic appearance is the same as normal renal cortex and normal renal sinus.
- Horseshoe kidney:
  - (a) The kidneys are connected, usually at the lower poles.
  - (b) Sonographic appearance is the same as normal renal cortex.
- Renal ectopia:
  - (a) One or both kidneys may be found outside the normal renal fossa.
  - (b) Other locations include lower abdominal to pelvic and rarely intrathoracic.

PATIENT PREP

- None.

PATIENT POSITION

Right Kidney

- **Supine.**
- Left posterior oblique, left lateral decubitus, and prone as needed.

Left Kidney

- **Right lateral decubitus.**
- Prone as needed.

N O T E :   Different patient positions should be used whenever the suggested position does not give the desired results.

TRANSDUCER

- **3.0 MHz or 3.5 MHz.**
- 5.0 MHz for very thin patient.

BREATHING TECHNIQUE

- **Deep, held inspiration.**

RENAL SURVEY

N O T E :   While surveying the kidneys, evaluate the perirenal regions for possible abnormalities.

Right Kidney Survey

≡ LONGITUDINAL SURVEY

Sagittal Plane • Anterior Approach

1. Begin with the transducer perpendicular, just inferior to the most lateral edge of the right costal margin.

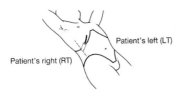

2. If the kidney is not seen here, move the transducer in medial and inferior sections until the kidney is located.

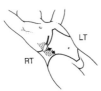

3. Once the kidney is located, rotate the transducer at varying degrees (to oblique the scanning plane according to the lie of the right kidney) to visualize the long axis of the kidney.

4. Once the long axis is located, slightly rock the transducer right to left and slide the transducer medially scanning through the kidney until you are beyond it.

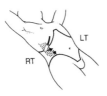

5. Move back onto the medial portion of the kidney. Rocking and sliding, scan through the lateral portion of the kidney until you are beyond it.

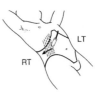

N O T E :   Longitudinal survey of the right kidney can be performed from a coronal plane, right lateral approach. Begin with the transducer perpendicular, midcoronal plane, just superior to the iliac crest. Move or angle the transducer superior to inferior or scan intercostal if necessary to locate the kidney.

Follow the above scanning methods. Note that this approach is generally easier when the patient is in the left lateral decubitus position.

☰ TRANSVERSE SURVEY

Transverse Plane • Anterior Approach

1. Still in the sagittal scanning plane, locate the long axis of the right kidney. Rotate the transducer 90 degrees into the transverse scanning plane and traverse the kidney.

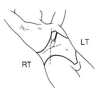

N O T E : Alternatively, begin the transverse survey in the transverse plane with the transducer perpendicular, just inferior to the costal margin of the medial angle of the ribs. Move the transducer in right lateral and inferior sections until the kidney is located.

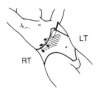

2. Once the kidney is located, move the transducer slightly superior and medial, to inferior and lateral, to find the midportion and hilum of the kidney. Slight and varying degrees of transducer obliques may be necessary to resolve the hilum. Note the renal artery and vein.

3. From the hilum, slightly rock the transducer superior to inferior and at the same time slide the transducer superior and medial through and beyond the superior pole of the kidney.

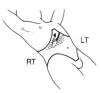

4. Continue rocking, and move the transducer back onto the superior pole. Slide the transducer inferior and lateral through midkidney and the inferior pole. Scan through and beyond the inferior pole.

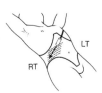

N O T E : Transverse survey of the right kidney can be performed from a right lateral approach. Use the same scanning approach mentioned for the coronal longitudinal survey and follow the above scanning methods.

Left Kidney Survey

≡ LONGITUDINAL SURVEY

Coronal Plane • Left Lateral Approach

N O T E :   Although this approach can be performed with the patient supine, it is generally easier with the patient in the right lateral decubitus position. Imaging quality might be improved by placing a sponge or rolled towel under the patient's right side. This opens up the rib spaces.

1. Begin with the transducer perpendicular, midcoronal plane, just superior to the iliac crest.

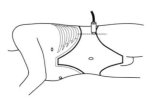

N O T E :   If the kidney is not seen in the midcoronal plane, try approaches just to the right and left of the midline.

2. Move or angle the transducer superior to inferior to locate the kidney. Once located, rotate the transducer at varying degrees (to oblique the scanning plane according to the lie of the left kidney) to visualize the long axis of the kidney.

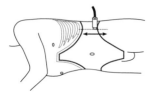

3. Once the long axis is located, slightly rock the transducer side to side and at the same time slide the

transducer toward the patient's front, scanning through the anterior portion of the kidney until you are beyond it.

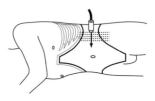

4. Move back onto the anterior portion of the kidney. Rocking and sliding, move toward the patient's back, scanning through the posterior portion of the kidney until you are beyond it.

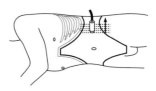

N O T E :   Longitudinal survey of the left kidney may have to be performed intercostally, depending on body habitus and the position of the kidney. Begin with the transducer perpendicular, midcoronal plane, in the first inferior intercostal space. Move to the adjacent intercostal spaces to evaluate the entire kidney. Varying respiration and angling the transducer within the intercostal spaces can aid evaluation. In some cases, only the superior pole will have to be evaluated intercostally.

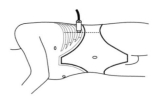

☰ TRANSVERSE SURVEY

Transverse Plane • Left Lateral Approach

1. Still in the coronal scanning plane, locate the long axis of the left kidney. Rotate the transducer 90 degrees into the transverse scanning plane and traverse the kidney.

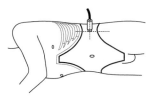

N O T E :   Alternatively, begin the transverse survey in the transverse plane with the transducer perpendicular, just superior to the iliac crest. Move or angle the transducer superior to inferior to locate the kidney.

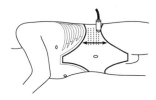

2. Once the kidney is located, move the transducer superior to inferior to find the midportion and hilum of the kidney. Slight and varying degrees of transducer obliques may be necessary to resolve the hilum. Note the renal artery and vein.

3. From the hilum, slightly rock the transducer superior to inferior and at the same time slide the transducer superior through and beyond the superior pole of the kidney.

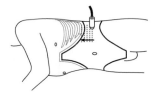

4. Continue rocking and move the transducer back onto the superior pole. Slide the transducer inferior through the midkidney and the inferior pole. Scan through and beyond the inferior pole.

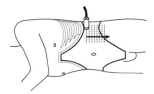

N O T E :   Transverse survey of the left kidney may have to be performed intercostally. Use the same approach mentioned for the intercostal coronal longitudinal survey and follow the above scanning methods.

REQUIRED IMAGES

Right Kidney

≡ LONGITUDINAL IMAGES

Sagittal Plane • Anterior Approach

1. Long axis image of the right kidney with *superior to inferior measurement.*

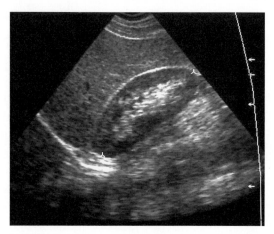

L A B E L E D :   RT KIDNEY SAG LONG AXIS

2. Same image as number 1 without calipers.

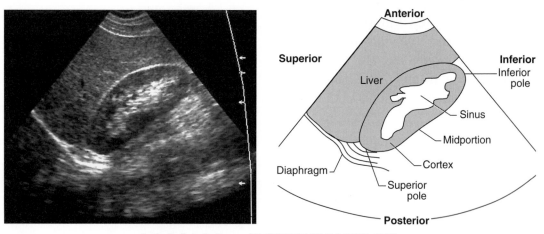

L A B E L E D :   RT KIDNEY SAG LONG AXIS

3. Long axis image of the right kidney with *superior to inferior measurement.*

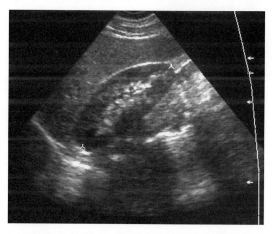

L A B E L E D :   RT KIDNEY SAG LONG AXIS

4. Same image as number 3 without calipers.

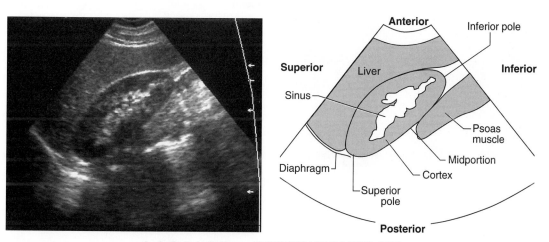

L A B E L E D :   RT KIDNEY SAG LONG AXIS

N O T E :   In many cases superior and/or inferior pole definition is sacrificed to achieve the long axis. If so, take those images here and label accordingly.

5. Longitudinal image of the right kidney superior pole.

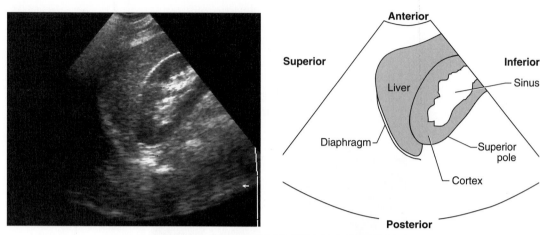

L A B E L E D :   RT KIDNEY SAG SUP POLE

6. Longitudinal image of the right kidney inferior pole.

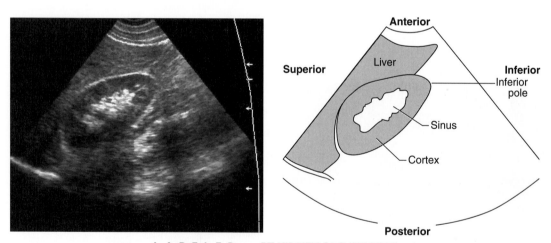

L A B E L E D :   RT KIDNEY SAG INF POLE

7. Longitudinal image of the right kidney just medial to the long axis.

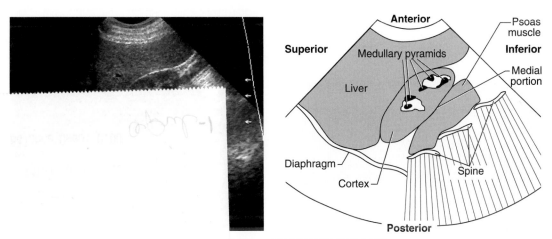

E D :   RT KIDNEY SAG MED

itudinal image of the right kidney just lateral to the axis to include part of the liver for parenchyma com-on.

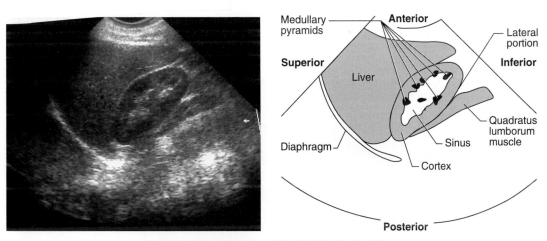

L A B E L E D :   RT KIDNEY SAG LAT

≡ TRANSVERSE IMAGES

Transverse Plane • Anterior Approach

9. Transverse image of the right kidney superior pole.

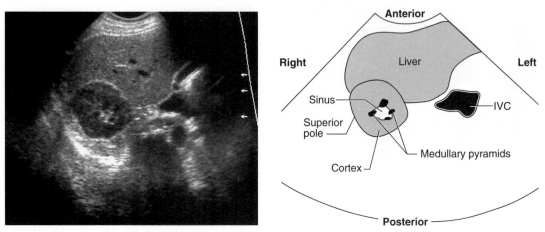

L A B E L E D :   RT KIDNEY TRV SUP POLE

10. Transverse image of the right kidney midportion to include the hilum with *anterior to posterior measurement.*

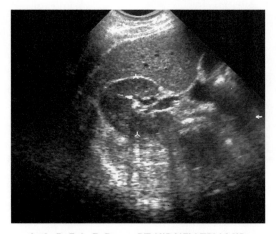

L A B E L E D :   RT KIDNEY TRV MID

11. Same image as number 10 without calipers.

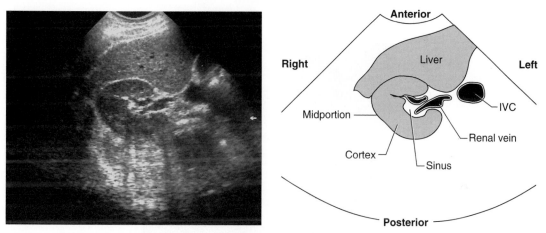

L A B E L E D : RT KIDNEY TRV MID

12. Transverse image of the right kidney inferior pole.

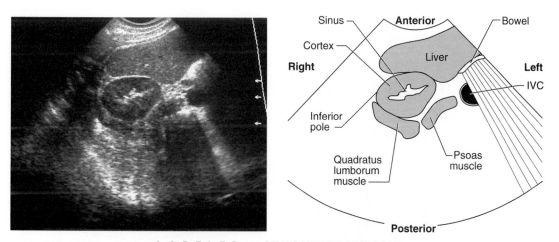

L A B E L E D : RT KIDNEY TRV INF POLE

Left Kidney

≡ LONGITUDINAL IMAGES

Coronal Plane • Left Lateral Approach

1. Long axis image of the left kidney with *superior to inferior measurement.*

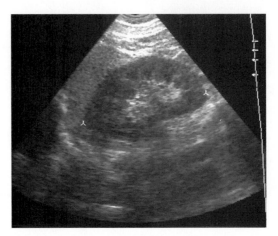

L A B E L E D :   LT KIDNEY COR LONG AXIS

2. Same image as number 1 without calipers.

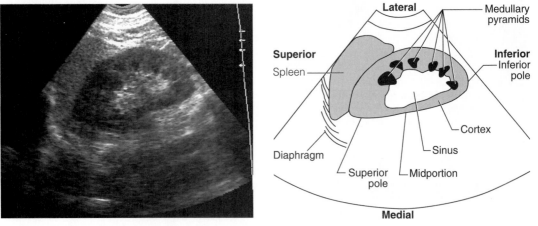

L A B E L E D :   LT KIDNEY COR LONG AXIS

3. Long axis image of the left kidney with *superior to inferior measurement.*

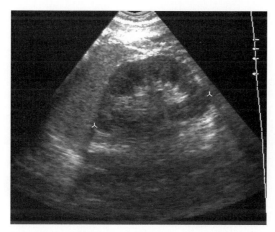

L A B E L E D :   LT KIDNEY COR LONG AXIS

4. Same image as number 3 without calipers.

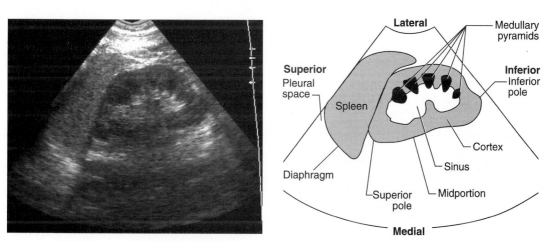

L A B E L E D :   LT KIDNEY COR LONG AXIS

N O T E :   In many cases, superior and/or inferior pole definition is sacrificed to achieve the long axis. If so, take those images here and label accordingly.

N O T E :   One of the long axis images or, if applicable, the superior pole image must include part of the spleen for parenchyma comparison.

5. Longitudinal image of the left kidney superior pole.

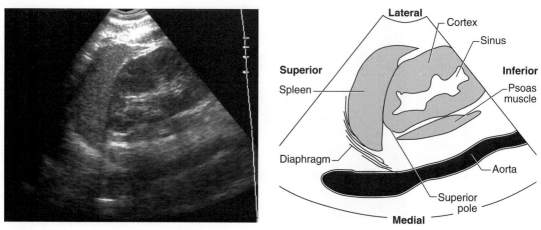

L A B E L E D :   LT KIDNEY COR SUP POLE

6. Longitudinal image of the left kidney inferior pole.

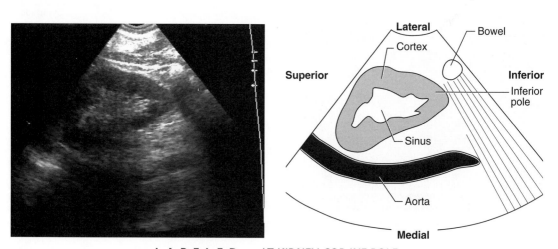

L A B E L E D :   LT KIDNEY COR INF POLE

7. Longitudinal image of the left kidney just anterior to the long axis.

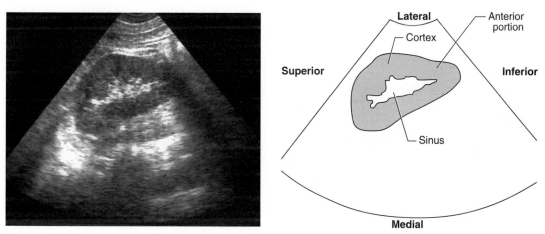

L A B E L E D : LT KIDNEY COR ANT

8. Longitudinal image of the left kidney just posterior to the long axis.

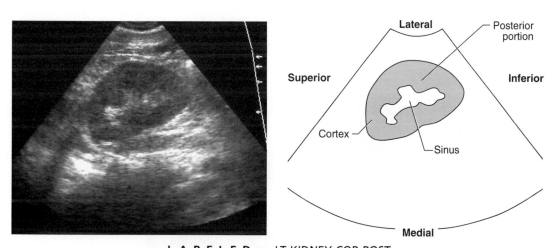

L A B E L E D : LT KIDNEY COR POST

≡ TRANSVERSE IMAGES

Transverse Plane • Left Lateral Approach

9. Transverse image of the left kidney superior pole.

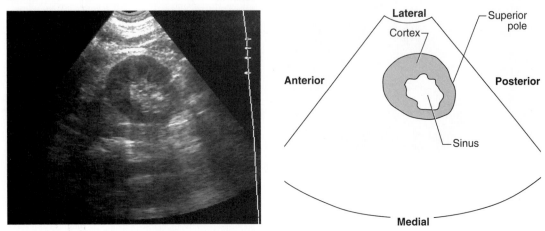

L A B E L E D :   LT KIDNEY LT TRV SUP POLE

10. Transverse image of the left kidney midportion to include the hilum with *anterior to posterior measurement.*

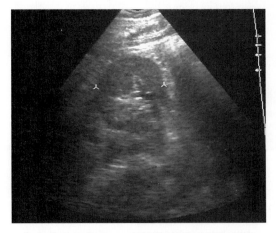

L A B E L E D :   LT KIDNEY LT TRV MID

11. Same image as number 10 without calipers.

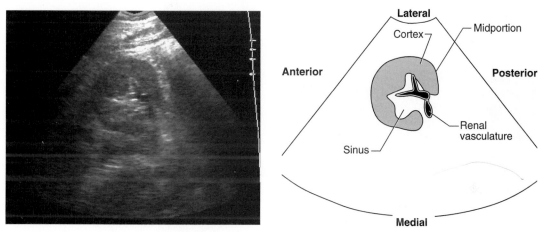

LABELED: LT KIDNEY LT TRV MID

12. Transverse image of the left kidney inferior pole.

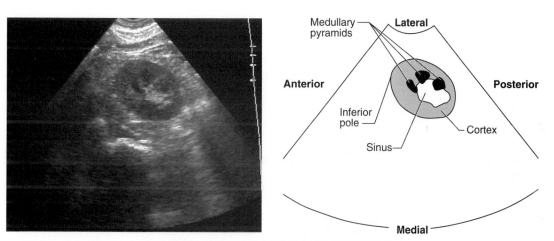

LABELED: LT KIDNEY LT TRV INF POLE

REQUIRED IMAGES WHEN THE KIDNEYS ARE NOT THE PRIMARY AREA OF INTEREST

Right Kidney

☰ LONGITUDINAL IMAGE(S)

Sagittal Plane • Anterior Approach

1. Long axis image of the right kidney.

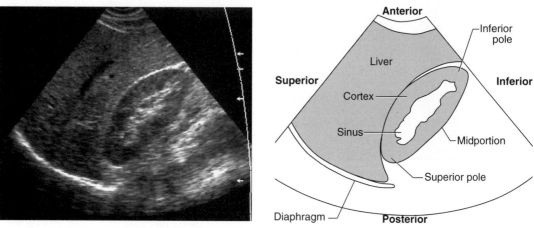

L A B E L E D :   RT KIDNEY SAG LONG AXIS

N O T E :   Take additional images of the superior and/or inferior poles if they are not clearly defined and label accordingly.

☰ TRANSVERSE IMAGE

Transverse Plane • Anterior Approach

2. Transverse image of the right kidney midportion to include the hilum.

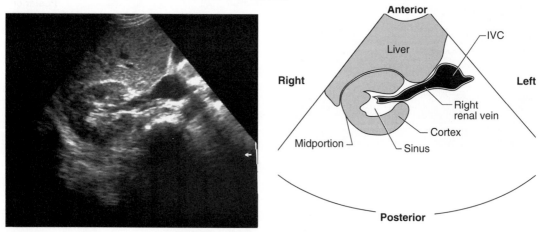

L A B E L E D :   RT KIDNEY TRV MID

Left Kidney

≡ LONGITUDINAL IMAGE(S)

Coronal Plane • Left Lateral Approach

3. Long axis image of the left kidney.

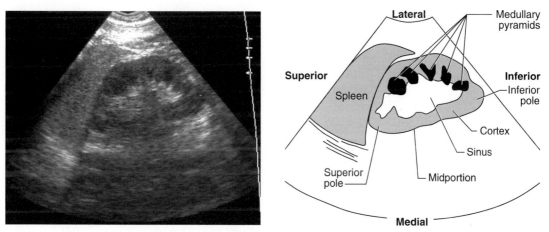

L A B E L E D :   LT KIDNEY COR LONG AXIS

N O T E :   Take additional images of the superior and/or inferior poles if they are not clearly defined and label accordingly.

≡ TRANSVERSE IMAGE

Transverse Plane • Left Lateral Approach

4. Transverse image of the left kidney midportion to include the hilum.

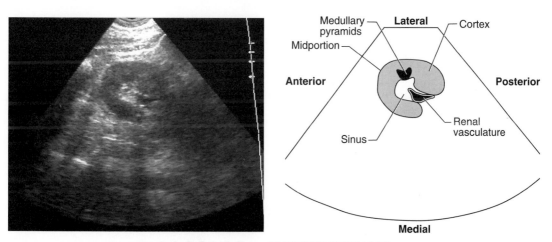

L A B E L E D :   LT KIDNEY LT TRV MID

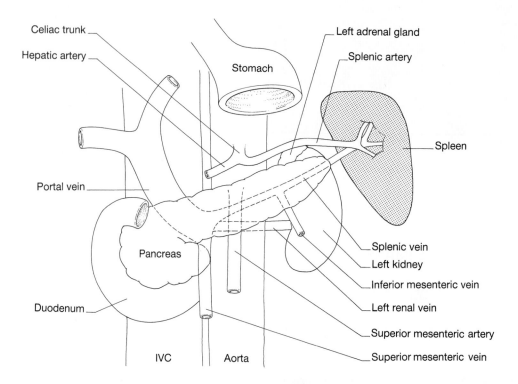

Location and anatomy of the spleen

Spleen Scanning Protocol

CHAPTER

9

LOCATION

- The spleen occupies the posterolateral section of the left upper quadrant.
- Intraperitoneal (except for its hilum).
- Immediately inferior and anterior to the diaphragm.
- Lateral to the stomach and, depending on its size, sometimes posterior to it.
- Lateral to the tail of the pancreas, left kidney, adrenal gland, and the splenic flexure of the colon.

ANATOMY

- Size is variable but is considered normal when it appears about the same size as the adjacent left kidney.
- Shape is variable but may resemble a half moon.
- The splenic vein and artery, lymphatic vessels, and nerves pass through the splenic hilum.
- The splenic vein passes through the splenic hilum and courses immediately posterior to the tail and body of the pancreas to join the superior mesenteric vein posterior to the pancreas neck to form the portal vein.
- The splenic artery courses from the celiac trunk of the aorta immediately superior to the body and tail of the pancreas to enter the splenic hilum.

PHYSIOLOGY

- The spleen is a large mass of lymphatic tissue that is part of the reticuloendothelial system.
- Although not essential to life, the spleen filters foreign material from the blood, and forms antibodies. It also breaks down hemoglobin, is a blood reservoir, and is important for blood formation in the fetus or when there is severe anemia.

SONOGRAPHIC APPEARANCE

- The parenchyma of the spleen is homogeneous, midgray, or medium-level echoes with even texture that is usually the same as the normal liver but may appear slightly less echogenic.
- Interspersed within the spleen are small vascular structures that are seen as branching, anechoic, and round or tubular. Closer to the hilum the larger venous structures can be distinguished from the smaller arterial branches.
- The outer contour of the normal spleen should appear smooth.

NORMAL VARIANTS

- Accessory spleen:
  (a) Splenic tissue found separate from the organ.
  (b) Found most often at the splenic hilum.
  (c) Sonographic appearance is the same as normal splenic tissue.
- Asplenia:
  (a) Rare absence of the spleen.
  (b) Often associated with congestive heart disease.

PATIENT PREP

- None.

PATIENT POSITION

- **Right lateral decubitus.**
- Supine, sitting semierect to erect and prone as needed.

N O T E :   Different patient positions should be used whenever the suggested position does not give the desired results.

TRANSDUCER

- **5.0 MHz** for intercostal or lateral subcostal scanning approaches.
- 3.0 or 3.5 MHz for anterior or posterior scanning approaches.

BREATHING TECHNIQUE

• **Deep, held inspiration.**

N O T E :   Different breathing techniques should be used whenever the suggested breathing technique does not give the desired results.

SPLEEN SURVEY

☰ LONGITUDINAL SURVEY

Coronal Plane • Left Lateral Approach

N O T E :   Although this approach can be performed with the patient supine, it is generally easier with the patient in the right lateral decubitus position. Imaging quality might be improved by placing a sponge or rolled towel under the patient's right side. This opens up the rib spaces.

1. Begin with the transducer perpendicular, midcoronal plane, in the most inferior intercostal space. In most cases the superior and inferior margins of the spleen can be visualized from this space. How much of the normal spleen you see, however, will depend on its shape and body habitus. If the spleen is not seen in the inferior intercostal space, move to adjacent superior intercostal spaces.

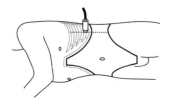

2. Once the spleen is located, rotate the transducer at varying degrees (to oblique the scanning plane according to the lie of the spleen) to visualize the long axis of the spleen.

Note the adjacent pleural space superiorly and the left kidney and per-inephric space inferiorly. The splenic hilum may also be seen medially. Slightly rotating the transducer can aid evaluation of the hilum.

3. While visualizing the long axis of the spleen, move or angle the transducer within the intercostal space toward the patient's front, scanning through the anterior portion of the spleen until you are beyond it.

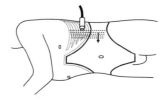

4. Move back onto the spleen and move or angle the transducer toward the patient's back, scanning through the posterior portion of the spleen until you are beyond it.

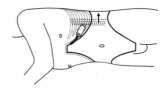

N O T E :   Rib shadows are a consequence of intercostal scanning and may obscure part of the spleen. In most cases, angling the transducer within the intercostal space toward the unseen area or moving to an adjacent rib space will aid visualization.

≡ TRANSVERSE SURVEY

Transverse Plane • Left Lateral Approach

1. Still in the coronal scanning plane, locate the long axis of the spleen, then rotate the transducer 90 degrees into the transverse scanning plane and traverse the spleen. Note the anterior and posterior margins of the spleen and the splenic hilum medially.

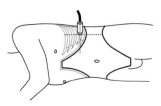

2. Move or angle the transducer superiorly, scanning through the superior portion of the spleen until you are beyond it. Note the adjacent pleural space.

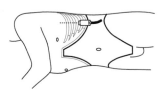

3. Move back onto the spleen and move or angle the transducer inferiorly, scanning through the inferior portion of the spleen until you are beyond it.

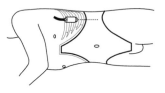

REQUIRED IMAGES

≡ LONGITUDINAL IMAGES

Coronal Plane • Left Lateral Approach

1. Long axis image of the spleen.

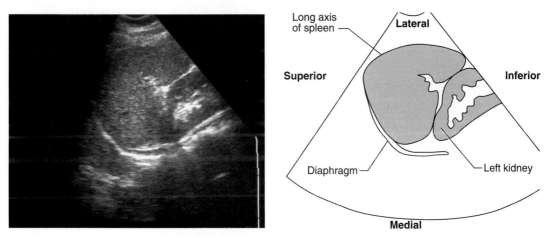

L A B E L E D :   SPLEEN COR LONG AXIS

2. Superior longitudinal image of the spleen to include the adjacent pleural space.

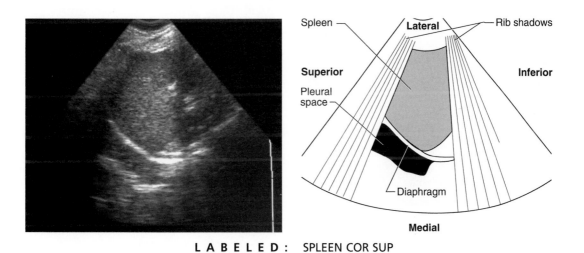

L A B E L E D :   SPLEEN COR SUP

3. Inferior longitudinal image of the spleen to include part of the left kidney for parenchyma comparison.

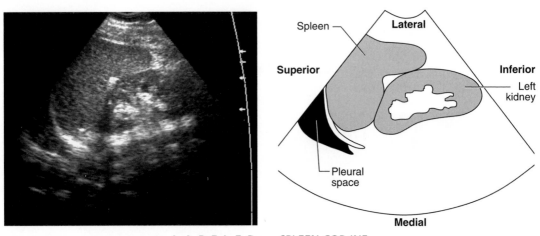

L A B E L E D :   SPLEEN COR INF

≡ TRANSVERSE IMAGES

Transverse Plane • Left Lateral Approach

4. Transverse image of the spleen to include both anterior and posterior margins.

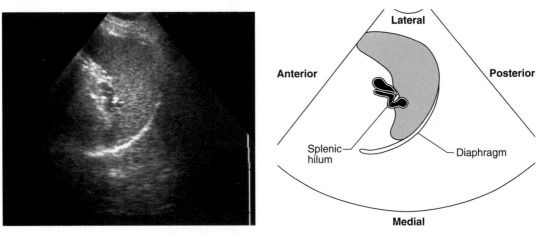

L A B E L E D :   SPLEEN LT TRV

5. Transverse image of the spleen to include the anterior margin and splenic hilum.

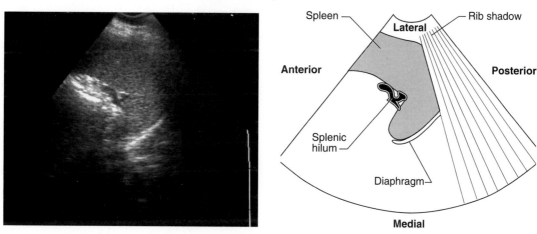

L A B E L E D :   SPLEEN LT TRV ANT

6. Transverse image of the spleen to include the posterior margin.

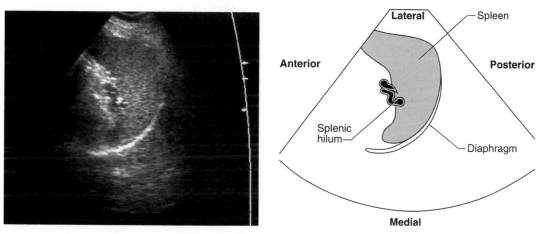

L A B E L E D :   SPLEEN LT TRV POST

REQUIRED IMAGES WHEN THE SPLEEN IS NOT THE PRIMARY AREA OF INTEREST

Required images are the same as the above except that:

1. The longitudinal images of the spleen that include the adjacent pleural space and part of the left kidney may be combined into one image if all of the structures are clearly seen. Label the image: **SPLEEN COR** In some cases these structures may also be seen on the long axis image. If so, label the image: **SPLEEN LONG AXIS**

2. Only one transverse image of the spleen is necessary as long as the anterior and posterior margins of the spleen are well visualized. Label the image: **SPLEEN LT TRV**

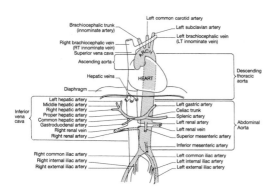

Location and anatomy of the aorta

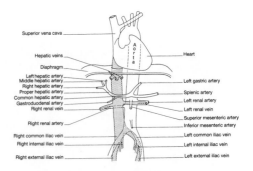

Location and anatomy of the inferior vena cava

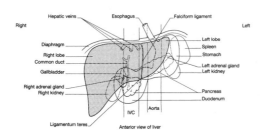

Anterior view of liver

Location and anatomy of the gallbladder and biliary tract

Location and anatomy of the pancreas

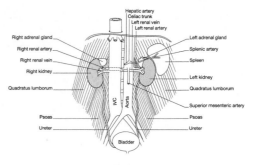

Location of the urinary system

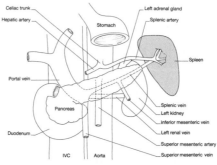

Location and anatomy of the spleen

Scanning Protocols for Full and Limited Studies of the Abdomen

CHAPTER

10

INTRODUCTION

- This chapter is a combination of images from Chapters 3-9. Combined, the images represent complete full and limited studies of the abdomen.
- Required images vary according to which abdominal structure is the area of interest.
- Surveys must precede images. Refer to Chapters 3-9 to review survey steps.
- Refer to Chapters 3-9 for study specifics such as patient preparation, choice of transducer(s), suggested patient position(s), "how to" survey steps, etc.
- Note that any image taken with a measurement or notation over any part of the image should be taken again without calipers and erased notations. Measurement calipers and notations can obscure some detail of interest to the interpreting physician.
- Required images are only a representation of what was determined during the survey; therefore, they should provide the physician with the most technically accurate information available.

N O T E : Images are included for the first study, "Liver Study with Full Abdomen." Figures for the remainder of the studies can be referenced in the chapters on specific abdominal organs (Chapters 3 through 9).

FULL ABDOMINAL STUDIES
I. Liver Study with Full Abdomen

≡ REQUIRED IMAGES

Liver

1. Longitudinal image of the left lobe to include the inferior margin and the aorta.

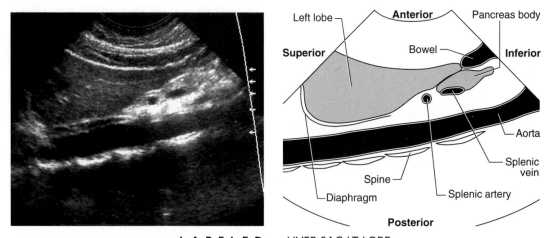

L A B E L E D :   LIVER SAG LT LOBE

2. Longitudinal image of the left lobe to include the diaphragm and caudate lobe.

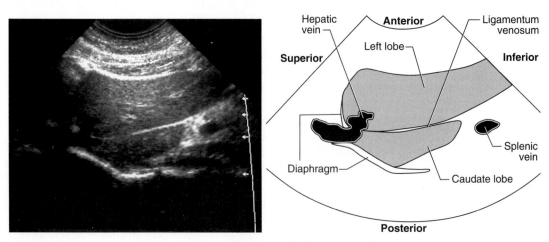

L A B E L E D :   LIVER SAG LT LOBE

3. Longitudinal image of the right lobe to include the IVC where it passes through the liver.

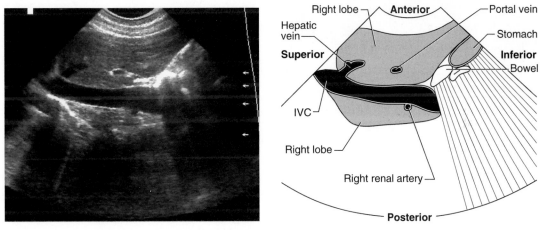

LABELED: LIVER SAG RT LOBE

4. Longitudinal image of the right lobe to include the main lobar fissure, gallbladder, and portal vein.

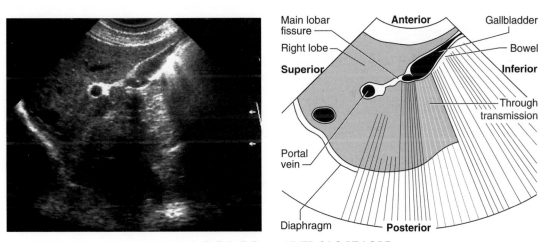

LABELED: LIVER SAG RT LOBE

5. Longitudinal image of the right lobe to include part of the right kidney for parenchyma comparison.

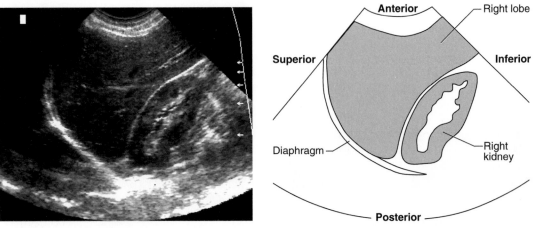

L A B E L E D :   LIVER SAG RT LOBE

6. Longitudinal image of the right lobe to include the dome and the adjacent pleural space.

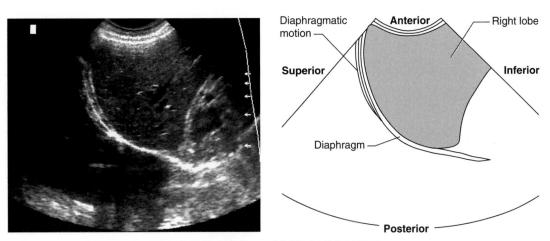

L A B E L E D :   LIVER SAG RT LOBE

7. Transverse image of the left lobe to include its lateral margin.

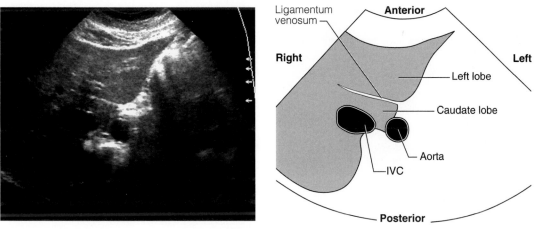

LABELED: LIVER TRV LT LOBE

8. Transverse image of the left lobe to include the ligamentum teres.

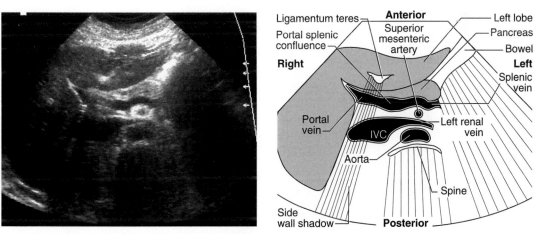

LABELED: LIVER TRV LT LOBE

9. Transverse image of the right lobe to include the hepatic veins.

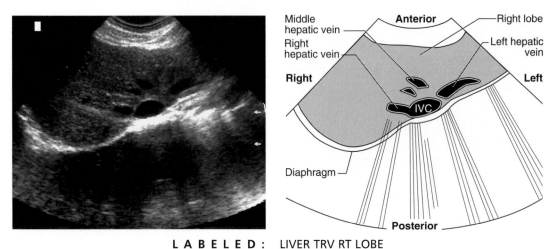

L A B E L E D :   LIVER TRV RT LOBE

10. Transverse image of the right lobe to include the right and left branches of the portal vein.

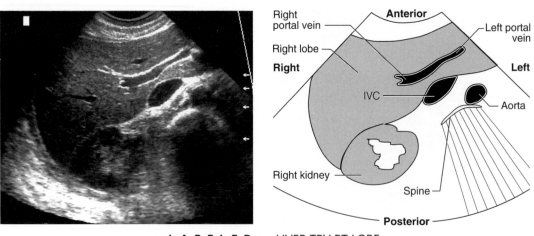

L A B E L E D :   LIVER TRV RT LOBE

11. Transverse image of the right lateral inferior lobe.

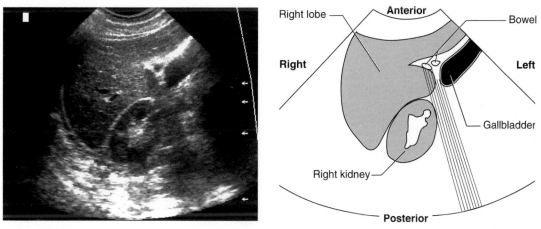

L A B E L E D :   LIVER TRV RT LOBE

12. Transverse image of the right lobe to include the dome and the adjacent pleural space.

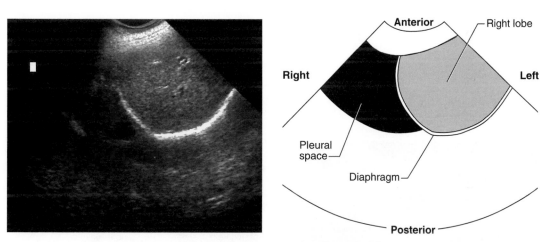

L A B E L E D :   LIVER TRV RT LOBE

Aorta

N O T E :   Images of the aorta can be included with the images of the liver if the aorta is well visualized.

13. Longitudinal image of the proximal and middle aorta.

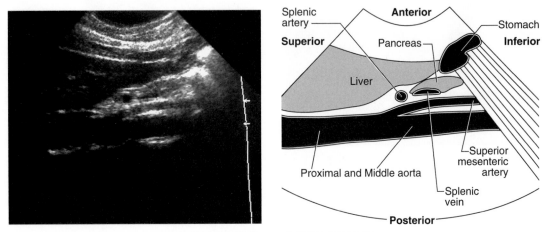

L A B E L E D :   AORTA SAG MID

14. Transverse image of the middle aorta at the level of the renal arteries.

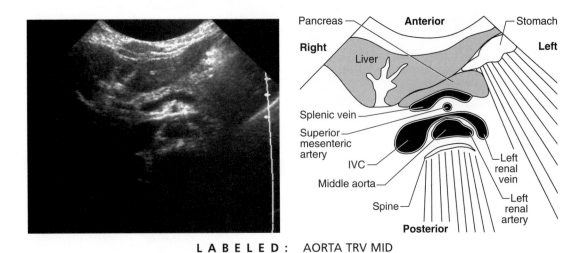

L A B E L E D :   AORTA TRV MID

Inferior Vena Cava

N O T E :   Images of the inferior vena cava can be included with the images of the liver if the inferior vena cava is well visualized.

15. Longitudinal image of the distal and middle IVC.

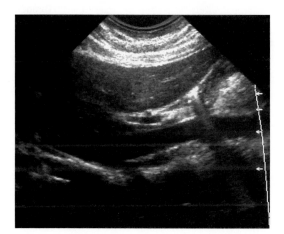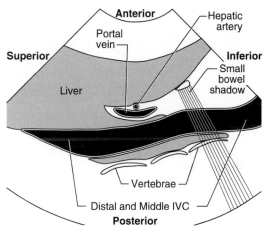

L A B E L E D :   IVC SAG DISTAL

16. Transverse image of the distal IVC to include the hepatic veins.

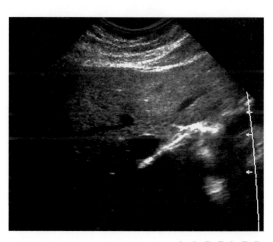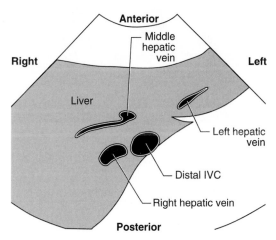

L A B E L E D :   IVC TRV DISTAL

Gallbladder and Biliary Tract

17. Long axis image of the gallbladder.

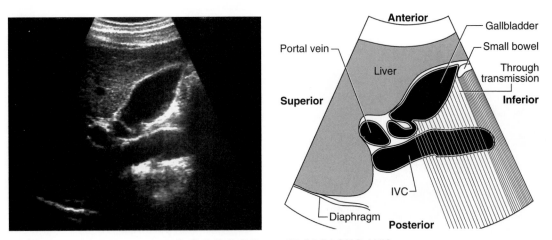

L A B E L E D :   GB SAG LONG AXIS

18. Transverse image of the gallbladder fundus.

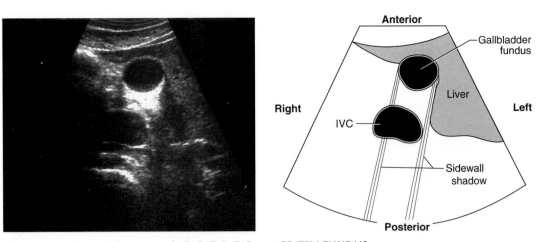

L A B E L E D :   GB TRV FUNDUS

19. Longitudinal image of the common hepatic duct.

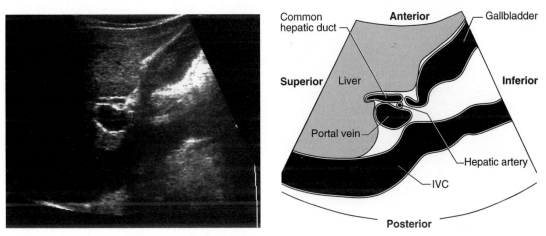

LABELED: SAG CHD

20. Longitudinal image of the common bile duct with *anterior to posterior measurement.*

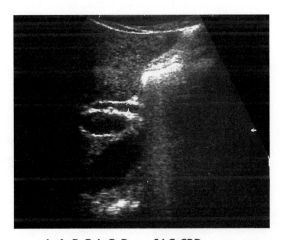

LABELED: SAG CBD

21. Same image as number 20 without calipers.

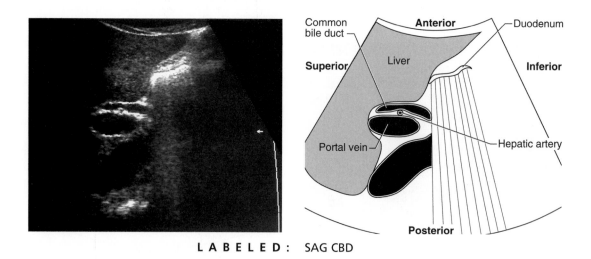

L A B E L E D :   SAG CBD

Pancreas

22. Long axis image of the pancreas to include as much head, uncinate, neck, body, tail, and pancreatic duct as possible.

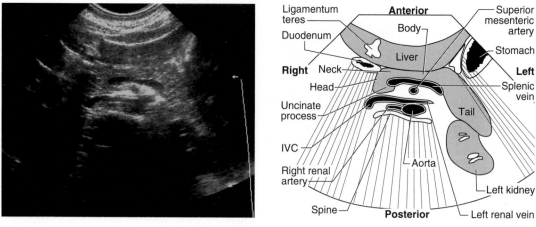

L A B E L E D :   PANCREAS TRV LONG AXIS

23. Longitudinal image of the pancreas head to include the uncinate process and common bile duct (if bile-filled).

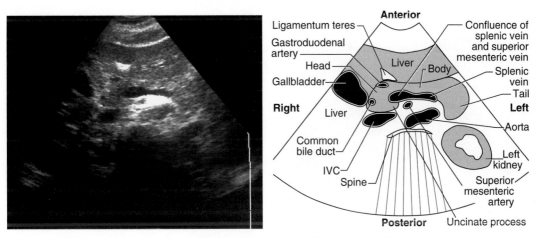

L A B E L E D :   PANCREAS TRV HEAD

24. Transverse image of the pancreas head to include the common bile duct (if bile-filled).

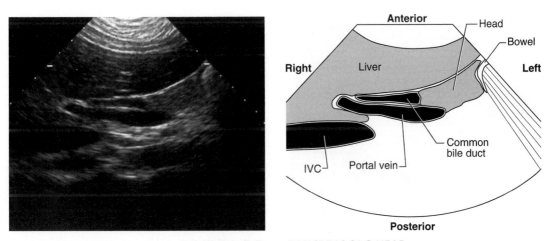

L A B E L E D :   PANCREAS SAG HEAD

Kidneys • Right Kidney

25. Long axis image of the right kidney.

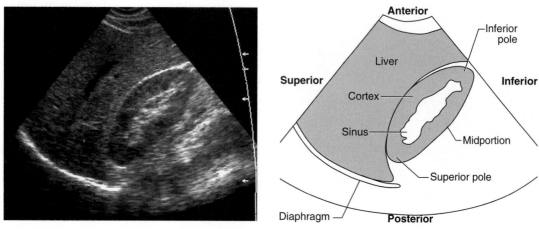

L A B E L E D :   RT KIDNEY SAG LONG AXIS

26. Transverse image of the right kidney midportion to include the hilum.

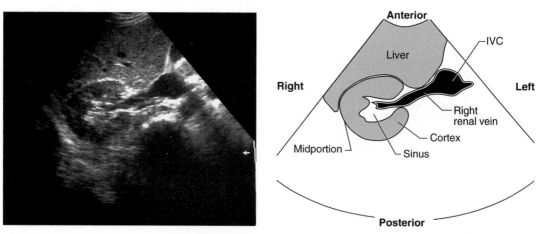

L A B E L E D :   RT KIDNEY TRV MID

Kidneys • Left Kidney

27. Long axis image of the left kidney.

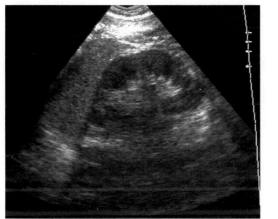 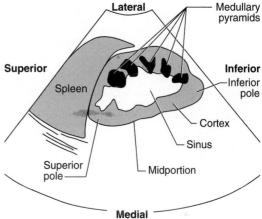

L A B E L E D :   LT KIDNEY COR LONG AXIS

28. Transverse image of the left kidney midportion to include the hilum.

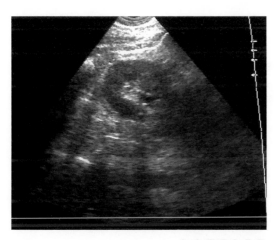 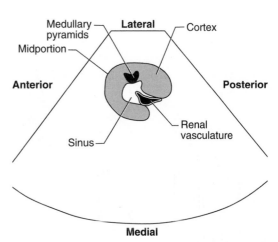

L A B E L E D :   LT KIDNEY LT TRV MID

Spleen

29. Long axis image of the spleen.

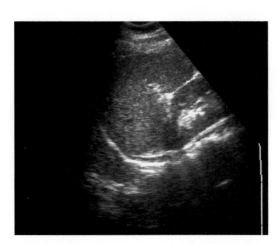
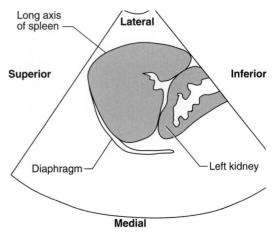

L A B E L E D :   SPLEEN COR LONG AXIS

30. Superior longitudinal image of the spleen to include the adjacent pleural space.

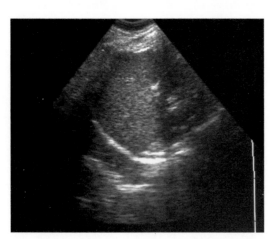
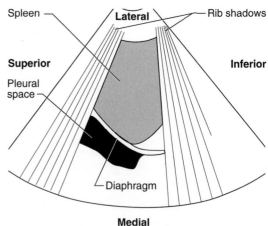

L A B E L E D :   SPLEEN COR SUP

31. Inferior longitudinal image of the spleen to include part of the left kidney for parenchyma comparison.

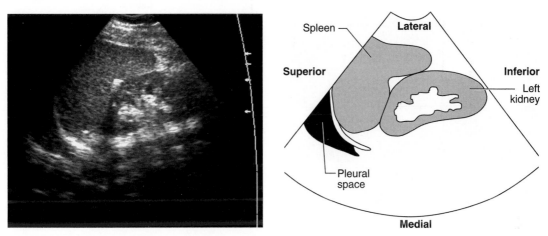

L A B E L E D :   SPLEEN COR INF

32. Transverse image of the spleen to include both anterior and posterior margins.

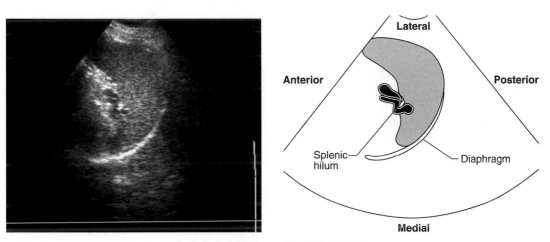

L A B E L E D :   SPLEEN LT TRV

33. Transverse image of the spleen to include the anterior margin and splenic hilum.

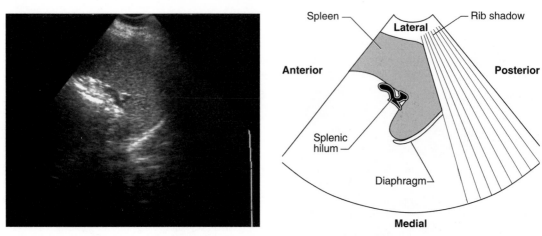

L A B E L E D :   SPLEEN LT TRV ANT

34. Transverse image of the spleen to include the posterior margin.

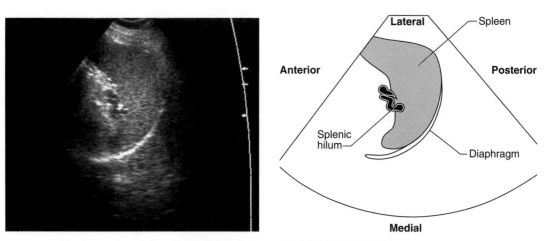

L A B E L E D :   SPLEEN LT TRV POST

N O T E :   The longitudinal images of the spleen that include the adjacent pleural space and part of the left kidney may be combined into one image if all of the structures are well visualized. Label the image: **SPLEEN COR** In some cases these structures may also be seen on the long axis image. If so, label the image: **SPLEEN LONG AXIS**

Only one transverse image of the spleen is necessary as long as the anterior and posterior margins of the spleen are well visualized. Label the image: **SPLEEN LT TRV**

II. *Gallbladder and Biliary Tract Study with Full Abdomen*

≡ REQUIRED IMAGES

Liver

1. Longitudinal image of the left lobe to include the inferior margin and the aorta.

   L A B E L E D :   LIVER SAG LT LOBE

2. Longitudinal image of the left lobe to include the diaphragm and caudate lobe.

   L A B E L E D :   LIVER SAG LT LOBE

3. Longitudinal image of the right lobe to include the IVC where it passes through the liver.

   L A B E L E D :   LIVER SAG RT LOBE

4. Longitudinal image of the right lobe to include the main lobar fissure, gallbladder, and portal vein.

   L A B E L E D :   LIVER SAG RT LOBE

5. Longitudinal image of the right lobe to include part of the right kidney for parenchyma comparison.

   L A B E L E D :   LIVER SAG RT LOBE

6. Longitudinal image of the right lobe to include the dome and the adjacent pleural space.

   L A B E L E D :   LIVER SAG RT LOBE

7. Transverse image of the left lobe to include its lateral margin.

   L A B E L E D :   LIVER TRV LT LOBE

8. Transverse image of the left lobe to include the ligamentum teres.

   L A B E L E D :   LIVER TRV LT LOBE

9. Transverse image of the right lobe to include the hepatic veins.

   L A B E L E D :   LIVER TRV RT LOBE

10. Transverse image of the right lobe to include the right and left branches of the portal vein.

   L A B E L E D :   LIVER TRV RT LOBE

11. Transverse image of the right lateral inferior lobe.

L A B E L E D :   LIVER TRV RT LOBE

12. Transverse image of the right lobe to include the dome and the adjacent pleural space.

L A B E L E D :   LIVER TRV RT LOBE

Aorta

N O T E :   Images of the aorta can be included with the images of the liver if the aorta is well visualized.

13. Longitudinal image of the proximal and middle aorta.

L A B E L E D :   AORTA SAG MID

14. Transverse image of the middle aorta at the level of the renal arteries.

L A B E L E D :   AORTA TRV MID

Inferior Vena Cava

N O T E :   Images of the inferior vena cava can be included with the images of the liver if the inferior vena cava is well visualized.

15. Longitudinal image of the distal and middle IVC.

L A B E L E D :   IVC SAG DISTAL

16. Transverse image of the distal IVC to include the hepatic veins.

L A B E L E D :   IVC TRV DISTAL

Gallbladder and Biliary Tract • First Position/Supine

17. Long axis image of the gallbladder.

L A B E L E D :   GB SAG LONG AXIS

18. Longitudinal image of the gallbladder fundus and body.

L A B E L E D :   GB SAG FUNDUS/BODY

19. Longitudinal image of the gallbladder neck.

L A B E L E D :   GB SAG NECK

20. Transverse image of the gallbladder fundus.

L A B E L E D :   GB TRV FUNDUS

21. Transverse image of the gallbladder body.

L A B E L E D :   GB TRV BODY

22. Transverse image of the gallbladder neck.

L A B E L E D :   GB TRV NECK

23. Longitudinal image of the common hepatic duct.

L A B E L E D :   SAG CHD

24. Longitudinal image of the common bile duct with *anterior to posterior measurement.*

L A B E L E D :   SAG CBD

25. Same image as number 24 without calipers.

L A B E L E D :   SAG CBD

Gallbladder and Biliary Tract • Second Position/ Left Lateral Decubitus

26. Long axis image of the gallbladder.

L A B E L E D :   GB SAG LONG AXIS

27. Transverse image of the gallbladder fundus.

L A B E L E D :   GB TRV FUNDUS

Pancreas

28. Long axis image of the pancreas to include as much head, uncinate, neck, body, tail, and pancreatic duct as possible.

L A B E L E D :   PANCREAS TRV LONG AXIS

29. Longitudinal image of the pancreas head to include the uncinate process and common bile duct (if bile-filled).

L A B E L E D :   PANCREAS TRV HEAD

30. Transverse image of the pancreas head to include the common bile duct (if bile-filled).

L A B E L E D :   PANCREAS SAG HEAD

Kidneys • Right Kidney

31. Long axis image of the right kidney.

L A B E L E D :   RT KIDNEY SAG LONG AXIS

32. Transverse image of the right kidney midportion to include the hilum.

L A B E L E D :   RT KIDNEY TRV MID

Kidneys • Left Kidney

33. Long axis image of the left kidney.

L A B E L E D :   LT KIDNEY COR LONG AXIS

34. Transverse image of the left kidney midportion to include the hilum.

L A B E L E D :   LT KIDNEY LT TRV MID

Spleen

35. Long axis image of the spleen.

L A B E L E D :   SPLEEN COR LONG AXIS

36. Superior longitudinal image of the spleen to include the adjacent pleural space.

L A B E L E D :   SPLEEN COR SUP

37. Inferior longitudinal image of the spleen to include part of the left kidney for parenchyma comparison.

L A B E L E D :   SPLEEN COR INF

38. Transverse image of the spleen to include both anterior and posterior margins.

L A B E L E D :   SPLEEN LT TRV

39. Transverse image of the spleen to include the anterior margin and splenic hilum.

L A B E L E D :   SPLEEN LT TRV ANT

40. Transverse image of the spleen to include the posterior margin.

L A B E L E D :   SPLEEN LT TRV POST

N O T E :   The longitudinal images of the spleen that include the adjacent pleural space and part of the left kidney may be combined into one image if all of the structures are well visualized. Label the image: SPLEEN COR In some cases these structures may also be seen on the long axis image. If so, label the image: SPLEEN LONG AXIS

Only one transverse image of the spleen is necessary as long as the anterior and posterior margins of the spleen are well visualized. Label the image: SPLEEN LT TRV

III. *Pancreas Study with Full Abdomen*

≡ REQUIRED IMAGES

Liver

1. Longitudinal image of the left lobe to include the inferior margin and the aorta.

   L A B E L E D :   LIVER SAG LT LOBE

2. Longitudinal image of the left lobe to include the diaphragm and caudate lobe.

   L A B E L E D :   LIVER SAG LT LOBE

3. Longitudinal image of the right lobe to include the IVC where it passes through the liver.

   L A B E L E D :   LIVER SAG RT LOBE

4. Longitudinal image of the right lobe to include the main lobar fissure, gallbladder, and portal vein.

   L A B E L E D :   LIVER SAG RT LOBE

5. Longitudinal image of the right lobe to include part of the right kidney for parenchyma comparison.

   L A B E L E D :   LIVER SAG RT LOBE

6. Longitudinal image of the right lobe to include the dome and the adjacent pleural space.

   L A B E L E D :   LIVER SAG RT LOBE

7. Transverse image of the left lobe to include its lateral margin.

   L A B E L E D :   LIVER TRV LT LOBE

8. Transverse image of the left lobe to include the ligamentum teres.

   L A B E L E D :   LIVER TRV LT LOBE

9. Transverse image of the right lobe to include the hepatic veins.

   L A B E L E D :   LIVER TRV RT LOBE

10. Transverse image of the right lobe to include the right and left branches of the portal vein.

    L A B E L E D :   LIVER TRV RT LOBE

11. Transverse image of the right lateral inferior lobe.

L A B E L E D :   LIVER TRV RT LOBE

12. Transverse image of the right lobe to include the dome and the adjacent pleural space.

L A B E L E D :   LIVER TRV RT LOBE

Aorta

N O T E :   Images of the aorta can be included with the images of the liver if the aorta is well visualized.

13. Longitudinal image of the proximal and middle aorta.

L A B E L E D :   AORTA SAG MID

14. Transverse image of the middle aorta at the level of the renal arteries.

L A B E L E D :   AORTA TRV MID

Inferior Vena Cava

N O T E :   Images of the inferior vena cava can be included with the images of the liver if the inferior vena cava is well visualized.

15. Longitudinal image of the distal and middle IVC.

L A B E L E D :   IVC SAG DISTAL

16. Transverse image of the distal IVC to include the hepatic veins.

L A B E L E D :   IVC TRV DISTAL

Gallbladder and Biliary Tract

17. Long axis image of the gallbladder.

L A B E L E D :   GB SAG LONG AXIS

18. Transverse image of the gallbladder fundus.

L A B E L E D :   GB TRV FUNDUS

19. Longitudinal image of the common hepatic duct.

L A B E L E D :   SAG CHD

20. Longitudinal image of the common bile duct with *anterior to posterior measurement.*

L A B E L E D :   SAG CBD

21. Same image as number 20 without calipers.

L A B E L E D :   SAG CBD

Pancreas

22. Long axis image of the pancreas to include as much head, uncinate, neck, body, tail, and pancreatic duct as possible.

L A B E L E D :   PANCREAS TRV LONG AXIS

23. Longitudinal image of the pancreas body and neck to include the splenic vein.

L A B E L E D :   PANCREAS TRV BODY/NECK

24. Longitudinal image of the pancreas tail.

L A B E L E D :   PANCREAS TRV TAIL

25. Longitudinal image of the pancreas head to include the uncinate process and common bile duct (if bile-filled).

L A B E L E D :   PANCREAS TRV HEAD

26. Transverse image of the pancreas head to include the common bile duct (if bile-filled).

L A B E L E D :   PANCREAS SAG HEAD

27. Transverse image of the pancreas neck and uncinate process to include the superior mesenteric vein.

L A B E L E D :   PANCREAS SAG NECK/UNCINATE

28. Transverse image of the pancreas body to include the splenic vein.

L A B E L E D :   PANCREAS SAG BODY

29. Transverse image of the pancreas tail.

L A B E L E D :   PANCREAS SAG TAIL

Kidneys • Right Kidney

30. Long axis image of the right kidney.

L A B E L E D :   RT KIDNEY SAG LONG AXIS

31. Transverse image of the right kidney midportion to include the hilum.

L A B E L E D :   RT KIDNEY TRV MID

Kidneys • Left Kidney

32. Long axis image of the left kidney.

L A B E L E D :   LT KIDNEY COR LONG AXIS

33. Transverse image of the left kidney midportion to include the hilum.

L A B E L E D :   LT KIDNEY LT TRV MID

Spleen

34. Long axis image of the spleen.

L A B E L E D :   SPLEEN COR LONG AXIS

35. Superior longitudinal image of the spleen to include the adjacent pleural space.

L A B E L E D :   SPLEEN COR SUP

36. Inferior longitudinal image of the spleen to include part of the left kidney for parenchyma comparison.

L A B E L E D :   SPLEEN COR INF

37. Transverse image of the spleen to include both anterior and posterior margins.

L A B E L E D :   SPLEEN LT TRV

38. Transverse image of the spleen to include the anterior margin and splenic hilum.

L A B E L E D :   SPLEEN LT TRV ANT

39. Transverse image of the spleen to include the posterior margin.

L A B E L E D :   SPLEEN LT TRV POST

N O T E :   The longitudinal images of the spleen that include the adjacent pleural space and part of the left kidney may be combined into one image if all of the structures are well visualized. Label the image: SPLEEN COR In some cases these structures may also be seen on the long axis image. If so, label the image: SPLEEN LONG AXIS

Only one transverse image of the spleen is necessary as long as the anterior and posterior margins of the spleen are well visualized. Label the image: SPLEEN LT TRV

IV. *Renal Study with Full Abdomen*

≡ REQUIRED IMAGES

Liver

1. Longitudinal image of the left lobe to include the inferior margin and the aorta.

L A B E L E D :   LIVER SAG LT LOBE

2. Longitudinal image of the left lobe to include the diaphragm and caudate lobe.

L A B E L E D :   LIVER SAG LT LOBE

3. Longitudinal image of the right lobe to include the IVC where it passes through the liver.

L A B E L E D :   LIVER SAG RT LOBE

4. Longitudinal image of the right lobe to include the main lobar fissure, gallbladder, and portal vein.

L A B E L E D :   LIVER SAG RT LOBE

5. Longitudinal image of the right lobe to include part of the right kidney for parenchyma comparison.

L A B E L E D :   LIVER SAG RT LOBE

6. Longitudinal image of the right lobe to include the dome and the adjacent pleural space.

L A B E L E D :   LIVER SAG RT LOBE

7. Transverse image of the left lobe to include its lateral margin.

L A B E L E D :   LIVER TRV LT LOBE

8. Transverse image of the left lobe to include the ligamentum teres.

L A B E L E D :   LIVER TRV LT LOBE

9. Transverse image of the right lobe to include the hepatic veins.

L A B E L E D :   LIVER TRV RT LOBE

10. Transverse image of the right lobe to include the right and left branches of the portal vein.

L A B E L E D :   LIVER TRV RT LOBE

11. Transverse image of the right lateral inferior lobe.

L A B E L E D :   LIVER TRV RT LOBE

12. Transverse image of the right lobe to include the dome and the adjacent pleural space.

L A B E L E D :   LIVER TRV RT LOBE

Aorta

N O T E :   Images of the aorta can be included with the images of the liver if the aorta is well visualized.

13. Longitudinal image of the proximal and middle aorta.

L A B E L E D :   AORTA SAG MID

14. Transverse image of the middle aorta at the level of the renal arteries.

L A B E L E D :   AORTA TRV MID

Inferior Vena Cava

N O T E :   Images of the inferior vena cava can be included with the images of the liver if the inferior vena cava is well visualized.

15. Longitudinal image of the distal and middle IVC.

L A B E L E D :   IVC SAG DISTAL

16. Transverse image of the distal IVC to include the hepatic veins.

L A B E L E D :   IVC TRV DISTAL

Gallbladder and Biliary Tract

17. Long axis image of the gallbladder.

L A B E L E D :   GB SAG LONG AXIS

18. Transverse image of the gallbladder fundus.

L A B E L E D :   GB TRV FUNDUS

19. Longitudinal image of the common hepatic duct.

L A B E L E D :   SAG CHD

20. Longitudinal image of the common bile duct with *anterior to posterior measurement.*

L A B E L E D :   SAG CBD

21. Same image as number 20 without calipers.

L A B E L E D :   SAG CBD

Pancreas

22. Long axis image of the pancreas to include as much head, uncinate, neck, body, tail, and pancreatic duct as possible.

L A B E L E D :   PANCREAS TRV LONG AXIS

23. Longitudinal image of the pancreas head to include the uncinate process and common bile duct (if bile-filled).

L A B E L E D :   PANCREAS TRV HEAD

24. Transverse image of the pancreas head to include the common bile duct (if bile-filled).

L A B E L E D :   PANCREAS SAG HEAD

Kidneys • Right Kidney

25. Long axis image of the right kidney with *superior to inferior measurement*.

L A B E L E D :   RT KIDNEY SAG LONG AXIS

26. Same image as number 25 without calipers.

L A B E L E D :   RT KIDNEY SAG LONG AXIS

27. Long axis image of the right kidney with *superior to inferior measurement*.

L A B E L E D :   RT KIDNEY SAG LONG AXIS

28. Same image as number 27 without calipers.

L A B E L E D :   RT KIDNEY SAG LONG AXIS

29. Longitudinal image of the right kidney superior pole.

L A B E L E D :   RT KIDNEY SAG SUP POLE

30. Longitudinal image of the right kidney inferior pole.

L A B E L E D :   RT KIDNEY SAG INF POLE

31. Longitudinal image of the right kidney just medial to the long axis.

L A B E L E D :   RT KIDNEY SAG MED

32. Longitudinal image of the right kidney just lateral to the long axis to include part of the liver for parenchyma comparison.

L A B E L E D :   RT KIDNEY SAG LAT

33. Transverse image of the right kidney superior pole.

L A B E L E D :   RT KIDNEY TRV SUP POLE

34. Transverse image of the right kidney midportion to include the hilum with *anterior to posterior measurement.*

L A B E L E D :   RT KIDNEY TRV MID

35. Same image as number 34 without calipers.

L A B E L E D :   RT KIDNEY TRV MID

36. Transverse image of the right kidney inferior pole.

L A B E L E D :   RT KIDNEY TRV INF POLE

Kidneys • Left Kidney

37. Long axis image of the left kidney with *superior to inferior measurement.*

L A B E L E D :   LT KIDNEY COR LONG AXIS

38. Same image as number 37 without calipers.

L A B E L E D :   LT KIDNEY COR LONG AXIS

39. Long axis image of the left kidney with *superior to inferior measurement.*

L A B E L E D :   LT KIDNEY COR LONG AXIS

40. Same image as number 39 without calipers.

L A B E L E D :   LT KIDNEY COR LONG AXIS

41. Longitudinal image of the left kidney superior pole.

L A B E L E D :   LT KIDNEY COR SUP POLE

42. Longitudinal image of the left kidney inferior pole.

L A B E L E D :   LT KIDNEY COR INF POLE

43. Longitudinal image of the left kidney just anterior to the long axis.

L A B E L E D :   LT KIDNEY COR ANT

44. Longitudinal image of the left kidney just posterior to the long axis.

L A B E L E D :   LT KIDNEY COR POST

45. Transverse image of the left kidney superior pole.

L A B E L E D :   LT KIDNEY LT TRV SUP POLE

46. Transverse image of the left kidney midportion to include the hilum with *anterior to posterior measurement.*

L A B E L E D :   LT KIDNEY LT TRV MID

47. Same image as number 46 without calipers.

L A B E L E D :   LT KIDNEY LT TRV MID

48. Transverse image of the left kidney inferior pole.

L A B E L E D :   LT KIDNEY LT TRV INF POLE

Spleen

49. Long axis image of the spleen.

L A B E L E D :   SPLEEN COR LONG AXIS

50. Superior longitudinal image of the spleen to include the adjacent pleural space.

L A B E L E D :   SPLEEN COR SUP

51. Inferior longitudinal image of the spleen to include part of the left kidney for parenchyma comparison.

L A B E L E D :   SPLEEN COR INF

52. Transverse image of the spleen to include both anterior and posterior margins.

L A B E L E D :   SPLEEN LT TRV

53. Transverse image of the spleen to include the anterior margin and splenic hilum.

L A B E L E D :   SPLEEN LT TRV ANT

54. Transverse image of the spleen to include the posterior margin.

L A B E L E D :   SPLEEN LT TRV POST

N O T E :   The longitudinal images of the spleen that include the adjacent pleural space and part of the left kidney may be combined into one image if all of the structures are well visualized. Label the image: **SPLEEN COR** In some cases these structures may also be seen on the long axis image. If so, label the image: **SPLEEN LONG AXIS**

Only one transverse image of the spleen is necessary as long as the anterior and posterior margin of the spleen are well visualized. Label the image: **SPLEEN LT TRV**

V. *Spleen Study with Full Abdomen*

≡ REQUIRED IMAGES

Liver

1. Longitudinal image of the left lobe to include the inferior margin and the aorta.

L A B E L E D :   LIVER SAG LT LOBE

2. Longitudinal image of the left lobe to include the diaphragm and caudate lobe.

L A B E L E D :   LIVER SAG LT LOBE

3. Longitudinal image of the right lobe to include the IVC where it passes through the liver.

L A B E L E D :   LIVER SAG RT LOBE

4. Longitudinal image of the right lobe to include the main lobar fissure, gallbladder, and portal vein.

L A B E L E D :   LIVER SAG RT LOBE

5. Longitudinal image of the right lobe to include part of the right kidney for parenchyma comparison.

L A B E L E D :   LIVER SAG RT LOBE

6. Longitudinal image of the right lobe to include the dome and the adjacent pleural space.

L A B E L E D :   LIVER SAG RT LOBE

7. Transverse image of the left lobe to include its lateral margin.

L A B E L E D :   LIVER TRV LT LOBE

8. Transverse image of the left lobe to include the ligamentum teres.

L A B E L E D :   LIVER TRV LT LOBE

9. Transverse image of the right lobe to include the hepatic veins.

L A B E L E D :   LIVER TRV RT LOBE

10. Transverse image of the right lobe to include the right and left branches of the portal vein.

L A B E L E D :   LIVER TRV RT LOBE

11. Transverse image of the right lateral inferior lobe.

L A B E L E D :   LIVER TRV RT LOBE

12. Transverse image of the right lobe to include the dome and the adjacent pleural space.

L A B E L E D :   LIVER TRV RT LOBE

Aorta

N O T E :   Images of the aorta can be included with the images of the liver if the aorta is well visualized.

13. Longitudinal image of the proximal and middle aorta.

L A B E L E D :   AORTA SAG MID

14. Transverse image of the middle aorta at the level of the renal arteries.

L A B E L E D :   AORTA TRV MID

Inferior Vena Cava

N O T E :   Images of the inferior vena cava can be included with the images of the liver if the inferior vena cava is well visualized.

15. Longitudinal image of the distal and middle IVC.

L A B E L E D :   IVC SAG DISTAL

16. Transverse image of the distal IVC to include the hepatic veins.

L A B E L E D :   IVC TRV DISTAL

Gallbladder and Biliary Tract

17. Long axis image of the gallbladder.

L A B E L E D :   GB SAG LONG AXIS

18. Transverse image of the gallbladder fundus.

L A B E L E D :   GB TRV FUNDUS

19. Longitudinal image of the common hepatic duct.

L A B E L E D :   SAG CHD

20. Longitudinal image of the common bile duct with *anterior to posterior measurement.*

L A B E L E D :   SAG CBD

21. Same image as number 20 without calipers.

L A B E L E D :   SAG CBD

Pancreas

22. Long axis image of the pancreas to include as much head, uncinate, neck, body, tail, and pancreatic duct as possible.

L A B E L E D :   PANCREAS TRV LONG AXIS

23. Longitudinal image of the pancreas head to include the uncinate process and common bile duct (if bile-filled).

L A B E L E D :   PANCREAS TRV HEAD

24. Transverse image of the pancreas head to include the common bile duct (if bile-filled).

L A B E L E D :   PANCREAS SAG HEAD

Kidneys • Right Kidney

25. Long axis image of the right kidney.

L A B E L E D :   RT KIDNEY SAG LONG AXIS

26. Transverse image of the right kidney midportion to include the hilum.

L A B E L E D :   RT KIDNEY TRV MID

Kidneys • Left Kidney

27. Long axis image of the left kidney.

L A B E L E D :   LT KIDNEY COR LONG AXIS

28. Transverse image of the left kidney midportion to include the hilum.

L A B E L E D :   LT KIDNEY LT TRV MID

Spleen

29. Long axis image of the spleen.

L A B E L E D :   SPLEEN COR LONG AXIS

30. Superior longitudinal image of the spleen to include the adjacent pleural space.

L A B E L E D :   SPLEEN COR SUP

31. Inferior longitudinal image of the spleen to include part of the left kidney for parenchyma comparison.

L A B E L E D :   SPLEEN COR INF

32. Transverse image of the spleen to include both anterior and posterior margins.

L A B E L E D :   SPLEEN LT TRV

33. Transverse image of the spleen to include the anterior margin and splenic hilum.

L A B E L E D :   SPLEEN LT TRV ANT

34. Transverse image of the spleen to include the posterior margin.

L A B E L E D :   SPLEEN LT TRV POST

N O T E :   The longitudinal images of the spleen that include the adjacent pleural space and part of the left kidney may be combined into one image if all of the structures are well visualized. Label the image: SPLEEN COR In some cases these structures may also be seen on the long axis image. If so, label the image: SPLEEN LONG AXIS

Only one transverse image of the spleen is necessary as long as the anterior and posterior margins of the spleen are well visualized. Label the image: SPLEEN LT TRV

LIMITED ABDOMINAL STUDIES

I. Right Upper Quadrant

☰ REQUIRED IMAGES

Liver

1. Longitudinal image of the left lobe to include the inferior margin and the aorta.

L A B E L E D :   LIVER SAG LT LOBE

2. Longitudinal image of the left lobe to include the diaphragm and caudate lobe.

L A B E L E D :   LIVER SAG LT LOBE

3. Longitudinal image of the right lobe to include the IVC where it passes through the liver.

L A B E L E D :   LIVER SAG RT LOBE

4. Longitudinal image of the right lobe to include the main lobar fissure, gallbladder, and portal vein.

L A B E L E D :   LIVER SAG RT LOBE

5. Longitudinal image of the right lobe to include part of the right kidney for parenchyma comparison.

L A B E L E D :   LIVER SAG RT LOBE

6. Longitudinal image of the right lobe to include the dome and the adjacent pleural space.

L A B E L E D :   LIVER SAG RT LOBE

7. Transverse image of the left lobe to include its lateral margin.

L A B E L E D :   LIVER TRV LT LOBE

8. Transverse image of the left lobe to include the ligamentum teres.

L A B E L E D :   LIVER TRV LT LOBE

9. Transverse image of the right lobe to include the hepatic veins.

L A B E L E D :   LIVER TRV RT LOBE

10. Transverse image of the right lobe to include the right and left branches of the portal vein.

L A B E L E D :   LIVER TRV RT LOBE

11. Transverse image of the right lateral inferior lobe.

L A B E L E D :   LIVER TRV RT LOBE

12. Transverse image of the right lobe to include the dome and the adjacent pleural space.

L A B E L E D :   LIVER TRV RT LOBE

Inferior Vena Cava

N O T E :   Images of the inferior vena cava can be included with the images of the liver if the inferior vena cava is well visualized.

13. Longitudinal image of the distal and middle IVC.

L A B E L E D :   IVC SAG DISTAL

14. Transverse image of the distal IVC to include the hepatic veins.

L A B E L E D :   IVC TRV DISTAL

Gallbladder and Biliary Tract • First Position/Supine

15. Long axis image of the gallbladder.

L A B E L E D :   GB SAG LONG AXIS

16. Longitudinal image of the gallbladder fundus and body.

L A B E L E D :   GB SAG FUNDUS/BODY

17. Longitudinal image of the gallbladder neck.

L A B E L E D :   GB SAG NECK

18. Transverse image of the gallbladder fundus.

L A B E L E D :   GB TRV FUNDUS

19. Transverse image of the gallbladder body.

L A B E L E D :   GB TRV BODY

20. Transverse image of the gallbladder neck.

L A B E L E D :   GB TRV NECK

21. Longitudinal image of the common hepatic duct.

L A B E L E D :   SAG CHD

22. Longitudinal image of the common bile duct with *anterior to posterior measurement.*

L A B E L E D :   SAG CBD

23. Same image as number 22 without calipers.

L A B E L E D :   SAG CBD

Gallbladder and Biliary Tract • Second Position/ Left Lateral Decubitus

24. Long axis image of the gallbladder.

L A B E L E D :   GB SAG LONG AXIS

25. Transverse image of the gallbladder fundus.

L A B E L E D :   GB TRV FUNDUS

Pancreas

26. Long axis image of the pancreas to include as much head, uncinate, neck, body, tail, and pancreatic duct as possible.

L A B E L E D :   PANCREAS TRV LONG AXIS

27. Longitudinal image of the pancreas head to include the uncinate process and common bile duct (if bile-filled).

L A B E L E D :   PANCREAS TRV HEAD

28. Transverse image of the pancreas head to include the common bile duct (if bile-filled).

L A B E L E D :   PANCREAS SAG HEAD

Kidneys • Right Kidney

29. Long axis image of the right kidney.

L A B E L E D :   RT KIDNEY SAG LONG AXIS

30. Transverse image of the right kidney midportion to include the hilum.

L A B E L E D :   RT KIDNEY TRV MID

II. Gallbladder and Biliary Tract

☰ REQUIRED IMAGES

Liver

1. Longitudinal image of the left lobe to include the inferior margin and the aorta.

L A B E L E D :   LIVER SAG LT LOBE

2. Longitudinal image of the left lobe to include the diaphragm and caudate lobe.

L A B E L E D :   LIVER SAG LT LOBE

3. Longitudinal image of the right lobe to include the IVC where it passes through the liver.

L A B E L E D :   LIVER SAG RT LOBE

4. Longitudinal image of the right lobe to include the main lobar fissure, gallbladder, and portal vein.

L A B E L E D :   LIVER SAG RT LOBE

5. Longitudinal image of the right lobe to include part of the right kidney for parenchyma comparison.

L A B E L E D :   LIVER SAG RT LOBE

6. Longitudinal image of the right lobe to include the dome and the adjacent pleural space.

L A B E L E D :   LIVER SAG RT LOBE

7. Transverse image of the left lobe to include its lateral margin.

L A B E L E D :   LIVER TRV LT LOBE

8. Transverse image of the left lobe to include the ligamentum teres.

L A B E L E D :   LIVER TRV LT LOBE

9. Transverse image of the right lobe to include the hepatic veins.

L A B E L E D :   LIVER TRV RT LOBE

10. Transverse image of the right lobe to include the right and left branches of the portal vein.

L A B E L E D :   LIVER TRV RT LOBE

11. Transverse image of the right lateral inferior lobe.

L A B E L E D :   LIVER TRV RT LOBE

12. Transverse image of the right lobe to include the dome and the adjacent pleural space.

L A B E L E D :   LIVER TRV RT LOBE

Gallbladder and Biliary Tract • First Position/Supine

13. Long axis image of the gallbladder.

L A B E L E D :   GB SAG LONG AXIS

14. Longitudinal image of the gallbladder fundus and body.

L A B E L E D :   GB SAG FUNDUS/BODY

15. Longitudinal image of the gallbladder neck.

L A B E L E D :   GB SAG NECK

16. Transverse image of the gallbladder fundus.

L A B E L E D :   GB TRV FUNDUS

17. Transverse image of the gallbladder body.

L A B E L E D :   GB TRV BODY

18. Transverse image of the gallbladder neck.

L A B E L E D :   GB TRV NECK

19. Longitudinal image of the common hepatic duct.

L A B E L E D :   SAG CHD

20. Longitudinal image of the common bile duct with *anterior to posterior measurement.*

L A B E L E D :   SAG CBD

21. Same image as number 20 without calipers.

L A B E L E D :   SAG CBD

Gallbladder and Biliary Tract • Second Position/ Left Lateral Decubitus

22. Long axis image of the gallbladder.

L A B E L E D :   GB SAG LONG AXIS

23. Transverse image of the gallbladder fundus.

L A B E L E D :   GB TRV FUNDUS

Pancreas

24. Long axis image of the pancreas to include as much head, uncinate, neck, body, tail, and pancreatic duct as possible.

L A B E L E D :   PANCREAS TRV LONG AXIS

25. Longitudinal image of the pancreas head to include the uncinate process and common bile duct (if bile-filled).

L A B E L E D :   PANCREAS TRV HEAD

26. Transverse image of the pancreas head to include the common bile duct (if bile-filled).

L A B E L E D :   PANCREAS SAG HEAD

III. Pancreas Study

☰ REQUIRED IMAGES

Liver

1. Longitudinal image of the left lobe to include the inferior margin and the aorta.

L A B E L E D :   LIVER SAG LT LOBE

2. Longitudinal image of the left lobe to include the diaphragm and caudate lobe.

L A B E L E D :   LIVER SAG LT LOBE

3. Longitudinal image of the right lobe to include the IVC where it passes through the liver.

L A B E L E D :   LIVER SAG RT LOBE

4. Longitudinal image of the right lobe to include the main lobar fissure, gallbladder, and portal vein.

L A B E L E D :   LIVER SAG RT LOBE

5. Longitudinal image of the right lobe to include part of the right kidney for parenchyma comparison.

L A B E L E D :   LIVER SAG RT LOBE

6. Longitudinal image of the right lobe to include the dome and the adjacent pleural space.

L A B E L E D :   LIVER SAG RT LOBE

7. Transverse image of the left lobe to include its lateral margin.

L A B E L E D :   LIVER TRV LT LOBE

8. Transverse image of the left lobe to include the ligamentum teres.

L A B E L E D :   LIVER TRV LT LOBE

9. Transverse image of the right lobe to include the hepatic veins.

L A B E L E D :   LIVER TRV RT LOBE

10. Transverse image of the right lobe to include the right and left branches of the portal vein.

L A B E L E D :   LIVER TRV RT LOBE

11. Transverse image of the right lateral inferior lobe.

L A B E L E D :   LIVER TRV RT LOBE

12. Transverse image of the right lobe to include the dome and the adjacent pleural space.

L A B E L E D :   LIVER TRV RT LOBE

Gallbladder and Biliary Tract

13. Long axis image of the gallbladder.

L A B E L E D :   GB SAG LONG AXIS

14. Transverse image of the gallbladder fundus.

L A B E L E D :   GB TRV FUNDUS

15. Longitudinal image of the common hepatic duct.

L A B E L E D :   SAG CHD

16. Longitudinal image of the common bile duct with *anterior to posterior measurement.*

L A B E L E D :   SAG CBD

17. Same image as number 16 without calipers.

L A B E L E D :   SAG CBD

Pancreas

18. Long axis image of the pancreas to include as much head, uncinate, neck, body, tail, and pancreatic duct as possible.

L A B E L E D :   PANCREAS TRV LONG AXIS

19. Longitudinal image of the pancreas body and neck to include the splenic vein.

L A B E L E D :   PANCREAS TRV BODY/NECK

20. Longitudinal image of the pancreas tail.

L A B E L E D :   PANCREAS TRV TAIL

21. Longitudinal image of the pancreas head to include the uncinate process and common bile duct (if bile-filled).

L A B E L E D :   PANCREAS TRV HEAD

22. Transverse image of the pancreas head to include the common bile duct (if bile-filled).

L A B E L E D :   PANCREAS SAG HEAD

23. Transverse image of the pancreas neck and uncinate process to include the superior mesenteric vein.

L A B E L E D :   PANCREAS SAG NECK/UNCINATE

24. Transverse image of the pancreas body to include the splenic vein.

L A B E L E D :   PANCREAS SAG BODY

25. Transverse image of the pancreas tail.

L A B E L E D :   PANCREAS SAG TAIL

IV. Renal Study

≡ REQUIRED IMAGES

Kidneys • Right Kidney

1. Long axis image of the right kidney with *superior to inferior measurement*.

L A B E L E D :   RT KIDNEY SAG LONG AXIS

2. Same image as number 1 without calipers.

L A B E L E D :   RT KIDNEY SAG LONG AXIS

3. Long axis image of the right kidney with *superior to inferior measurement*.

L A B E L E D :   RT KIDNEY SAG LONG AXIS

4. Same image as number 3 without calipers.

L A B E L E D :   RT KIDNEY SAG LONG AXIS

5. Longitudinal image of the right kidney superior pole.

L A B E L E D :   RT KIDNEY SAG SUP POLE

6. Longitudinal image of the right kidney inferior pole.

L A B E L E D :   RT KIDNEY SAG INF POLE

7. Longitudinal image of the right kidney just medial to the long axis.

L A B E L E D :   RT KIDNEY SAG MED

8. Longitudinal image of the right kidney just lateral to the long axis to include part of the liver for parenchyma comparison.

L A B E L E D :   RT KIDNEY SAG LAT

9. Transverse image of the right kidney superior pole.

L A B E L E D :   RT KIDNEY TRV SUP POLE

10. Transverse image of the right kidney midportion to include the hilum with *anterior to posterior measurement*.

L A B E L E D :   RT KIDNEY TRV MID

11. Same image as number 10 without calipers.

L A B E L E D :   RT KIDNEY TRV MID

12. Transverse image of the right kidney inferior pole.

L A B E L E D :   RT KIDNEY TRV INF POLE

Kidneys • Left Kidney

13. Long axis image of the left kidney with *superior to inferior measurement.*

L A B E L E D :   LT KIDNEY COR LONG AXIS

14. Same image as number 13 without calipers.

L A B E L E D :   LT KIDNEY COR LONG AXIS

15. Long axis image of the left kidney with *superior to inferior measurement.*

L A B E L E D :   LT KIDNEY COR LONG AXIS

16. Same image as number 15 without calipers.

L A B E L E D :   LT KIDNEY COR LONG AXIS

17. Longitudinal image of the left kidney superior pole to include part of the spleen for parenchyma comparison.

L A B E L E D :   LT KIDNEY COR SUP POLE

18. Longitudinal image of the left kidney inferior pole.

L A B E L E D :   LT KIDNEY COR INF POLE

19. Longitudinal image of the left kidney just anterior to the long axis.

L A B E L E D :   LT KIDNEY COR ANT

20. Longitudinal image of the left kidney just posterior to the long axis.

L A B E L E D :   LT KIDNEY COR POST

21. Transverse image of the left kidney superior pole.

L A B E L E D :   LT KIDNEY LT TRV SUP POLE

22. Transverse image of the left kidney midportion to include the hilum with *anterior to posterior measurement.*

L A B E L E D :   LT KIDNEY LT TRV MID

23. Same image as number 22 without calipers.

L A B E L E D :   LT KIDNEY LT TRV MID

24. Transverse image of the left kidney inferior pole.

L A B E L E D :   LT KIDNEY LT TRV INF POLE

V. *Spleen Study*

≡ REQUIRED IMAGES

Spleen

1. Long axis image of the spleen.

L A B E L E D :   SPLEEN COR LONG AXIS

2. Superior longitudinal image of the spleen to include the adjacent pleural space.

L A B E L E D :   SPLEEN COR SUP

3. Inferior longitudinal image of the spleen to include part of the left kidney for parenchyma comparison.

L A B E L E D :   SPLEEN COR INF

4. Transverse image of the spleen to include both anterior and posterior margins.

L A B E L E D :   SPLEEN LT TRV

5. Transverse image of the spleen to include the anterior margin and splenic hilum.

L A B E L E D :   SPLEEN LT TRV ANT

6. Transverse image of the spleen to include the posterior margin.

L A B E L E D :   SPLEEN LT TRV POST

N O T E :   The longitudinal images of the spleen that include the adjacent pleural space and part of the left kidney may be combined into one image if all of the structures are well visualized. Label the image: SPLEEN COR In some cases these structures may also be seen on the long axis image. If so, label the image: SPLEEN LONG AXIS

Only one transverse image of the spleen is necessary as long as the anterior and posterior margins of the spleen are well visualized. Label the image: SPLEEN LT TRV

Kidneys • Left Kidney

7. Long axis image of the left kidney.

L A B E L E D :   LT KIDNEY COR LONG AXIS

8. Transverse image of the left kidney midportion to include the hilum.

L A B E L E D :   LT KIDNEY LT TRV MID

VI. *Abdominal Aorta*

≡ REQUIRED IMAGES

Aorta

1. Longitudinal image of the proximal aorta (inferior to the diaphragm and superior to the celiac trunk).

L A B E L E D :　AORTA SAG PROX

2. Longitudinal image of the middle aorta (inferior to the celiac trunk and along the length of the SMA).

L A B E L E D :　AORTA SAG MID

3. Longitudinal image of the distal aorta (inferior to the SMA and superior to the bifurcation).

L A B E L E D :　AORTA SAG DISTAL

4. Longitudinal image of the aorta bifurcation (common iliac arteries).

L A B E L E D :　AORTA SAG BIF RT or LT OBL (depending on the lateral aspect you angle the transducer from) or AORTA LT or RT COR BIF

5. Transverse image of the proximal aorta with *anterior to posterior measurement (calipers outside wall to outside wall)*. (Inferior to the diaphragm and superior to the celiac trunk).

L A B E L E D :　AORTA TRV PROX

6. Same image as number 5 without calipers.

L A B E L E D :　AORTA TRV PROX

7. Transverse image of the middle aorta with *anterior to posterior measurement (calipers outside wall to outside wall)*. (Inferior to the celiac trunk, *at the level of the renal arteries,* and along the length of the SMA.)

L A B E L E D :　AORTA TRV MID

8. Same image as number 7 without calipers.

L A B E L E D :　AORTA TRV MID

N O T E :　If the renal arteries are not represented on the above images, an additional image(s) of the renal arteries should be taken here and labeled accordingly:

L A B E L E D :　RT RENAL ART TRV
　　　　　　　　and
L A B E L E D :　LT RENAL ART TRV
　　　　　　　　or
L A B E L E D :　RT & LT RENAL ARTS TRV

9. Transverse image of the distal aorta with *anterior to posterior measurement (calipers outside wall to outside wall).* (Inferior to the SMA and superior to the bifurcation.)

L A B E L E D :   AORTA TRV DISTAL

10. Same image as number 9 without calipers.

L A B E L E D :   AORTA TRV DISTAL

11. Transverse image of the bifurcation (common iliac arteries).

L A B E L E D :   AORTA TRV BIF

VII. Inferior Vena Cava

≡ REQUIRED IMAGES

Inferior Vena Cava

1. Longitudinal image of the distal IVC to include the diaphragm and hepatic vein(s).

L A B E L E D :   IVC SAG DISTAL

2. Longitudinal image of the middle IVC at the level of the head of the pancreas.

L A B E L E D :   IVC SAG MID

3. Longitudinal image of the proximal IVC.

L A B E L E D :   IVC SAG PROX

4. Longitudinal image of the IVC bifurcation (common iliac veins).

L A B E L E D :   IVC SAG BIF RT or LT OBL (depending on the lateral aspect you angle the transducer from) or IVC RT COR BIF

5. Transverse image of the distal IVC to include the hepatic veins.

L A B E L E D :   IVC TRV DISTAL

6. Transverse image of the middle IVC at the level of the renal veins.

L A B E L E D :   IVC TRV MID

7. Transverse image of the proximal IVC.

L A B E L E D :   IVC TRV PROX

8. Transverse image of the IVC bifurcation (common iliac veins).

L A B E L E D :   IVC TRV BIF

Pelvic Scanning Protocols

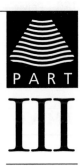

PART

III

Overview

STANDARDS

- No single organ exams.
- Protocols provide specific survey steps with "how-to" illustrations.
- Protocols provide image specifications.
- Patient care and safety are always a priority.
- Use good clinical skills and always practice professional behavior.
- Use real time, transabdominal or endocavital scanners with sector or curved linear transducers.
- Verbal or preferably written consent from the patient is required for endocavital studies. The examination should be witnessed by another health care professional and his or her initials should be labeled on the film(s).
- Transabdominal pelvic studies require a full urinary bladder to better delineate pelvic structures. This can cause the patient discomfort; therefore, every effort should be made to perform the study as quickly as possible.
- **Only physicians can give a legal diagnostic impression.**
- **Only physicians can give a diagnosis.**

SURVEYS

- Studies begin with surveys or evaluations of the pelvic organs and adjacent structures in at least two scanning planes.
- Surveys are used to set correct imaging techniques, to rule out pathologies, and to recognize any normal variants.
- If an abnormality is identified, it is surveyed in at least two scanning planes *following* the completed survey of the

pelvic organs and adjacent structures. Refer to Chapter 2 for specifics on how to survey pathology.

- Images are not taken during a survey.

IMAGE DOCUMENTATION

- Images are taken following the completed survey.
- As with the survey, documented areas of interest must be represented in at least two scanning planes. Single-plane representation is not enough confirmation.
- Documented areas of interest must be done so in a logical sequence. Follow imaging protocol examples.
- After an abnormality is identified and surveyed, it must be documented in at least two scanning planes *following* the completed survey and completed images of the pelvic organs and adjacent structures even if the abnormality is demonstrated on the standard set of required images. Refer to Chapter 2 for specifics on how to document pathology.

OTHER CONSIDERATIONS

- Patient comfort and the amount of transabdominal transducer pressure on the skin is always an important consideration. Experiment using different amounts of transducer pressure on the skin surface. More often than not, beginning sonographers can usually apply more pressure than they realize and in turn improve image quality. However, always make sure the patient is comfortable, especially if he or she has a full urinary bladder.
- Echo textures of pelvic organ parenchyma should be homogeneous with ranges in echogenicity. Note that parenchymal patterns change with disease processes.
- Normal sonographic patterns in the pelvis:
  - (a) Organ parenchyma, muscles, and tissues: homogeneous echo textures.
  - (b) Endometrial cavity and vaginal canal: compared to uterine parenchyma they are hyperechoic the majority of time and exhibit variations in echogenicity during the menstrual cycle.
  - (c) Fluid-filled structures such as blood vessels, ovarian follicles, and urinary bladder: anechoic central portions surrounded by hyperechoic walls.
  - (d) Gastrointestinal tract: presentation varies depending on content. Walls are usually hypoechoic to surrounding structures. Lumens can present as highly reflective areas filled with gas or air or have a heterogeneous appearance from a combination of fluid and gas or air, or

as a fluid-filled, homogeneous, anechoic presentation (in this case, walls are hyperechoic to the fluid).

(e) Bone: sound waves do not penetrate bone; therefore, it is highly reflective and hyperechoic to adjacent structures.

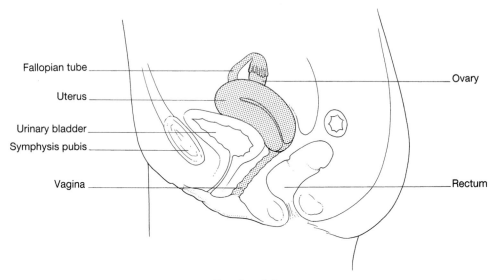

Female pelvis

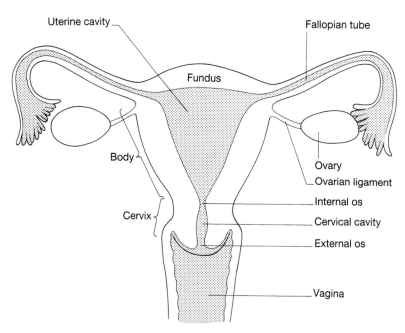

**Anatomy of uterus, fallopian tubes,
ovaries, and vagina**

Female Pelvis Scanning Protocol

CHAPTER 11

B.B. Tempkin and Deborah D. Werneburg

LOCATION

- The urinary bladder is posterior to the symphysis pubis.
- The uterus, cervix, and vagina are posterior to the distended bladder and anterior to the rectum.
- The fundus of the uterus usually lies just to the right or left of midline.
- The cervix and vagina usually lie in the midline of the pelvic cavity.
- The ovaries are lateral to the uterus and lie against the pelvic side walls.
- The ureter and internal iliac vessels are posterior to the ovary.

ANATOMY

- The female pelvic cavity consists of the female reproductive organs, a portion of the ureters, the urinary bladder, musculature, and intestinal tract.
- The female reproductive system consists of the vagina, uterus, two fallopian tubes, and two ovaries.
- The adnexa consist of the ovaries, fallopian tubes, pelvic ligaments, and pelvic side walls.
- The vagina is a muscular, tubular structure that extends for 3 to 5 inches from the cervix of the uterus to the vulva.
- The uterus is a muscular, hollow organ. The size of the uterus is variable depending on patient parity and age. Postpubertal size is usually 7 to 8 cm long, 3 to 5 cm wide, and 3 to 5 cm thick.
- The uterus consists of three muscle layers:
  - (a) Endometrium: The inner mucous layer.
  - (b) Myometrium: The middle, smooth muscle, thickest layer.

(c) Serous: The outer peritoneal layer.

- The uterus is pear-shaped; its rounded superior portion is the fundus and its inferior tapering portion is the cervix or neck. The middle portion of the uterus is referred to as its body.

- The uterus has a centrally located endometrial cavity. The cervical portion of the cavity where it meets the vagina is referred to as the external os and where it meets the uterine body is referred to as the internal os.

- The uterine cavity is continuous with the centrally located vaginal canal.

- The fallopian tubes arise from the uterus and course within the broad ligament for about 10 cm (4 in.) toward the ovaries.

- The ovaries are oval-shaped organs that lie within the ovarian fossae against the pelvic side walls. The size of the ovaries is variable and depends on age. Postpubertal size is approximately 2.5-5 cm long, 1.5-3 cm wide, and .6 cm to 2.2 cm thick.

- The two ureters are long, narrow tubular structures that extend from the hilum of each kidney to the urinary bladder. The ureters are less than 1.4 in. wide and 10 to 12 in. long. The ureters decrease in diameter as they course to the bladder.

- The urinary bladder is a symmetrical, hollow, muscular organ. Bladder shape is variable depending on distention. The bladder can hold as much as 16 to 18 ounces of urine. The normal distended urinary bladder wall measures 1 cm or less.

- Pelvic side wall musculature includes:
  (a) Obturator internus muscle.
  (b) Iliopsoas muscle.
  (c) Piriformis muscle.
  (d) Pubococcygeal sling muscle.

PHYSIOLOGY

- The function of the uterus, vagina, and ovaries is reproduction.

- The function of the ureters is to carry urine from the hilum of each kidney to the urinary bladder.

- The function of the urinary bladder is to store urine until the urge to void is felt.

SONOGRAPHIC APPEARANCE

- The uterine myometrium is midgray or medium-level echoes with even texture. The contour of the normal myometrium should appear smooth. Occasionally round, anechoic venous structures may be seen along the uterine periphery.

- The endometrial cavity is a thin echogenic line that varies in intensity and thickness depending on the menstrual phase and patient age.
- The vaginal walls are midgray or medium-level echoes with even texture that is equal to the normal uterus. The vaginal canal is hyperechoic.
- The ovaries are midgray or medium-level echoes with even texture that is equal to or more echogenic than the normal uterus. Uterine follicles are seen as round or oval anechoic structures along the ovarian periphery.
- The fallopian tubes are not normally seen.
- The ureters are not normally seen.
- The urinary bladder cavity is not seen if it is collapsed; otherwise it appears anechoic. The bladder wall appears as a smooth, thin echogenic line. Distended bladder shape is variable but transversely it may appear somewhat squared.
- The pelvic side wall musculature is midgray or medium-level echoes with even texture that is less echogenic than the normal uterus and ovaries.
- The cul-de-sac or pouch of Douglas is a recessed portion of the peritoneum posterior to the uterus that is seen when it contains fluid or blood. It is normal to see a small amount of anechoic free fluid between the echogenic walls of the cul-de-sac and the myometrium of the uterus.

NORMAL VARIANTS

- Retroverted uterus:
  (a) The entire uterus is tilted posteriorly.
  (b) Sonographic appearance is the same as that of the normal uterus.
- Retroflexed uterus:
  (a) Only the uterine fundus and body are tilted posteriorly.
  (b) Sonographic appearance is the same as that of the normal uterus.
- Didelphia uterus:
  (a) Developmental variant causing two uterine bodies, two cervices, and two vaginas.
  (b) Sonographic appearance is the same as that of the normal uterus, cervix, and vagina, but anatomy is duplicated.
- Bicornuate uterus:
  (a) Developmental variant causing two uterine bodies (divided) or two uterine horns (septated) with one vagina and one or two cervices.

(b) Sonographic appearance is the same as that of the normal uterus, cervix, and vagina, with duplication of the uterus.

PATIENT PREP

- Full urinary bladder.
- 32 to 40 ounces of clear fluid should be ingested one hour before the exam and finished within a 15- to 20-minute time period.
- If for any reason the patient cannot have fluids, sterile water can be used to fill the bladder through a Foley catheter.

N O T E : The fully distended urinary bladder displaces the bowel and brings the pelvic organs into view. Note that an overfilled bladder can actually push the pelvic contents out of view. If so, have the patient partially void.

N O T E : Normal bowel can mimic pathology. To distinguish between the two, the patient can be given a water enema that will clarify the bowel.

PATIENT POSITION

Supine.

TRANSDUCER

- **3.0 MHz** or **3.5 MHz.**
- 5.0 MHz for thin patients.

BREATHING TECHNIQUE

- **Normal respiration.**

FEMALE PELVIS SURVEY

N O T E : Prior to the examination a patient history should be taken to include the date of the first day of the patient's last period, parity, gravidity (pregnancy test results if available), symptoms, pelvic exam results, and history of pelvic surgery. Most sonography departments have standard forms where this information is recorded.

N O T E :   Survey of the female pelvis begins with longitudinal and transverse surveys of the uterus and pelvic cavity followed by longitudinal and transverse surveys of the ovaries.

UTERUS AND PELVIC CAVITY SURVEY

≡ LONGITUDINAL SURVEY

Sagittal Plane • Anterior Approach

1. Begin with the transducer perpendicular, at the midline of the body, just superior to the symphysis pubis. In most cases the vagina and cervix will be visualized here and possibly the body and fundus of the uterus depending on their lie. If the vagina is not seen, angle the transducer inferiorly and rotate the transducer varying degrees (to oblique the scanning plane according to the lie of the vagina) to visualize the vagina and its long axis.

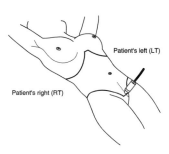

Note the bladder anteriorly.

2. Once the long axis of the vagina is located, angle the transducer inferiorly to scan through the vagina until you are beyond it.

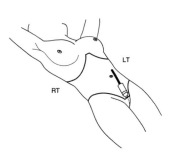

3. Return to the midline just superior to the symphysis pubis. With the transducer perpendicular, locate the long axis of the uterus. It may be necessary to rotate the transducer varying degrees (to oblique the scanning plane according to uterine lie) to visualize the long axis of the uterus.

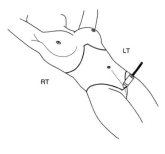

4. Once the long axis of the uterus is located, slowly move the transducer toward the patient's right, scanning laterally through the uterus and vagina until you are just beyond them.

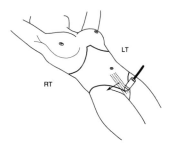

Note the bladder anteriorly.

5. Continue to scan right lateral through the pelvic side wall until you are beyond it.

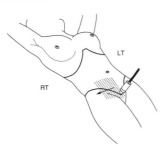

Note the bladder anteriorly and the location of the right ovary.

6. Return to midline, just superior to the symphysis pubis, and locate the long axis of the uterus.

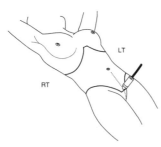

7. Once the long axis is located, slowly move the transducer toward the pa-tient's left, scanning laterally through the uterus and vagina until you are just beyond them.

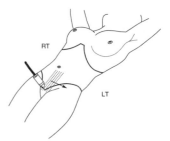

Note the bladder anteriorly.

8. Continue to scan left lateral through the pelvic side wall until you are beyond it.

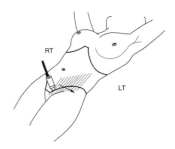

Note the bladder anteriorly and the location of the left ovary.

≡ TRANSVERSE SURVEY

Transverse Plane • Anterior Approach

1. Still in the sagittal plane, locate the long axis of the uterus. Rotate the transducer 90 degrees into the transverse scanning plane to traverse the uterus.

2. Begin with the transducer angled inferiorly, at the midline of the body, just superior to the symphysis pubis.

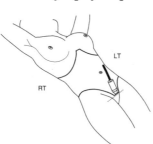

3. Angle the transducer inferiorly enough that you are out of the pelvis. *Slowly* angle the transducer back into the pelvis, looking first for the vagina.

Note the bladder anteriorly, rectum posteriorly, and the side walls.

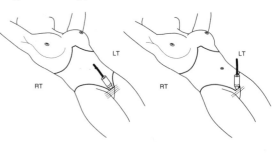

N O T E :   The normal traversed vagina, cervix, uterus body, and fundus appear as smooth, oval, organ textures with hyperechoic to hypoechoic centers. They gradually increase in size from the vagina to uterine fundus. Note that these structures lie between the distended anterior bladder and posterior bowel.

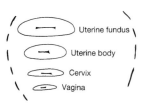

4. With the transducer becoming perpendicular, scan superiorly through the vagina and onto the cervix.

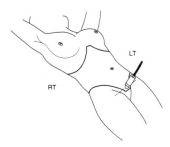

Note the bladder anteriorly, area of the cul-de-sac posteriorly, and the side wall.

5. Scanning perpendicular and superiorly through the cervix, move onto the body of the uterus.

Note the bladder anteriorly, the side walls, and the location of the ovaries.

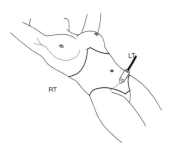

6. Continue scanning superiorly through the body of the uterus and onto the fundus. Scan superiorly through the fundus and superior bladder walls to the level of the umbilicus.

Note the bladder anteriorly, the side walls, and the location of the ovaries. As you scan beyond the bladder, adjust technique according to bowel appearance.

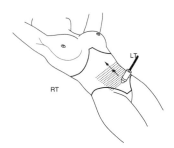

OVARIES SURVEY

N O T E :   The location of the ovaries is variable. They are generally lateral to the body or fundus of the uterus but may be found tucked in close to the side of the uterus. Other locations include posterior or superior to the uterus. If the ovaries are not identified during the following surveys, every effort must be made to locate them, including endovaginal sonography.

Right Ovary Survey

≡ LONGITUDINAL SURVEY

Sagittal Plane • Anterior Approach

1. Begin with the transducer perpendicular, at the midline of the body, just superior to the symphysis pubis. Recall the location of the right ovary from the pelvic cavity survey.

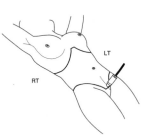

2. Locate the long axis of the uterus, then slowly move the transducer right lateral until the right ovary is located. Look for the longitudinal internal iliac vessels immediately posterior to the ovary. It may be necessary to slightly rotate the transducer to resolve the lie of the ovary.

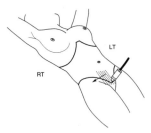

N O T E :   If the ovary cannot be seen because of overlying bowel, angle the transducer right lateral toward the right ovary from the midline of the pelvic cavity or just to the left of the midline.

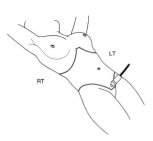

3. Once the ovary is located, move or angle the transducer right lateral, scanning through and beyond the lateral margin of the ovary.

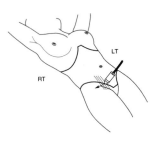

4. Move back onto the ovary and move or angle the transducer toward the midline of the pelvic cavity, scanning through and beyond the medial margin of the ovary.

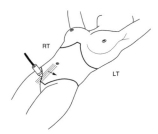

5. Move back onto the right ovary.

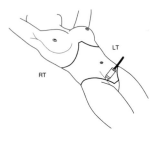

≡ TRANSVERSE SURVEY

Transverse Plane • Anterior Approach

1. Still viewing the longitudinal right ovary in the sagittal plane, rotate the transducer 90 degrees into the transverse scanning plane to traverse the right ovary.

Note the traversed internal iliac vessels posterior to the ovary.

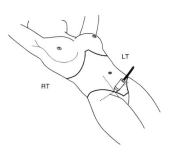

2. Move or angle the transducer superiorly, scanning through and beyond the superior margin of the ovary.

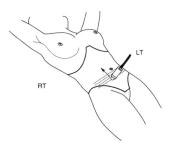

3. Move back onto the ovary and move or angle the transducer inferiorly, scanning through and beyond the inferior margin of the ovary.

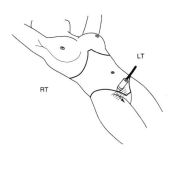

Left Ovary Survey

Use the same survey scanning methods as those for the right ovary.

REQUIRED IMAGES

Pelvic Cavity and Uterus

≡ LONGITUDINAL IMAGES

Sagittal Plane • Anterior Approach

N O T E :   Longitudinal images begin with survey images of the pelvic cavity to be followed by a long axis image of the uterus.

1. Longitudinal image of the midline of the pelvic cavity just superior to the symphysis pubis.

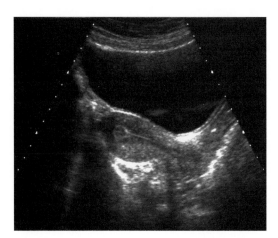 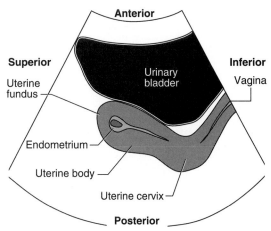

L A B E L E D :   PELVIS SAG ML

2. Longitudinal image of the right adnexa that may include part of the uterus depending on its lie.

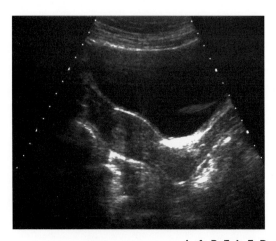 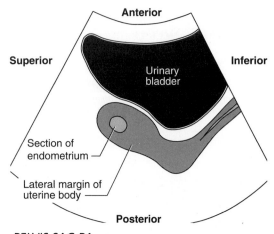

L A B E L E D :   PELVIS SAG R1

3. Longitudinal image to include the right lateral wall of the bladder and pelvic side wall.

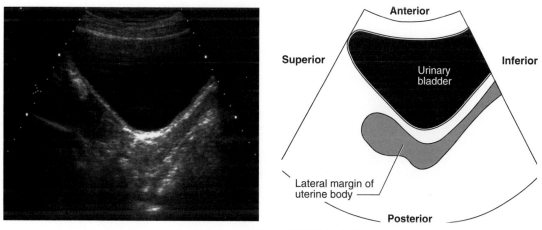

L A B E L E D :   PELVIS SAG R2

4. Longitudinal image of the left adnexa that may include part of the uterus depending on its lie.

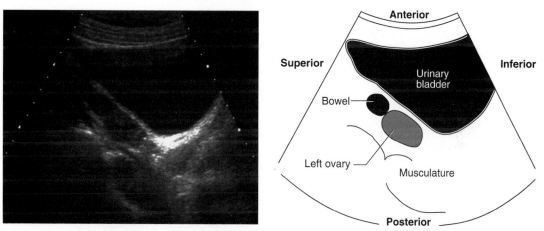

L A B E L E D :   PELVIS SAG L1

5. Longitudinal image to include the left lateral wall of the bladder and pelvic side wall.

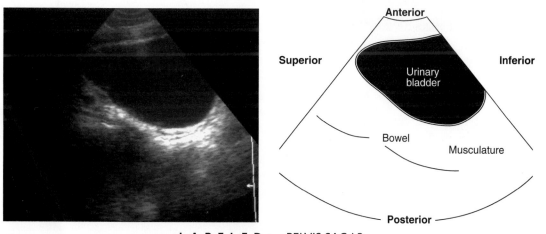

L A B E L E D :   PELVIS SAG L2

6. Long axis image of the uterus to include as much endometrial cavity as possible with uterine *length (superior to inferior) and height (anterior to posterior) measurements.*

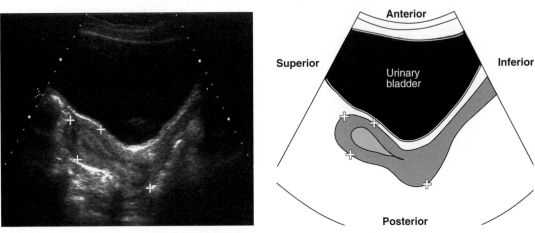

L A B E L E D :   UT SAG LONG AXIS

7. Same image as number 6 without calipers.

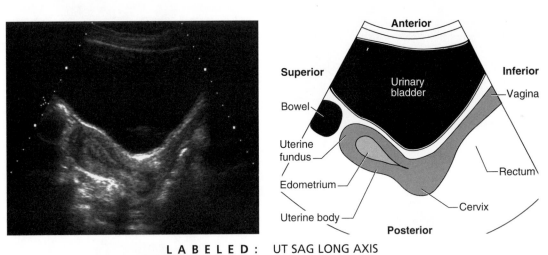

L A B E L E D :   UT SAG LONG AXIS

N O T E :   It may be necessary to take a separate image of the endometrial cavity. If so, label: **UT SAG**

≡ TRANSVERSE IMAGES

Transverse Plane • Anterior Approach

8. Transverse image of the vagina.

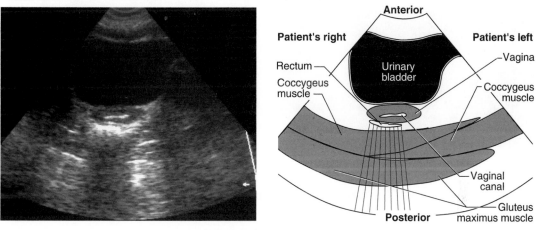

L A B E L E D :   TRV VAG

9. Transverse image of the cervix.

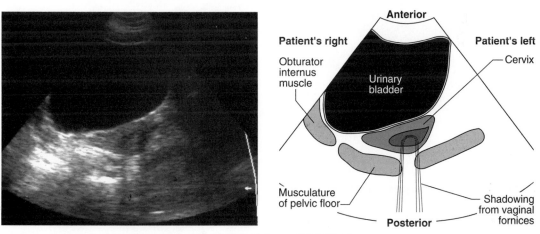

L A B E L E D :   TRV CERX

10. Transverse image of the uterus body.

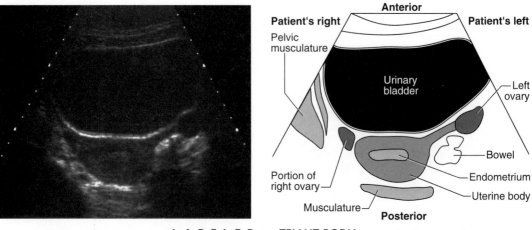

LABELED: TRV UT BODY

11. Transverse image of the uterus fundus *measuring uterine width (right to left).*

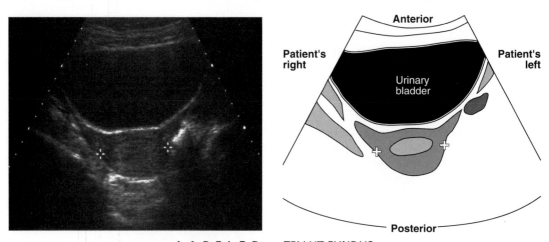

LABELED: TRV UT FUNDUS

12. Same image as number 11 without calipers.

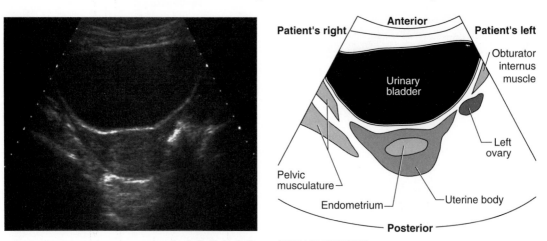

LABELED: TRV UT FUNDUS

Right Ovary

N O T E :   Due to the variability of the location and lie of the ovaries, the long axis can lie in any scanning plane. The following images reflect the long axis in the sagittal plane.

☰ LONGITUDINAL IMAGES

Sagittal Plane • Anterior Approach

13. Long axis image of the right ovary *measuring length (superior to inferior) and height (anterior to posterior).*

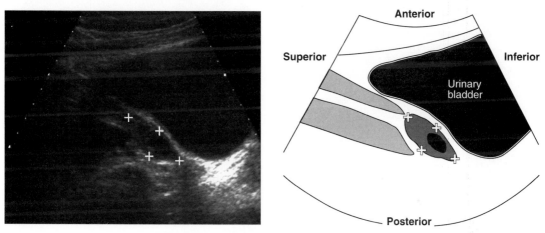

L A B E L E D :   RT OV SAG LONG AXIS

N O T E :   If this image of the ovary was angled from midline, then the image is obliqued and must be labeled: **RT OV SAG OBL LONG AXIS**

14. Same image as number 13 without calipers.

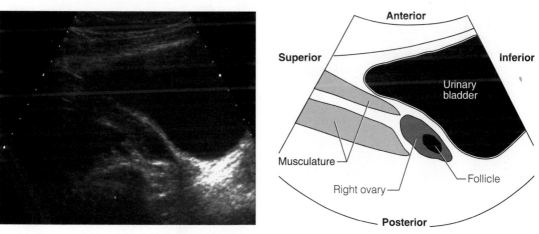

L A B E L E D :   RT OV SAG LONG AXIS

☰ TRANSVERSE IMAGES

Transverse Plane • Anterior Approach

15. Transverse image of the right ovary with *width (right to left) measurement.*

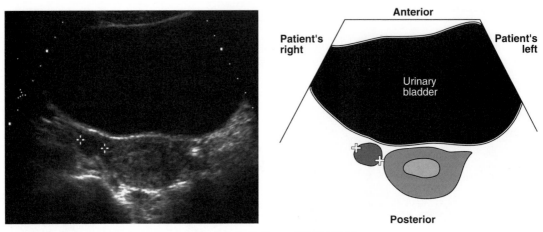

L A B E L E D :   RT OV TRV

N O T E :   If this is an oblique image, then label: **RT OV TRV OBL**

16. Same image as number 15 without calipers.

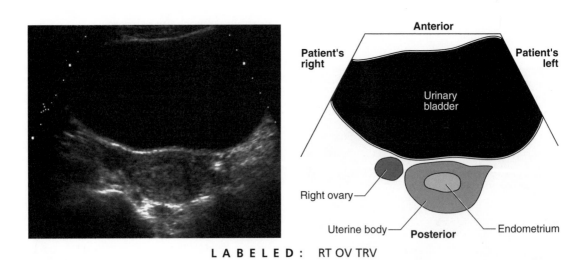

L A B E L E D :   RT OV TRV

Left Ovary

≡ LONGITUDINAL IMAGES

Sagittal Plane • Anterior Approach

17. Long axis image of the left ovary *measuring length (superior to inferior) and height (anterior to posterior)*.

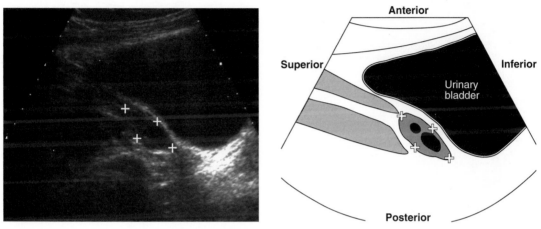

L A B E L E D :   LT OV SAG LONG AXIS

N O T E :   If this is an oblique image, then label: **LT OV SAG OBL LONG AXIS**

18. Same image as number 17 without calipers.

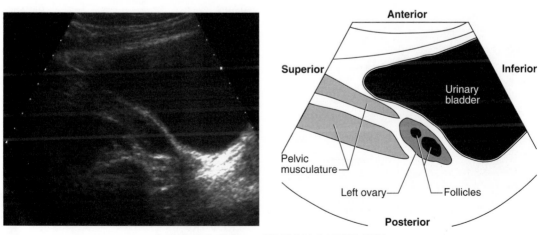

L A B E L E D :   LT OV SAG LONG AXIS

≡ TRANSVERSE IMAGES

Transverse Plane • Anterior Approach

19. Transverse image of the left ovary with *width (right to left) measurement.*

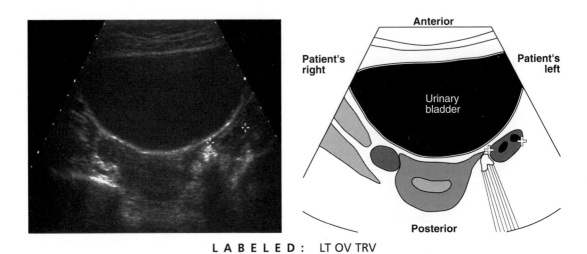

L A B E L E D :   LT OV TRV

N O T E :   If this is an obliqued image, then label: **LT OV OBL TRV**

20. Same image as number 19 without calipers.

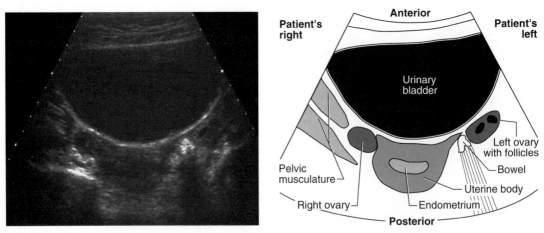

L A B E L E D :   LT OV TRV

Endovaginal Sonography

B.B. Tempkin, Deborah D. Werneburg, and
Kristin Dykstra-Downey

N O T E :   In most cases endovaginal sonography is used in conjunction with transabdominal sonography when pelvic contents require further evaluation. If the transabdominal scan provides the diagnosis, then the endovaginal scan is not necessary.

PATIENT PREP

- Explain the examination to the patient. Inform the patient that the exam is virtually painless, that the inserted transducer feels like a tampon, and the exam is necessary for an accurate diagnosis. Verbal or written consent is required, and the exam should be witnessed by a female health care professional. Note that the initials of the witness should be included as part of the film labeling.
- Empty urinary bladder.
- The transducer may be inserted by the patient, sonographer, or physician.

PATIENT POSITION

- Transducer design determines patient position so ideally having a gynecological examining table and the ability to put the patient in lithotomy position is optimal.
- Another option is positioning the patient at the end of the examining table or stretcher with the hips elevated by a pillow or foam cushion.

TRANSDUCER

- **5 MHz to 7.5 MHz.**
- Apply gel to the end of the transducer, then cover it with a condom or sheath. Make sure there are no air bubbles at the tip, then apply additional gel to the outside of the condom before insertion. If infertility is a consideration, then water or nonspermicidal gel may be used.

ORIENTATION

- Endovaginal scanning utilizes sagittal and coronal planes, both from the inferior approach. In the normal anteverted uterine position, these scanning planes demonstrate sagittal and transverse sections of the uterus and the ovaries (organ-oriented planes). Normal variations in organ position may result in a coronal section of the ovary when imaging in the coronal scanning plane, or, less frequently, a coronal section of the uterus (such as with a retroverted, retroflexed uterine position) in the coronal scanning plane.

- All endovaginal images should be labeled **EV SAG** or **EV COR,** depicting the scanning plane. Additional labeling may be used to indicate organ-oriented planes, which may vary with anatomic positioning.

- Proper image orientation is challenging in endovaginal scanning due to the narrow field of view, the inferior scanning approach, and normal positional variations of the reproductive organs. Therefore, it is important to determine proper positioning of the probe prior to insertion at the beginning of the exam. Proper positioning of the probe in the sagittal plane is confirmed when touching the edge of the probe which is directed toward the ceiling creates visible motion at the left of the image. From this position, the probe can be rotated 90 degrees counterclockwise in order to scan in the coronal plane.

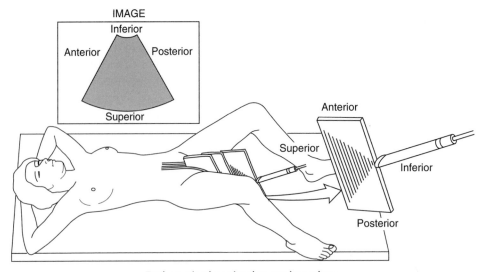

Endovaginal sagittal scanning place

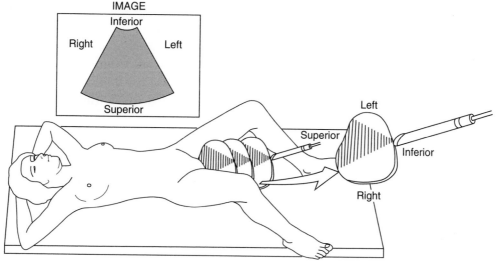

Endovaginal coronal scanning place

UTERUS AND PELVIC CAVITY SURVEY

N O T E :   The inserted transducer must be slightly angled in different directions to visualize the uterus and adnexa.

☰ LONGITUDINAL SURVEY

Sagittal Plane • Vaginal Approach

1. Begin by slowly lowering the transducer handle toward the floor to view the fundus of the uterus. Slightly move the transducer to the right and left to evaluate the lateral margins.

Note the endometrial cavity. If the bladder contains any urine, note it anteriorly (on the left side of the imaging screen).

2. Withdraw the transducer slightly, and slowly lift the handle toward the ceiling to view the body of the uterus, cervix, and cul-de-sac. Move the transducer to the right and left to evaluate the lateral margins.

Note the endometrial cavity.

3. After evaluating the uterus, continue the longitudinal survey to the adnexal regions. In the sagittal scanning plane, lower the transducer handle toward the floor to view the uterine fundus and the pelvic region superior to the uterus. Now slowly move the transducer handle toward the patient's left thigh in order to scan through the right adnexa. Return to midline, then move the transducer handle toward the patient's right thigh to visualize the left adnexa.

N O T E :   For the retroverted uterus, the uterine fundus is visualized by lifting the transducer handle towards the ceiling. It may also be helpful to rotate the probe 180 degrees and invert image orientation.

4. Repeat these lateral sweeps through the adnexal regions at the levels of the uterine body and cervix. These surveys will help to identify both normal anatomy and pathology within the pelvic cavity.

≡ TRANSVERSE SURVEY

Coronal Plane • Vaginal Approach

1. Rotate the transducer counterclockwise into the coronal plane.

2. Begin by slowly lowering the transducer handle toward the floor to evaluate the uterine fundus.

3. Withdraw the transducer slightly and slowly lift the handle toward the ceiling. Scan through the uterine body, cervix, and posterior cul-de-sac.

4. After evaluating the uterus in the coronal scanning plane, which affords transverse sections of this organ, survey the adnexal regions in the coronal scanning plane. Moving the transducer handle toward the floor, identify the uterine fundus. Now slowly move the transducer handle toward the patient's left thigh to visualize the right adnexa.

Now slowly move the transducer handle toward the ceiling in order to sweep through the right adnexa in the coronal plane.

5. Return to midline, then move the transducer handle toward the patient's right thigh to visualize the left adnexa. By slowly moving the transducer handle up and down, sweep through the left adnexa in the coronal plane.

OVARIES SURVEY

Right Ovary Survey

☰ TRANSVERSE SURVEY

Coronal Plane • Vaginal Approach

1. The ovaries are most easily evaluated by beginning in the coronal scanning plane. From initial insertion of the probe in the sagittal plane, the transducer handle should be rotated 90 degrees counterclockwise.

2. Begin by putting the transducer in a right oblique position. This is done by moving the transducer handle against the patient's left thigh, which angles the beam toward the right adnexa.

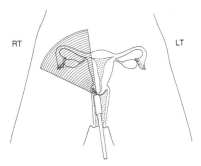

3. Find the ovary by slightly moving the transducer handle up and down.

Note the adjacent iliac vessels.

4. Once the ovary is located, move the transducer handle up and down to scan through the anterior and posterior margins.

☰ LONGITUDINAL SURVEY

Sagittal Plane • Vaginal Approach

1. Still viewing the ovary in the coronal plane, rotate the transducer 90 degrees clockwise into the sagittal plane.

2. Begin by very slightly moving the transducer handle to the right and left to scan through the lateral and medial margins.

Note the adjacent iliac vessels laterally.

Left Ovary Survey

1. Go back to the coronal scanning plane by rotating the transducer 90 degrees counterclockwise.

2. Put the transducer in a left oblique position by moving the transducer handle against the patient's right thigh. Follow the same survey methods as for the right ovary for transverse and longitudinal surveys.

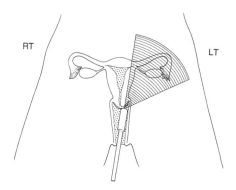

REQUIRED IMAGES

Uterus

≡ LONGITUDINAL IMAGES

Sagittal Plane • Vaginal Approach

1. Longitudinal image of the uterus usually obtained in a midline sagittal scanning plane. The long axis of the uterus should include *measurements of uterine length and height.*

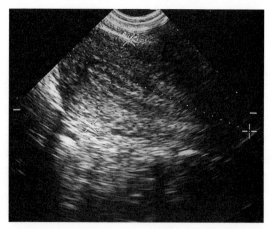

L A B E L E D :   EV SAG ML OR EV SAG ML UT LONG AXIS ("EV" INDICATES ENDOVAGINAL)

N O T E :   If the long axis is not imaged at midline, it should be taken here and labeled: EV SAG UT LONG AXIS.

2. Same image as number 1 without calipers.

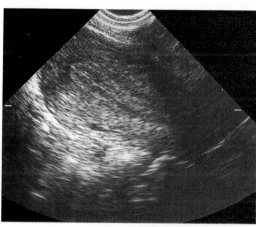 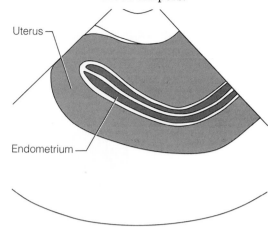

L A B E L E D :   EV SAG ML UT LONG AXIS

3. Longitudinal image of the uterus fundus to include the endometrial cavity.

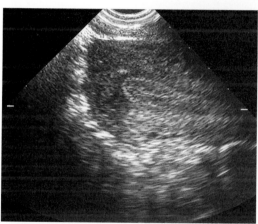 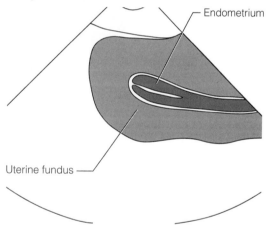

L A B E L E D :   EV SAG FUNDUS

4. Longitudinal image of the uterus body and cervix to include the endometrial cavity.

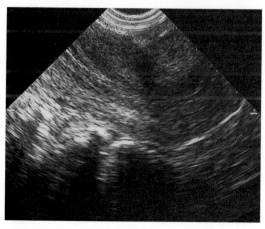 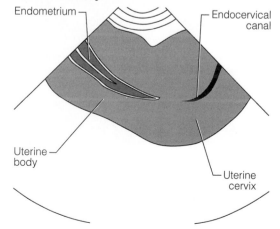

L A B E L E D :   EV SAG BODY CERX

≡ TRANSVERSE IMAGES

Coronal Plane • Vaginal Approach

5. Transverse image of the uterine fundus *measuring uterine width.*

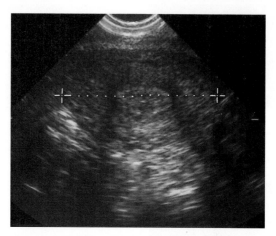

LABELED: EV COR FUNDUS

6. Same image as number 5 without calipers.

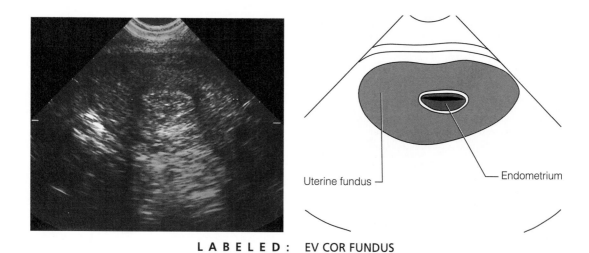

Uterine fundus ⏌   ⎾ Endometrium

LABELED: EV COR FUNDUS

7. Transverse image of the uterine body.

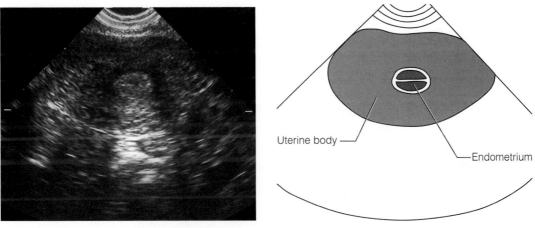

L A B E L E D :   EV COR BODY

8. Transverse image of the cervix.

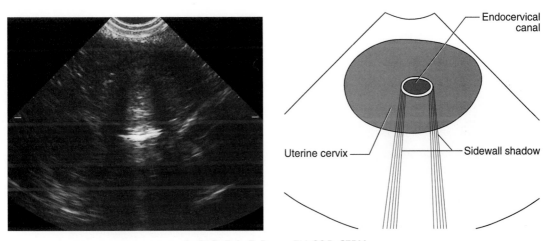

L A B E L E D :   EV COR CERX

Right Ovary

> **N O T E :**   Due to the variability of the location and lie of the ovaries, the long axis can lie in any scanning plane. The following images reflect the long axis in the sagittal plane.

≡ TRANSVERSE IMAGES

Coronal Plane • Vaginal Approach

9. Transverse image of the right ovary *measuring ovarian width (right to left).*

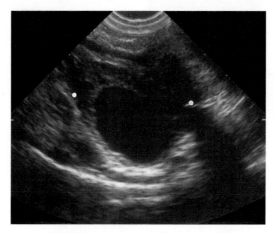

L A B E L E D :   EV COR RT OV

10. Same image as number 9 without calipers.

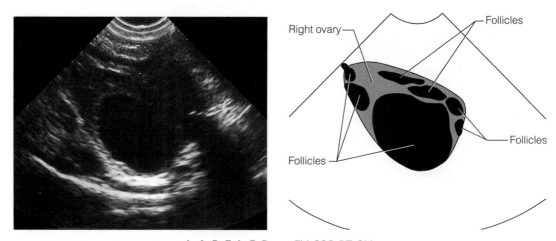

Right ovary

Follicles

Follicles

Follicles

Follicles

L A B E L E D :   EV COR RT OV

≡ LONGITUDINAL IMAGES

Sagittal Plane • Vaginal Approach

11. Long axis image of the right ovary *measuring ovarian length and height.*

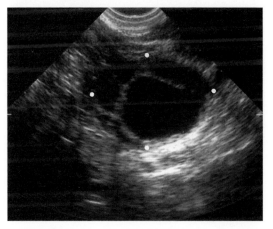

L A B E L E D :   EV SAG RT OV LONG AXIS

12. Same image as number 11 without calipers.

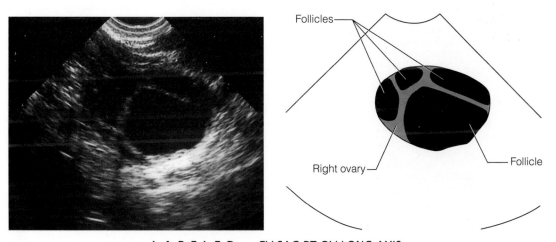

L A B E L E D :   EV SAG RT OV LONG AXIS

Left Ovary

≡ TRANSVERSE IMAGES

Coronal Plane • Vaginal Approach

13. Transverse image of the left ovary *measuring ovarian width (right to left).*

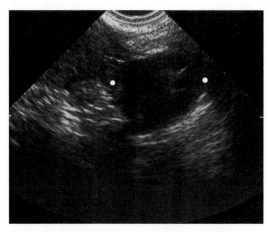

L A B E L E D :   EV COR LT OV

14. Same image as number 13 without calipers.

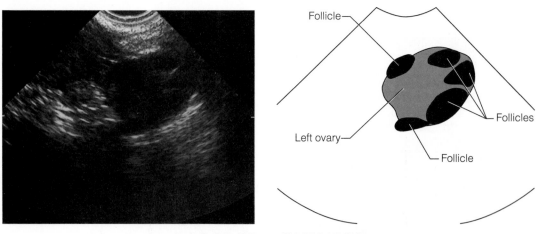

L A B E L E D :   EV COR LT OV

≡ LONGITUDINAL IMAGES

Sagittal Plane • Vaginal Approach

15. Long axis image of the left ovary *measuring ovarian length and height.*

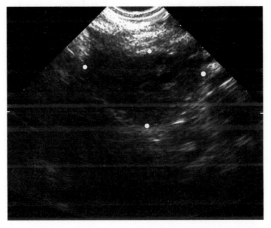

L A B E L E D :   EV SAG LT OV LONG AXIS

16. Same image as number 15 without calipers.

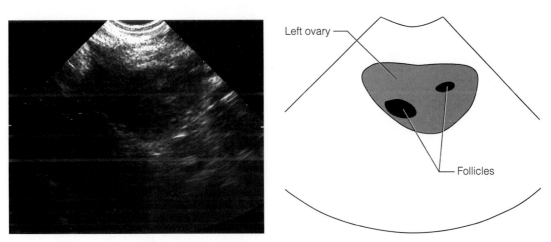

L A B E L E D :   EV SAG LT OV LONG AXIS

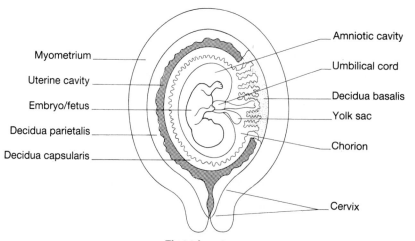

Myometrium

Uterine cavity

Embryo/fetus

Decidua parietalis

Decidua capsularis

Amniotic cavity

Umbilical cord

Decidua basalis

Yolk sac

Chorion

Cervix

First trimester

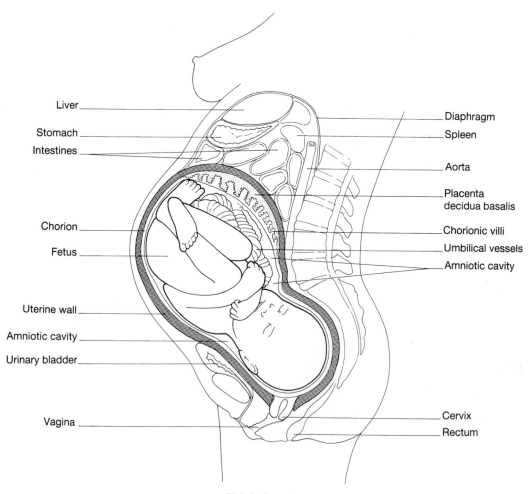

Liver

Stomach

Intestines

Chorion

Fetus

Uterine wall

Amniotic cavity

Urinary bladder

Vagina

Diaphragm

Spleen

Aorta

Placenta
decidua basalis

Chorionic villi

Umbilical vessels

Amniotic cavity

Cervix

Rectum

Third trimester

Obstetrical Scanning Protocol

CHAPTER

12

B.B. Tempkin and G. William Shepherd

ANATOMY

Maternal Anatomy

- Maternal pelvic cavity includes the vagina, uterus, two ovaries, two fallopian tubes, a portion of the ureters, the urinary bladder, musculature, and intestinal tract. Refer to Chapter 11 for anatomical specifics.

First Trimester Anatomy and Sonographic Appearance

- Gestational sac. Represents the anechoic, fluid-filled chorionic cavity surrounded by the echogenic trophoblastic ring. Normal locations include middle and fundal portions of the uterus. Early in the first trimester, the echogenic embyro and the yolk sac may be visualized within the gestational sac. The yolk sac disappears between the 10th and 12th weeks of the trimester.
- Fetal cardiac activity may be visible as early as 5 weeks and 2 days by transvaginal examination and is usually demonstrable before 6 weeks by transabdominal examination. The embryonic heart will appear small and pulsatile. Cardiac activity may be noticeable as a pulsation within a thickened wall of the yolk sac even before the embryo per se is clearly visible. The anechoic chambers and echogenic walls and contour may be discernable by the end of the first trimester.
- Later in the trimester the echogenic cranium, abdomen, and fetal limbs can be visualized.

Second and Third Trimester Anatomy and Sonographic Appearance

- The parenchyma of the placenta appears midgray to low gray with relatively even texture. As the gestation advances, the parenchyma is interrupted by echogenic calcium deposits and/or sonolucent vessels. The fetal and maternal placental surfaces appear echogenic. The position of the placenta is variable within the uterus and may change as the uterus expands to accommodate the growing fetus.
- The fetal skeleton and extremities appear echogenic.
- The normal fetal spine will appear as an echogenic closed circle when traversed. Longitudinally it appears as two echogenic, curvilinear lines that widen at the skull and narrow at the sacrum.
- The fetal diaphragm appears as an echogenic, thin, curvilinear line that is easiest to visualize when you scan along the longitudinal axis of the fetus.
- The parenchyma of the fetal organs appears as midgray echo textures.
- The fetal urinary bladder, gallbladder, and stomach appear anechoic if fluid-filled surrounded by echogenic walls. If collapsed, they are not visualized. The fetal intestine appears anechoic if fluid-filled; otherwise, echogenic.
- The umbilical cord and other fetal vessels appear as echogenic walls with anechoic lumina.
- The walls and contour of the heart appear echogenic. The chambers of the heart appear anechoic.
- The contour of the normal fetal head is smooth, echogenic, and elliptical in shape.
- Intracranial anatomy from superior to inferior:

  (a) Interhemispheric fissure:

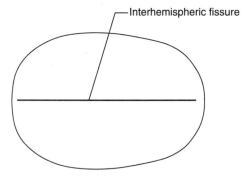

  Is a fissure that separates the cerebral hemispheres.

  It appears as a single, linear, echogenic structure visualized at the midline of the brain. Located within the fissure is the falx cerebrei, a fold of dura mater. It is not sonographically distinguishable from the fissure.

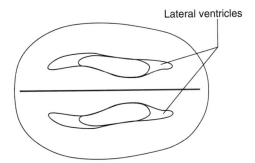

(b) Lateral ventricles:

The lateral walls appear as echogenic, linear structures lying the same distance from the interhemispheric fissure. The medial walls when visualized appear echogenic. The chambers of the ventricles appear anechoic. Ventricular width is normal up to 10 mm.

The echogenic choroid plexus can be seen within the ventricular chambers.

(c) Thalamus, third ventricle, cavum septum pellucidi, and frontal horns of the lateral ventricles.

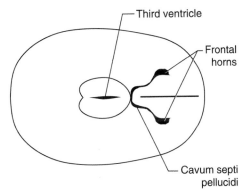

The thalamus is somewhat diamond shaped and is composed of 2 halves that lie on each side of and form a portion of the lateral wall of the third ventricle. They appear midgray or as medium to low-level echoes.

The third ventricle lies at the midline and appears as a bright line parallel to the interhemispheric fissure. Occasionally the small anechoic cavity can be visualized.

The cavum septum pellucidi lies at the midline between the anterior border of the thalami and the frontal horns of the lateral ventricles. It appears as an anechoic rectangular structure with two parallel hyperechoic lines on each side.

The frontal horns of the lateral ventricles can be seen anteriorly (occipital horns posteriorly).

(d) Cerebral peduncles, choroid plexus and the atrium of the lateral ventricles:

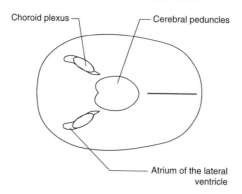

The cerebral peduncles are two heart-shaped masses that lie on each side of the midline. They appear similar in shape and texture to the thalami, but they are smaller and more rounded. Peduncle parenchyma is midgray with medium to low-level echoes.

Two parallel bright lines may be seen in the far-field of the section and sometimes in the near-field as well. These lines are the medial and lateral walls of the atrium of the lateral ventricle.

The hyperechoic choroid plexus can usually be seen between the ventricle walls and should nearly fill the space.

The basilar artery can be seen pulsating at the midline between the anterior portions of the peduncles.

The circle of Willis can be seen pulsating at the midline anterior to the peduncles.

(e) Base of the skull:

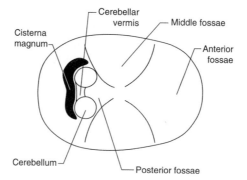

The anechoic anterior, middle, and posterior fossae are divided from one another by the echogenic petrous ridges of the skull posteriorly and the sphenoid bones anteriorly. The posterior fossa contains the two round halves of the cerebellum which appear midgray and the more echoic vermis which connects them at midline. Posterior to the cerebellum is the anechoic cisterna magnum.

PATIENT PREP

- Full urinary bladder.
- 32 to 40 ounces of clear fluid should be ingested 1 hour before the exam and finished within a 15- to 20-minute time period.
- If for any reason the patient cannot have fluids, sterile water can be used to fill the bladder through a Foley catheter.

N O T E : The fully distended urinary bladder displaces the bowel and brings the pelvic organs into view. Note that an overfilled bladder can actually push the pelvic contents out of view. If so, have the patient partially void.

ENDOVAGINAL PATIENT PREP

- See Chapter 11 for patient prep specifics.

PATIENT POSITION

- **Supine.**
- Right lateral decubitus or left lateral decubitus.
- During the third trimester if the fetal head is in the lower uterine segment, it may be helpful to elevate the patient's hips with a pillow or foam cushion.

ENDOVAGINAL PATIENT POSITION

- See Chapter 11 for patient position specifics.

TRANSDUCER

- **3.0 MHz or 3.5 MHz.**
- 2.5 MHz for very large patients. 5.0 MHz for thinner patients or earlier gestational ages.
- Sector, curvolinear, and linear transducers may be required for an adequate examination. It is not unusual to use two or even three transducers for an obstetric ultrasound exam.

ENDOVAGINAL TRANSDUCER

- See Chapter 11 for transducer specifics.

OBSTETRICAL SURVEY

N O T E :   Prior to the examination, a patient history should be taken to include the date of the first day of the patient's last period, gravidity, parity, and history of pelvic surgery. Most sonography departments have standard forms where this information is recorded.

N O T E :   The obstetrical survey begins with longitudinal and transverse surveys of the uterus and adnexa to be followed by longitudinal and transverse surveys of the fetus.

Uterus and Adnexa Survey

≡ LONGITUDINAL SURVEY

Sagittal Plane • Anterior Approach

N O T E :   While surveying the uterus and adnexa also verify **fetal life** and note if the pregnancy is **multiple.** Determine the fetal **lie and presentation.** Note the location of the **placenta**. Evaluate **amniotic fluid volume** subjectively; extremes are obvious.

N O T E :   Fetal lie is determined by comparing the long axis of the fetus to the long axis of the uterus. Presentation refers to the fetal part closest to the cervix.

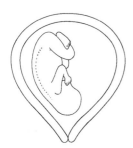

Longitudinal lie/cephalic presentation

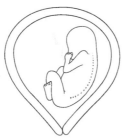

Longitudinal lie/breech presentation

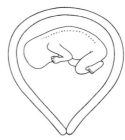

Transverse lie/head maternal right

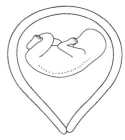

Transverse lie/head maternal left

1. Begin with the transducer perpendicular, at the midline of the body, just superior to the symphysis pubis. In most cases the vagina and cervix will be located here and possibly the body and fundus of the uterus, depending on their lie and their size according to the trimester. If the vagina is not seen, angle the transducer inferiorly and rotate the transducer to resolve the vagina and its long axis.

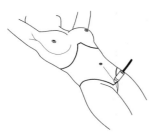

2. Once the vagina is located, angle the transducer inferiorly to scan through the vagina until you are beyond it.

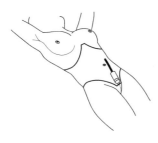

3. Return to the midline just superior to the symphysis pubis.

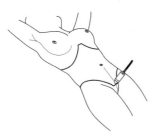

Evaluate the cervix and the area of the cul-de-sac posteriorly. Slightly rotating the transducer may help resolve the cervix.

4. Move superiorly through the cervix and along the midline to the level of the umbilicus. Evaluate whatever part of the uterus that may lie here.

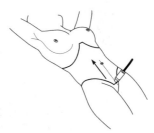

5. Return to the midline just superior to the symphysis pubis. Keep the transducer perpendicular and slowly move the transducer toward the patient's right side, scanning through the uterus and the adnexa until you are beyond it.

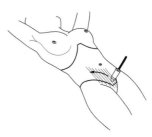

N O T E :   As you scan laterally note the ovaries. Also, move the transducer superiorly as necessary to evaluate the entire uterine fundus and its contents. Uterine lie is normally variable and its size is dependent on the trimester.

6. Return to the midline and move the transducer toward the patient's left side, scanning through the uterus and the adnexa until you are beyond it.

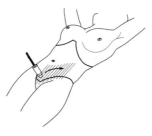

☰ TRANSVERSE SURVEY

Transverse Plane • Anterior Approach

1. Begin with the transducer angled inferiorly, at the midline, just superior to the symphysis pubis.

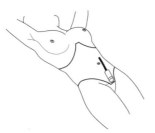

2. Angle the transducer inferiorly enough that you are out of the pelvis. *Slowly* angle the transducer back into the pelvis looking first for the vagina.

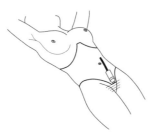

Note the bladder anteriorly, rectum posteriorly, and the side walls.

3. With the transducer becoming perpendicular, scan superiorly through the vagina and onto the cervix.

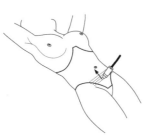

Note the area of the cul-de-sac posteriorly and the side walls.

4. Continue to scan superiorly through the cervix, body, and fundus of the uterus. As you move superiorly, also evaluate the adnexa.

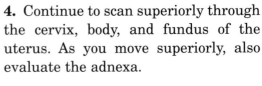
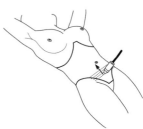

5. Scan superiorly through and beyond the fundus to the level of the umbilicus or further according to uterine size.

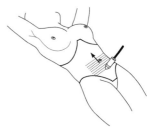

N O T E : As you scan superiorly also move laterally to completely evaluate the uterus and adnexa as the gestation progresses and the uterus becomes larger.

FETAL SURVEY

First Trimester Survey

☰ LONGITUDINAL SURVEY

Sagittal Plane • Anterior Approach

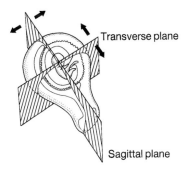

Transverse plane

Sagittal plane

1. Begin by resolving the long axis of the uterus and locating the gestational sac within.

2. Move the transducer right lateral through and beyond the gestational sac, then left lateral through and beyond the sac.

Note and evaluate any contents. Very early in the gestation the sac will normally appear empty. As the gestation progresses the small yolk sac, developing amniotic sac, developing embryo, developing placenta, and umbilical cord can be visualized.

N O T E : When a yolk sac is visualized early in the first trimester, inspect the areas adjacent to the yolk sac for cardiac activity. This may be more apparent than the fetal pole itself. Late in the first trimester, M-mode or Doppler ultrasound may be used to document viability if required by the hospital or clinic where the exam is performed.

☰ TRANSVERSE SURVEY

Transverse Plane • Anterior Approach

1. Still viewing the gestational sac in the sagittal plane, rotate the transducer 90 degrees into the transverse plane.

2. With the transducer perpendicular, begin by moving superiorly through and beyond the gestational sac, then inferior through and beyond the sac. Note and evaluate any contents.

Second and Third Trimester Survey

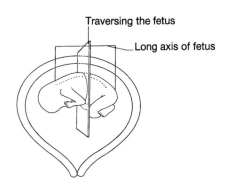

Traversing the fetus

Long axis of fetus

N O T E : Begin in the scanning plane where you visualized the long axis of the fetus during the survey of the uterus. Fetal position is variable, so the lie of the long axis may change. Change the scanning plane accordingly.

1. Locate the long axis of the fetus. Slowly move through the fetus noting the fetal heart, lungs, and diaphragm. Also evaluate the abdominopelvic contents including the kidneys, liver, IVC, and aorta. The gallbladder, stomach, and urinary bladder can be examined if fluid-filled. Note the bowel.

N O T E : The examination is not complete until a significant amount of time has been given to visualize the fetal urinary bladder. Nonvisualization may be interpreted as nonfunctioning fetal kidneys.

2. Locate the long axis of the fetal spine. Rotating the transducer slightly may aid visualization. Keep the transducer perpendicular and slowly move along the spine through the sacral end, then through the superior end to the skull. Note that the spine narrows at the sacrum and widens at the skull. Any other deviations seen along the "double line"-appearing spine indicate abnormality.

3. Rotate the transducer 90 degrees to traverse the spine. The normal spine appears as a closed circle. Beginning at the skull move inferiorly along the spine through the thoracic cavity. Note the fetal heart and lungs.

4. Continue to move inferiorly along the spine into and through the abdominopelvic cavity to the sacrum.

Note the fetal liver, IVC, aorta, kidneys, and adrenal glands. Also evaluate the umbilical cord and insertion site. The stomach, gallbladder, and urinary bladder can be examined if fluid-filled. Note the bowel. At the level of the sacrum look for the genitalia.

5. Locate the long axis of the fetal spine again and scan superiorly through to the base of the skull. Scan through the fetal cranium until you are beyond it.

Note the contour of the cranium, intracranial anatomy, and any facial features.

6. Return to the base of the skull and rotate the transducer 90 degrees. Again scan through the fetal cranium until you are beyond it.

Note the contour of the cranium and intracranial anatomy.

REQUIRED IMAGES

Early First Trimester/ *Gestational Sac/Embryo*

≡ LONGITUDINAL IMAGES

Sagittal Plane • Anterior Approach

N O T E :   Images of the gestational sac with measurements are taken whether an embryo is identified or not. Depending on how early the gestation is, it may be helpful to magnify the field of view for the gestational sac images.

1. Long axis image of the uterus showing the location of the gestational sac.

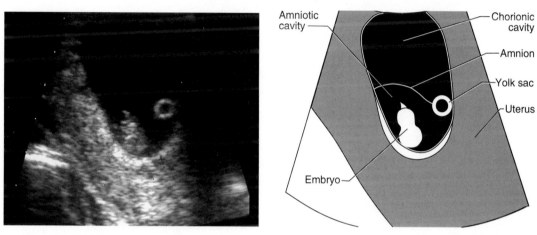

L A B E L E D :   UTERUS SAG LONG AXIS

2. Longitudinal image of the gestational sac with *length (superior to inferior) and height (anterior to posterior) measurements (calipers inside wall to inside wall).*

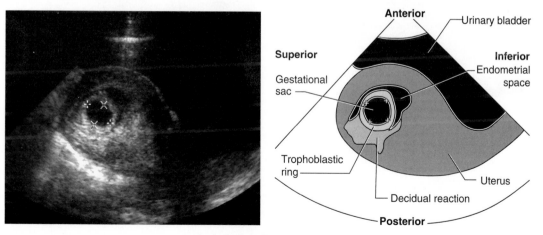

L A B E L E D :   GS SAG

3. Same image as number 2. without calipers.

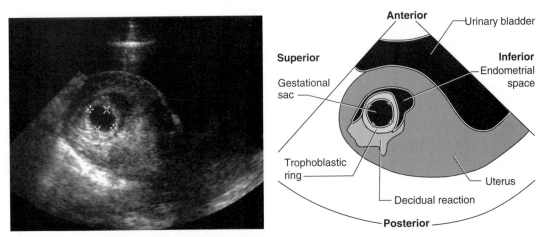

L A B E L E D :   GS SAG

N O T E :   If an embryo is present but not clearly represented on the gestational sac measurement images, an additional image of the embryo should be taken here and labeled accordingly.

4. Longitudinal image of the gestational sac with *superior to inferior measurement* of the fetal pole.

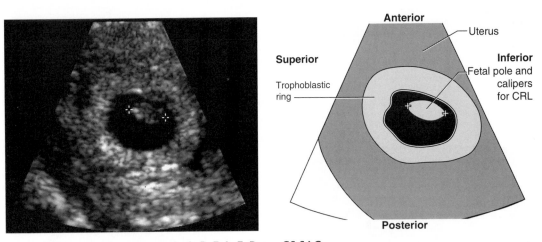

L A B E L E D :   GS SAG

5. Same image as number 4. without calipers.

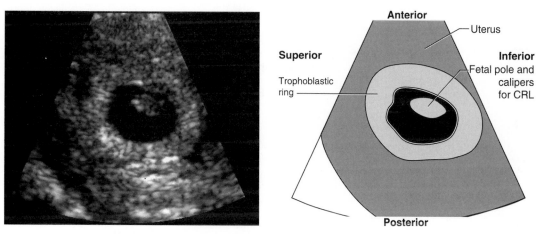

L A B E L E D :   GS SAG

≡ TRANSVERSE IMAGES

Transverse Plane • Anterior Approach

6. Transverse image of the gestational sac with *width (right to left) measurement (calipers inside wall to inside wall).*

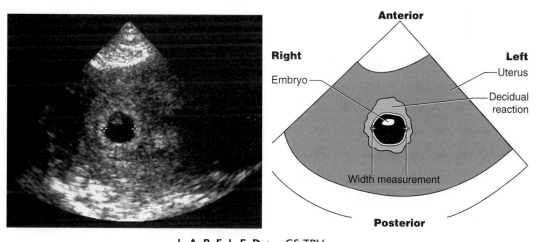

L A B E L E D :   GS TRV

7. Same image as number 6. without calipers.

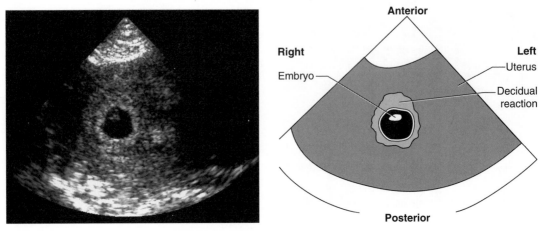

L A B E L E D :   GS TRV

8. Transverse image of the gestational sac and the yolk sac (optional magnified view).

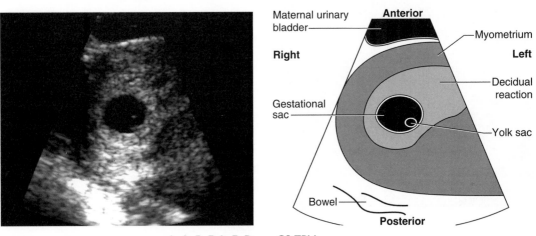

L A B E L E D :   GS TRV

9. Transverse image of the fetal pole (magnified view) with *width (right to left) measurement.*

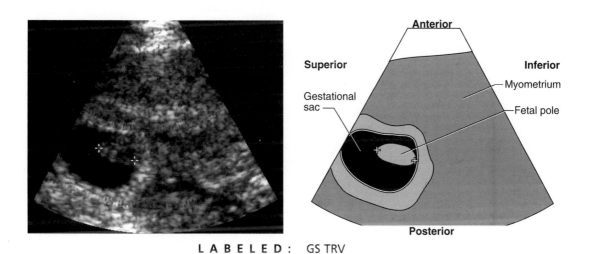

L A B E L E D :   GS TRV

10. Same image as number 9. without calipers.

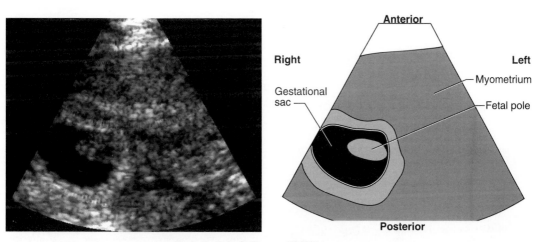

L A B E L E D :   GS TRV

11. Doppler documentation of viability.

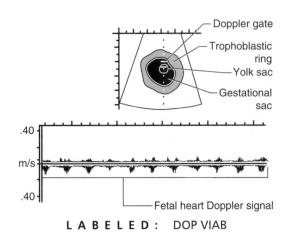

L A B E L E D :   DOP VIAB

Late First Trimester/ *Gestational Sac and Fetus*

N O T E :   The embryo is usually referred to as a fetal pole (or embryo) prior to 10 weeks' gestation. After 10 weeks it is called a fetus.

≡ LONGITUDINAL IMAGES

Sagittal Plane • Anterior Approach

1. Long axis image of the uterus showing the location of the gestational sac.

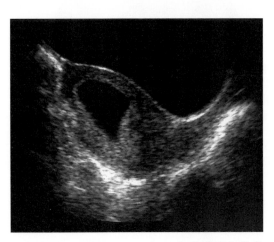 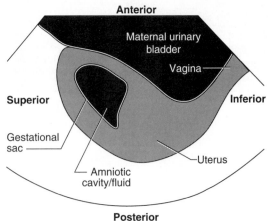

L A B E L E D :   UTERUS SAG LONG AXIS

2. Longitudinal image of the gestational sac to include the fetus and placenta location (if distinguishable).

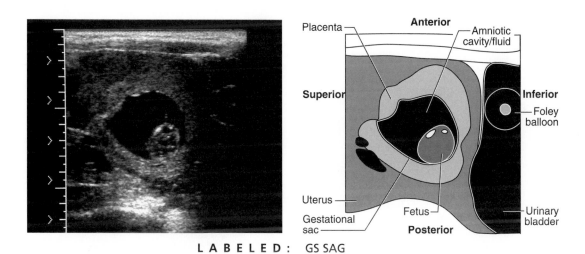

LABELED: GS SAG

≡ TRANSVERSE IMAGE

Transverse Plane • Anterior Approach

3. Transverse image of the gestational sac to include the fetus and placenta location (if distinguishable).

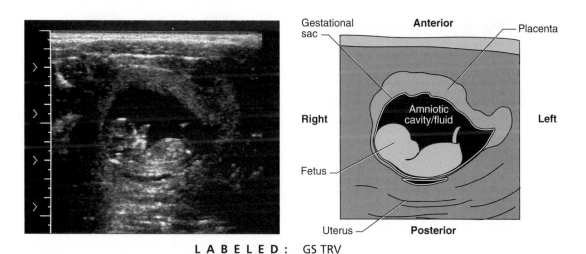

LABELED: GS TRV

N O T E : Because of the variability of the position of the fetus, scanning plane is not included as part of the film labeling on fetal measurement images.

4. Longitudinal image of the fetus with *measurement from fetal crown to rump.*

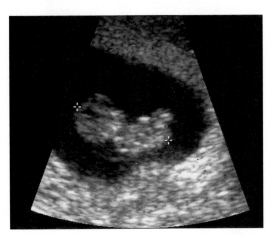 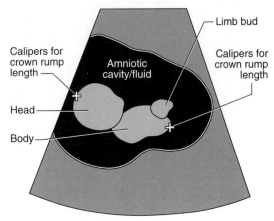

L A B E L E D : CR

5. Same image as number 4. without calipers.

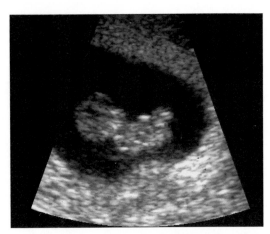 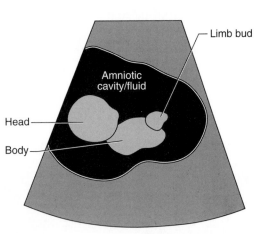

L A B E L E D : CR

N O T E : Depending on how early the gestation is, it may be helpful to magnify the field of view for the gestational sac and fetus.

N O T E : During the later part of the first trimester, measurements should include biparietal diameter, abdominal circumference, and other fetal measurements. See specifics for second and third trimester measurement images.

6. An optional magnified view of the fetus demonstrating limbs.

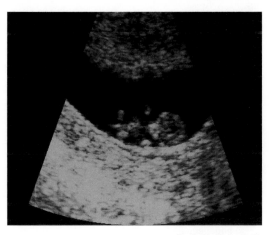
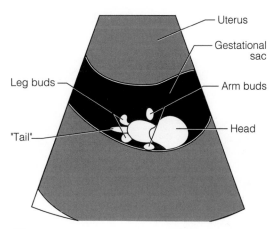

L A B E L E D : CR

Second and Third Trimesters

N O T E : Because of the variability of fetal position and movement, the following images may be taken in any sequence. An ultrasound examination during the second and third trimesters requires the documentation of a very large number of structures. The required structures will be shown in this chapter one or two at a time, but under some circumstances, two or more structures will often be documented on a single image. The suggested images are for a first-time ultrasound examination of a fetus. Repeat exams for growth measurements may require a reduced number of images.

1. When the trimester allows: long axis image of the uterus and contents.

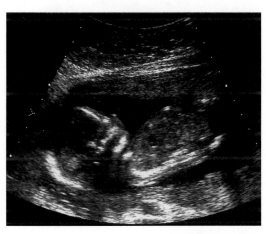
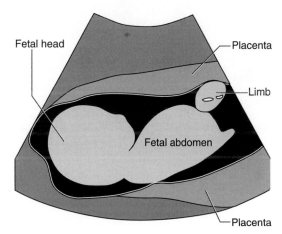

L A B E L E D : UTERUS SAG LONG AXIS

N O T E : In this case the trimester was too advanced to image the entire uterus on a single view.

2. Longitudinal image of the placenta.
   2A-2D are provided to aide identification of the different placental grades.

2A. Longitudinal image of a grade 0 placenta.

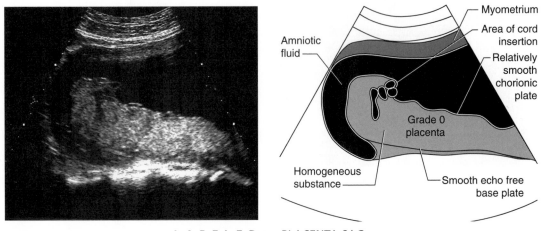

L A B E L E D :   PLACENTA SAG

2B. Longitudinal image of a grade I placenta.

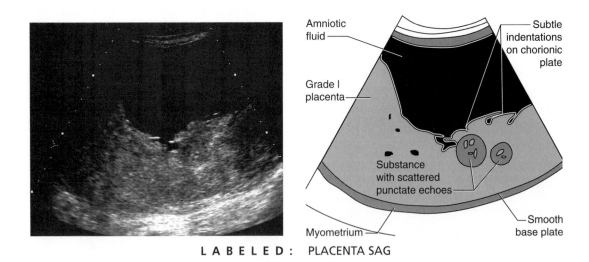

L A B E L E D :   PLACENTA SAG

2C. Longitudinal image of a grade II placenta.

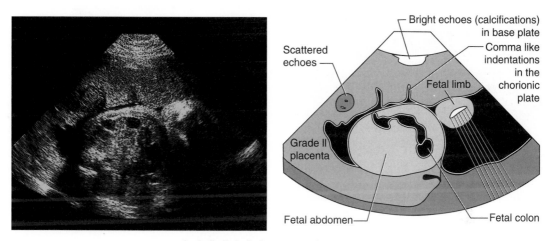

L A B E L E D :   PLACENTA SAG

2D. Longitudinal image of a grade III placenta.

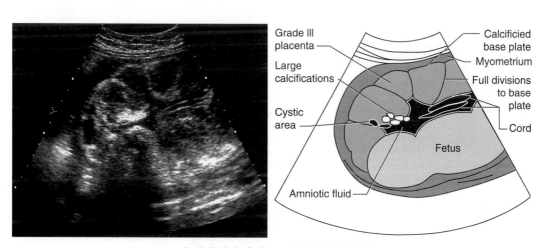

L A B E L E D :   PLACENTA SAG

3. Transverse image of placenta location.

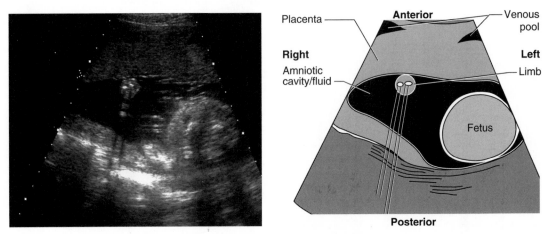

LABELED: PLACENTA TRV

4. Longitudinal image of the cervix to include the internal os.

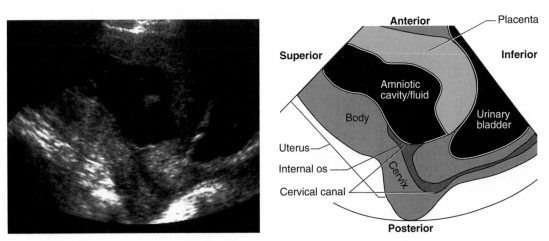

LABELED: CERVX SAG

NOTE: At times the head of the fetus or the mother's body habitus may inhibit imaging of the lower uterine segment. This image is required to rule out placental previa and to document the cervix. This situation requires either an endovaginal or translabial image. The translabial image is obtained with an empty or nearly empty bladder. The transducer is covered with a condom, glove, or even a food baggy and placed between the labia. The transducer is angled so that the cervix is nearly perpendicular to the ultrasound beam.

5. Longitudinal translabial image of the lower uterine segment.

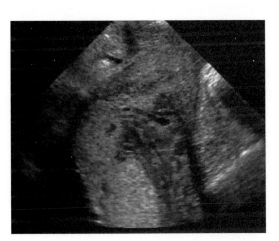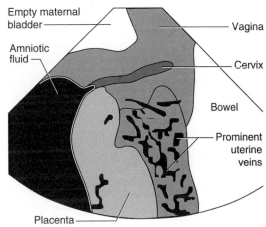

L A B E L E D :   CERVX SAG TRLAB

6. Depending on the stage of gestation, an overall longitudinal image of amniotic fluid or the largest pocket with *superior to inferior measurement.*

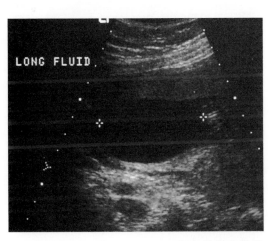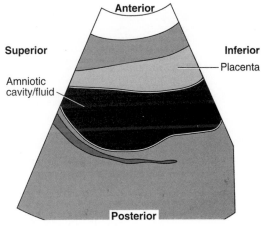

L A B E L E D :   FLUID SAG

7. Depending on the stage of gestation, an overall transverse image of amniotic fluid or the largest pocket with *anterior to posterior and right to left measurements.*

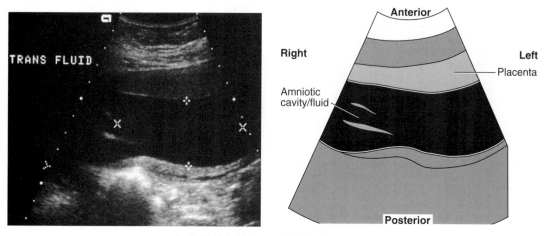

L A B E L E D :   FLUID TRV

N O T E :   At times a quantitative measurement of amniotic fluid is required. AP measurements are obtained for the right and left upper and lower quadrants. The sum of these AP measurements is called the amniotic fluid index (AFI). Fluid pockets that contain primarily cord or fetal parts are not included in the measurement.

8. Longitudinal image of the cervical spine.

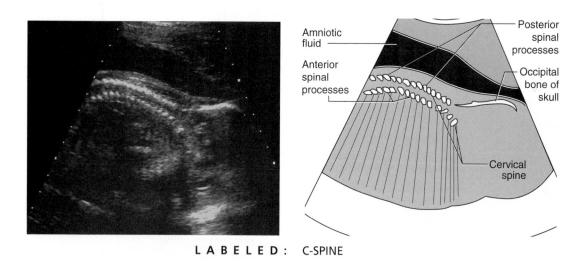

L A B E L E D :   C-SPINE

N O T E :   Because of the variability of the position of the fetus, the scanning plane is not included as part of the film labeling.

9. Longitudinal image of the thoracic spine.

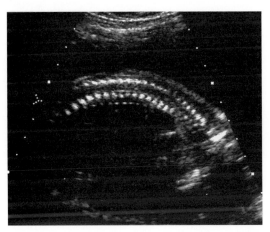 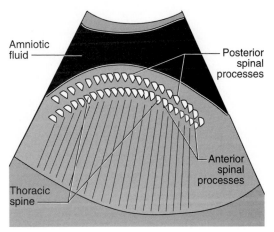

L A B E L E D :   T-SPINE

10. Longitudinal image of the lumbar spine.

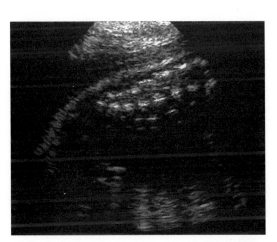 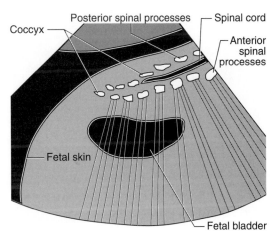

L A B E L E D :   L-SPINE

11. Longitudinal image of the sacral spine.

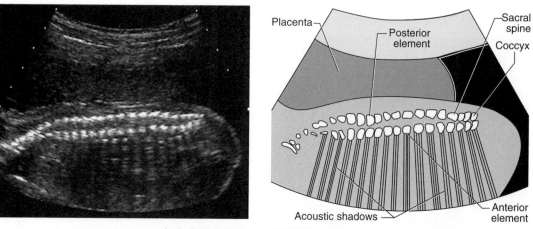

LABELED: S-SPINE

NOTE: In some cases the entire spine can be imaged. If so, take the image and label: **SPINE.**

12. Transverse image of the cervical spine.

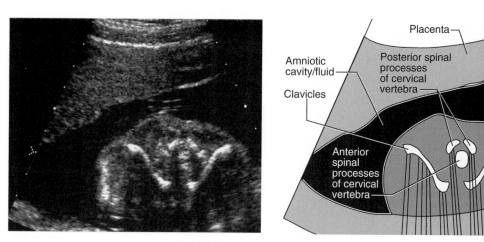

LABELED: C-SPINE

13. Transverse image of the thoracic spine.

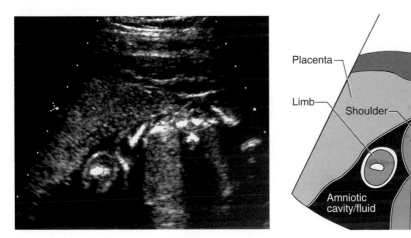

L A B E L E D :   T-SPINE

14. Transverse image of the lumbar spine.

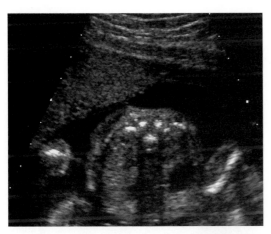
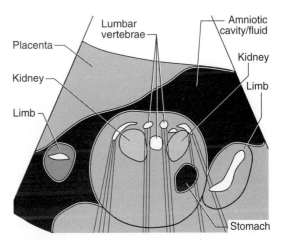

L A B E L E D :   L-SPINE

15. Four-chamber view of the fetal heart to include its location within the thorax.

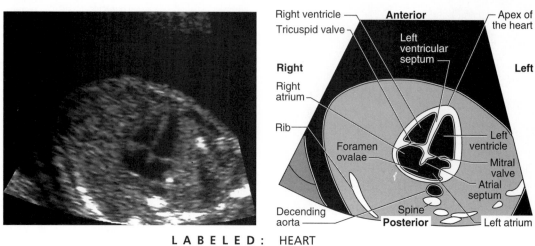

L A B E L E D :   HEART

16. An optional image showing the normal crossing of the cardiac outflow tracts.

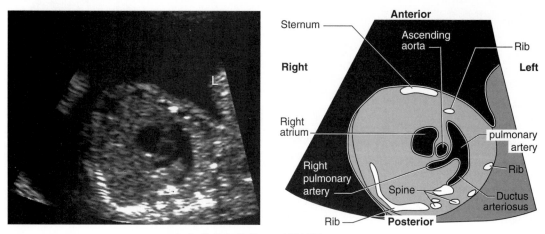

L A B E L E D :   HEART

17. Transverse image to include both fetal kidneys if possible.

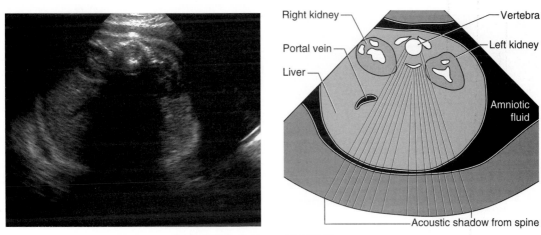

L A B E L E D :   KIDNEYS

N O T E :   When the kidneys cannot be imaged together because of fetal position or movement, take separate transverse images of each kidney and label accordingly.

18. Longitudinal image of the right kidney.

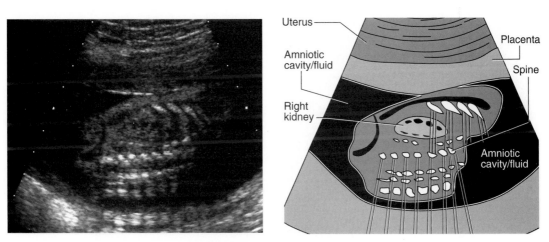

L A B E L E D :   RT KID

19. Longitudinal image of the left kidney.

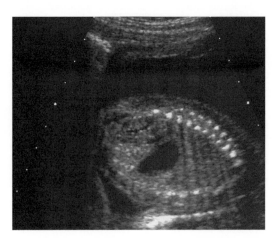 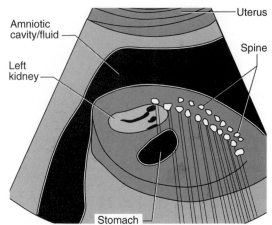

L A B E L E D :   LT KID

20. Image of the urinary bladder.

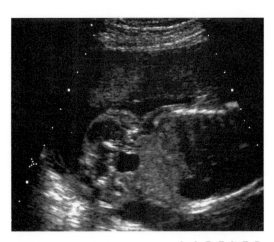 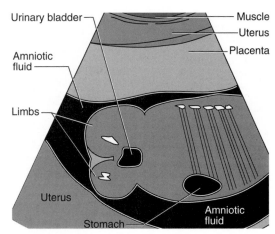

L A B E L E D :   UR BLADDER

21. Image of the umbilical cord insertion site on the anterior abdominal wall.

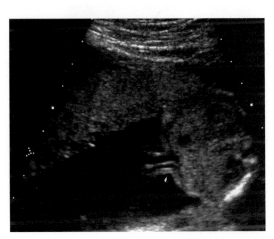 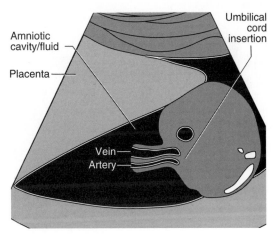

L A B E L E D :   CORD

N O T E :   If the insertion site image does not distinguish the three vessels of the cord, take an additional image and label accordingly.

22. A magnified view of a cross-section of a three-vessel cord.

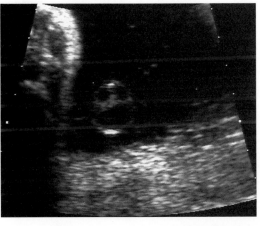 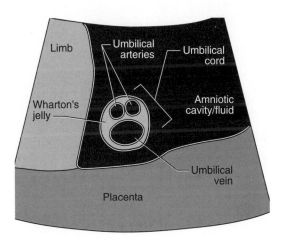

L A B E L E D :   CORD

23. Image of the stomach if visualized.

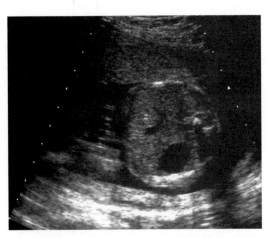

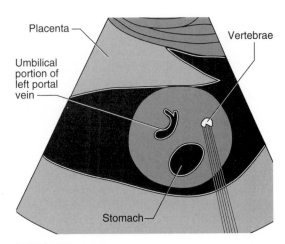

L A B E L E D :   STOMACH

N O T E :   The image of the stomach is not necessary if the stomach is visualized on any other image.

24. Image of genitalia.
   24A and 24B are provided to aide identification of the different genitalia.

24A. Image of male genitalia.

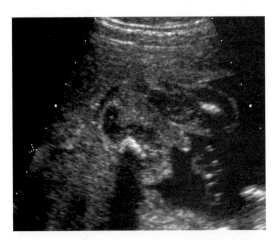

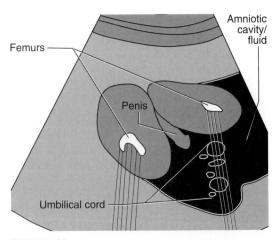

L A B E L E D :   GENITALIA

24B. Image of female genitalia.

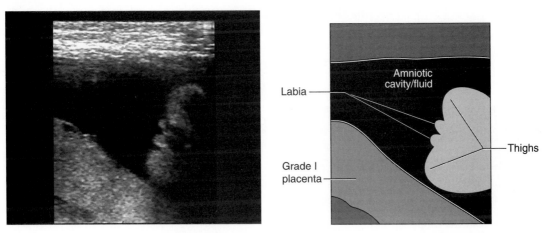

L A B E L E D :   GENITALIA

25. Longitudinal image of the fetus to include the diaphragm.

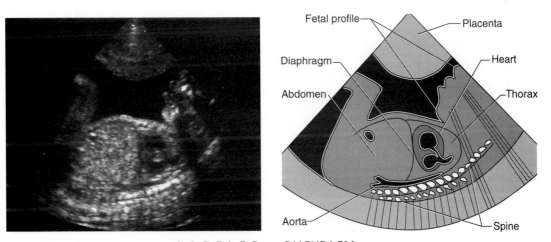

L A B E L E D :   DIAPHRAGM

N O T E : Because of the obvious nature of the fetal measurements, specifics are not included as part of the film labeling.

26. Biparietal diameter (BPD) image at the level of the thalamus and the cavum septi pellucidi. *Measurement is from the outside of the near cranium to the inside of the far cranium (leading to leading edge).*

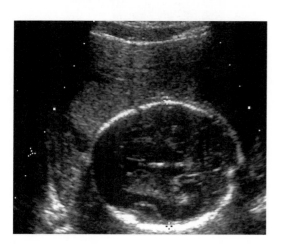
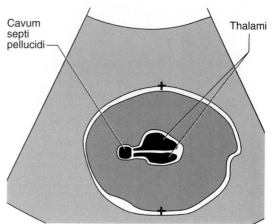

27. Cerebellum with *measurement.*

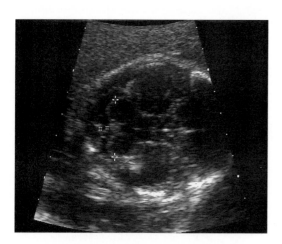
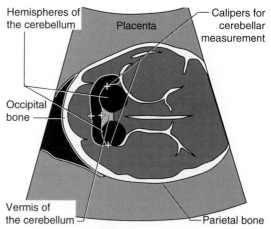

28. Cisterna magnum with *measurement*.

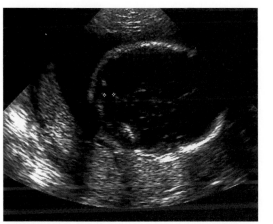
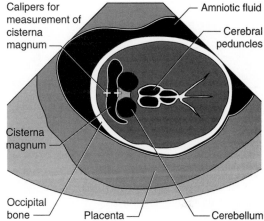

Calipers for measurement of cisterna magnum

Amniotic fluid

Cerebral peduncles

Cisterna magnum

Occipital bone

Placenta

Cerebellum

29. Nuchal fold (done between 16 and 24 weeks) with *measurement*.

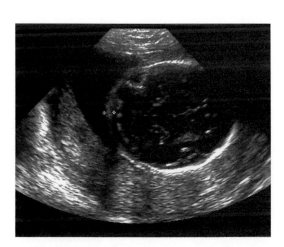
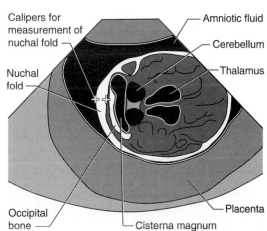

Calipers for measurement of nuchal fold

Amniotic fluid

Cerebellum

Nuchal fold

Thalamus

Occipital bone

Cisterna magnum

Placenta

N O T E : The measurement of the nuchal fold is not always routinely performed but should be considered in all patients over 35 or when a lower-than-normal serum AFP level has been detected in the mother.

30. Head circumference image at the same level as the biparietal diameter or use the BPD image. *Measurement is around the outline of the cranium.* Up-to-date ultrasound equipment provides tracking balls to trace the cranium or calipers that open to outline the cranium.

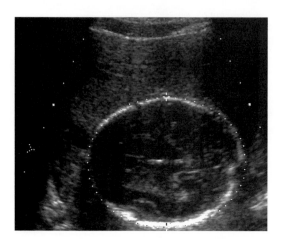
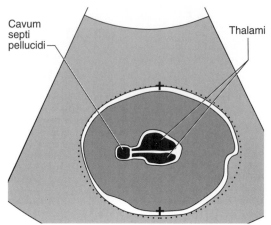

Cavum septi pellucidi

Thalami

31. Image of the choroid plexus.

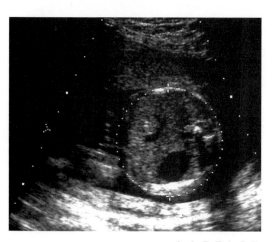
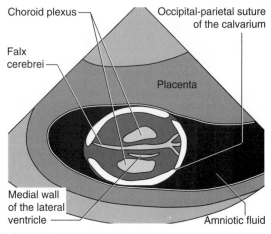

Choroid plexus

Occipital-parietal suture of the calvarium

Falx cerebrei

Placenta

Medial wall of the lateral ventricle

Amniotic fluid

L A B E L E D :   CH PLX

32. Lateral ventricle with *measurement.*

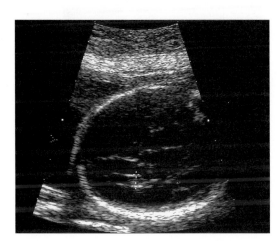
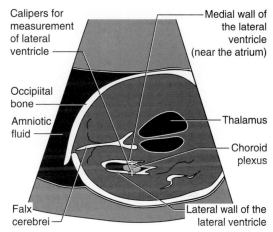

Calipers for measurement of lateral ventricle

Occipiital bone

Amniotic fluid

Falx cerebrei

Medial wall of the lateral ventricle (near the atrium)

Thalamus

Choroid plexus

Lateral wall of the lateral ventricle

33. Abdominal circumference image at the level of the junction of the umbilical vein and portal vein sinus. *Measurement is around the outline of the abdomen.* The abdomen should appear round.

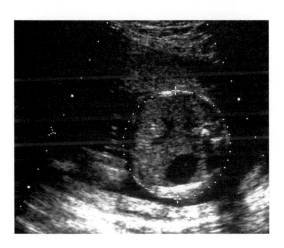
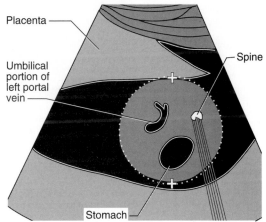

Placenta

Umbilical portion of left portal vein

Spine

Stomach

34. Long axis image of the fetal femur. *Measurement is from one end of the femur to the other.*

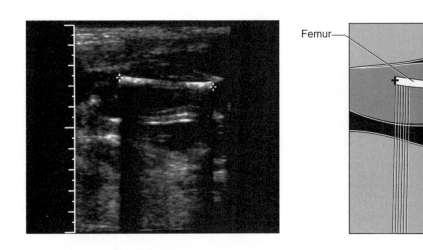

35. Humerus with *measurement.*

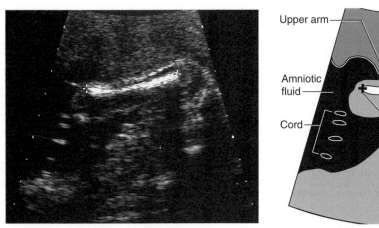
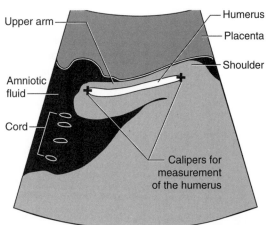

36. Image of the lower portion of the leg.

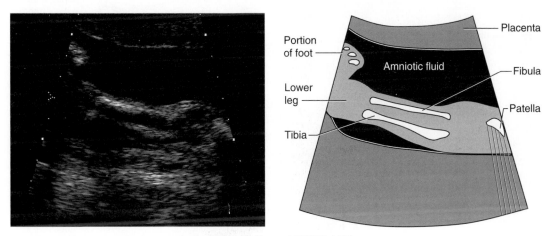

L A B E L E D :   LOWER LEG

37. Image of the radius and ulna.

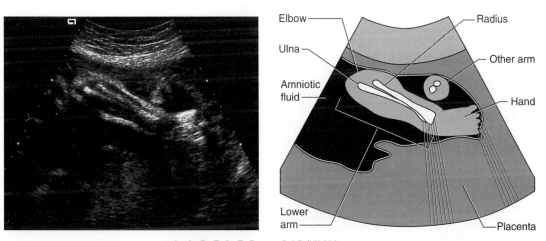

L A B E L E D :   RAD/ULNA

38. Image of a hand.

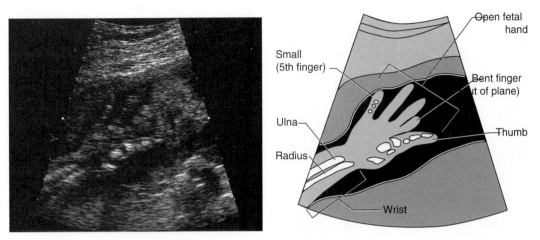

L A B E L E D :   HAND

39. Image of the feet.

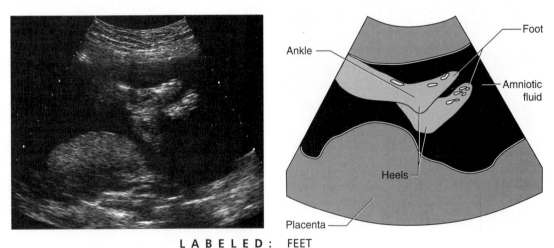

L A B E L E D :   FEET

N O T E :   Some physicians only require images of one hand, foot, arm, and leg based on the assumption that both were evaluated during the survey.

40. Profile of the fetal face.

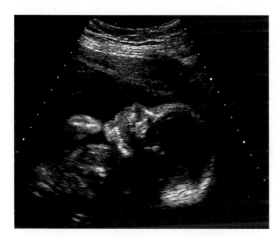
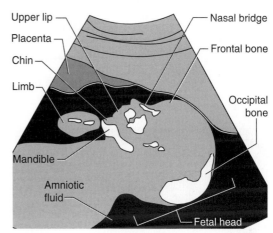

Upper lip
Placenta
Chin
Limb
Mandible
Amniotic fluid
Nasal bridge
Frontal bone
Occipital bone
Fetal head

L A B E L E D :   PROFILE

41. Coronal image of the nostrils and lips.

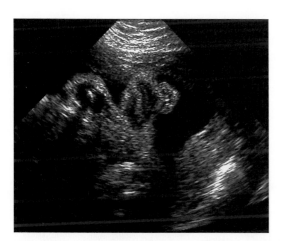
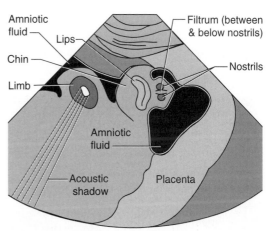

Amniotic fluid
Lips
Chin
Limb
Amniotic fluid
Acoustic shadow
Filtrum (between & below nostrils)
Nostrils
Placenta

L A B E L E D :   NOSTRILS/LIPS

MULTIPLE GESTATIONS: ADDITIONAL VIEWS REQUIRED

N O T E :   Each fetus of a multiple gestation should be imaged as previously described for singleton pregnancies; however, there are some additional views that should be obtained.

1. Image of a twin pregnancy demonstrating separate sacs.

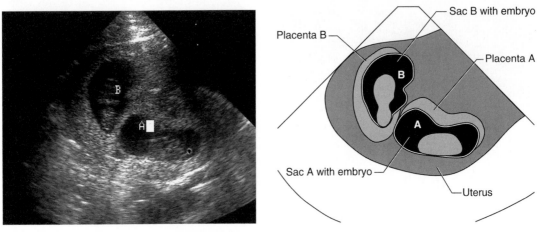

L A B E L E D :   TWINS/SEP SACS

2. Image of second trimester twins demonstrating the presence of a separating membrane.

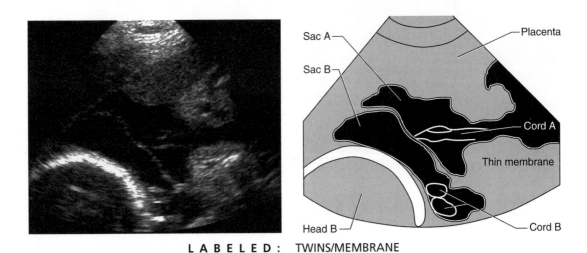

L A B E L E D :   TWINS/MEMBRANE

3. Image of triplets.

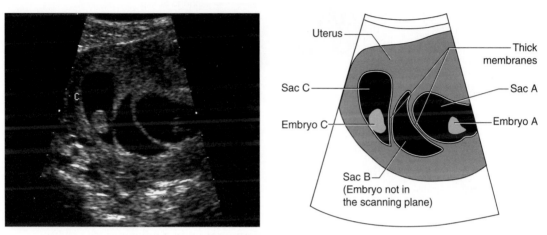

L A B E L E D :   TRIPLETS

A. A depiction of diamnionic–dichorionic twins.

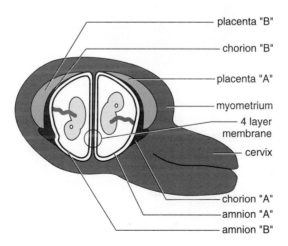

B. A depiction of diamnionic–monochorionic twins.

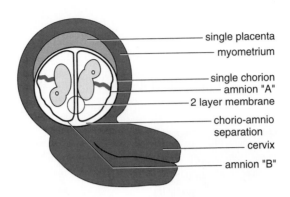

- single placenta
- myometrium
- single chorion
- amnion "A"
- 2 layer membrane
- chorio-amnio separation
- cervix
- amnion "B"

C. A depiction of monoamnionic–monochorionic twins.

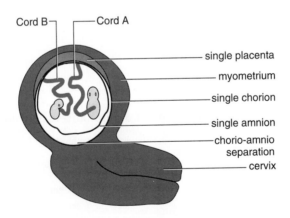

Cord B   Cord A

- single placenta
- myometrium
- single chorion
- single amnion
- chorio-amnio separation
- cervix

(note: dischordant growth)

N O T E :   It is important to demonstrate the position of the presenting fetus. This is the fetus that is lower in the uterus and will be delivered first. This fetus is labeled "A" and the other twin is labeled "B." If there are more than 2 (as in number 3) then "C," "D," etc., will be used. This labeling allows individual growth rates to be determined. If possible, determine the sex of each fetus. This information may help determine whether they are fraternal or identical.

THE BIOPHYSICAL PROFILE

An examination that is often performed during the late third trimester is the biophysical profile. This test measures fetal well being and consists of five parameters. The first part of the test involves a nonstress test. This test is performed in the delivery room or in an obstetrician's office and measures spontaneous heart rate accelerations. This part of the biophysical profile (BPP) is not performed by the sonographer. The remaining four parameters of the BPP are measured by the sonographer. They are: 1. fluid, 2. fetal respiration, 3. fetal tone, and 4. gross body motion. These parameters and scoring of this test are described in Table 12-1.

TABLE 12-1 Biophysical Profile Scoring

	CRITERION	SCORE (PTS)
Part I Nonstress test	2 Accelerations of 15 beats per minute in 30-min test	2
Part II Ultrasound Examination		
Gross movement	3 Separate flexions and extensions in 30-min examination	2
Tone	1 episode of fetal opening and closing of hand or clenching of foot in 30-min examination	2
Respiration	At least 60 seconds of fetal breathing in 30-min examination	2
Fluid	At least 1 pocket of amniotic fluid of at least 1 cm in 2 dimensions	2
	Unqualified pass	8 or more
	Maximum total	10

Data from Manning, E.A., Platt, L.D., Sipos, L. (1980). Antenatal fetal evaluation: development of a fetal biophysical profile. *Am J Obstet Gynecol* 136:787–795.

1. Demonstration of a pocket of fluid.

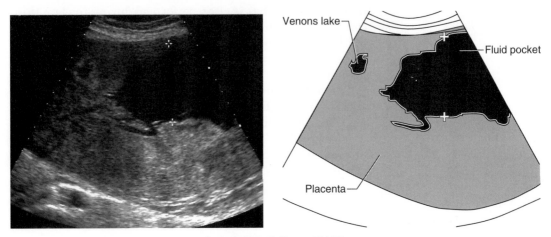

L A B E L E D :   FLUID

2. Demonstration of fetal respiration.

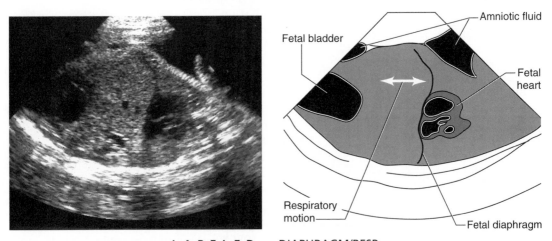

L A B E L E D :   DIAPHRAGM/RESP

3. Demonstration of fetal tone.

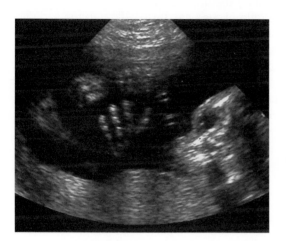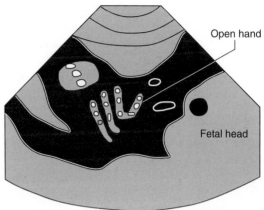

L A B E L E D :   HAND

4. Demonstration of fetal gross body motion.

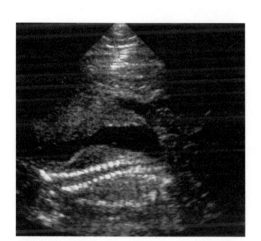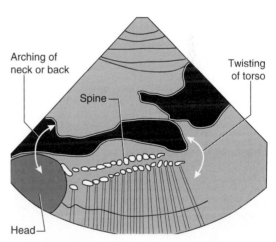

L A B E L E D :   MOTION

N O T E :   At times it is necessary to measure the resistance to blood flow within the umbilical arteries. This measurement is obtained by interrogating the umbilical cord artery with low power Doppler. The ratio of the peak systolic flow to the end diastolic flow is calculated (SD ratio). This number varies with the age of the fetus and charts are available to determine if blood flow through the cord is adequate.

5. Umbilical artery Doppler measurement and determination of the SD ratio.

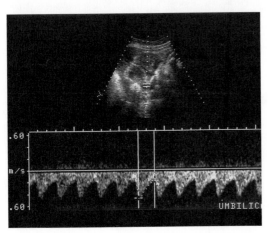

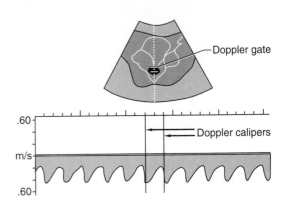

L A B E L E D :   DOP/UMB ART

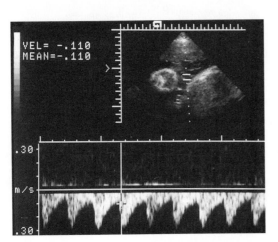

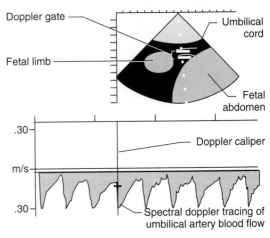

L A B E L E D :   DOP UMB/ART

N O T E :   At times the physician may also want to determine if the blood flow to the placenta from the mother's circulation is adequate, so another Doppler measurement is made at the interface between the placenta and uterus or in the uterine artery if possible. The SD ratio for the Doppler wave form is calculated and checked against a chart value for the appropriate gestational age.

6. Uterine artery Doppler measurement and determination of the SD ratio.

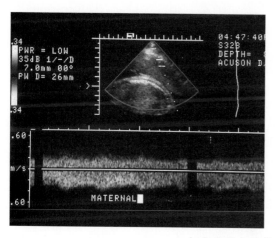 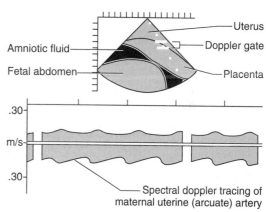

L A B E L E D :   DOP/UT ART

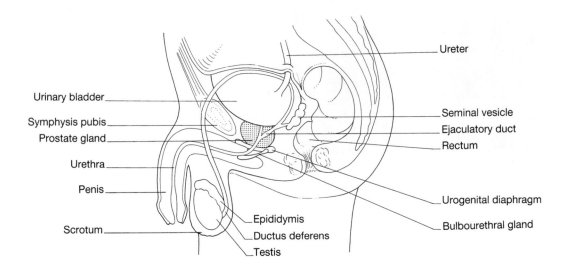

Ureter

Urinary bladder

Symphysis pubis

Prostate gland

Seminal vesicle

Ejaculatory duct

Rectum

Urethra

Penis

Urogenital diaphragm

Bulbourethral gland

Epididymis

Scrotum

Ductus deferens

Testis

Male pelvis

Male Pelvis Scanning Protocol

ENDORECTAL SONOGRAPHY

- Transabdominal male pelvis examinations are rarely performed anymore. The prostate gland is the primary interest of the male pelvis and is better evaluated by endorectal sonography.
- Male pelvis transabdominal studies are systematically evaluated and documented in the same manner as the female pelvis transabdominal studies. Longitudinal surveys extend from one side of the pelvic cavity to the other. Transverse surveys extend from the symphysis pubis to the umbilicus. The prostate gland is examined from an inferior transducer angle at the level of the symphysis pubis. Patient prep, patient position, and transducer are the same as those for the female pelvis. See Chapter 12 for specifics.

LOCATION

- The urinary bladder is posterior to the symphysis pubis.
- The prostate gland is retroperitoneal. It lies anterior to the rectum and inferior to the urinary bladder.

ANATOMY

- The prostate gland is about the size of a chestnut and conical in shape. It is approximately 3.5 cm long, 4.0 cm wide, and 2.5 cm anterior to posterior. The base, its broadest aspect, is superior to its apex.

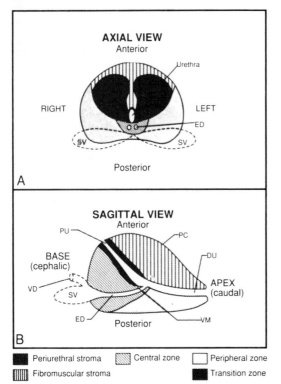

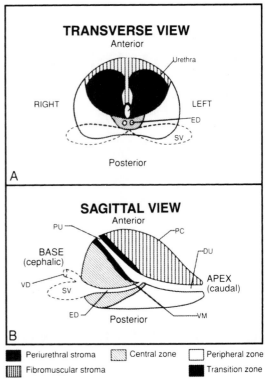

- The prostate consists of fibromuscular and glandular tissue that surrounds the neck of the bladder and urethra.
- The seminal vesicles are two sac-like structures that lie superior to the prostate and posterior to the bladder. Size is variable.
- The seminal vesicles join the vas deferens to form the ejaculatory ducts.
- The ejaculatory ducts enter the base of the prostate and pass through to the prostatic urethra at the verumontanum.
- The urethra runs back from the neck of the bladder through the prostate to the base of the penis. The proximal portion of the prostatic urethra extends from the bladder neck to the verumontanum and the distal portion extends from the verumontanum to the apex of the prostate.
- The vermontanum is the area where the ejaculatory ducts join the urethra.
- The glandular portion of the prostate is divided into zones:
  (a) Peripheral zone: located posterior and lateral to the distal prostatic urethra. Normally, it is the largest zone.
  (b) Central zone: extends from the base of the prostate to the verumontanum and surrounds the ejaculatory ducts.
  (c) Transition zone: located on both sides of the proximal urethra. Normally, it is the smallest zone.

PHYSIOLOGY

- The function of the male reproductive organs is reproduction.

SONOGRAPHIC APPEARANCE

- The majority of the parenchyma of the prostate gland appears as homogeneous, midgray, medium-level echoes. The periurethral glandular stroma that surrounds the urethra is slightly hypoechoic compared with surrounding tissue. The contour of the gland should appear smooth and the margins well defined. Calcifications may be seen throughout the gland in older patients. The normal prostate should appear symmetrical.
- The seminal vesicles appear as symmetrical midgray or medium- to low-level echo textures, superior to the prostate. They are easier to visualize when the urinary bladder is partially filled. They are seen in long axis on transverse scans.
- The prostatic urethra walls appear echogenic at the midline of the gland.
- The vas deferens and ejaculatory ducts may be difficult to distinguish from surrounding structures. However, when seen, the vas deferens are medial to, and have an echo texture similar to, the seminal vesicles. The ejaculatory ducts will appear as echogenic double lines.
- Normally, the central and transition zones are not sonographically distinctive. The peripheral zone appears homogeneous and slightly hyperechoic to adjacent parenchyma.

PATIENT PREP

- Self-administered enema prior to the exam. If for some reason the patient cannot have the enema, still attempt the exam.
- Explain the examination to the patient. Verbal or written consent is required and the exam should be witnessed by another health care professional. The initials of the witness should be part of the film labeling.
- The transducer may be inserted by the sonographer or physician.

PATIENT POSITION

- **Left lateral decubitus with knees bent toward the chest.**
- Lithotomy position.

TRANSDUCER

- **5 to 10 MHz.**
- Preparing the transducer includes providing a water path. Preparation options include:
  - (a) Some transducer manufacturers provide a finger-like sheath that slides onto the transducer head. The sheath is secured by a small rubber band, and 20 or 30 ml of nonionized water is injected into the sheath through a pathway inside the transducer handle. Tip the transducer down and tap the water-filled sheath so any air bubbles rise to the top and can be aspirated. Fill a condom half full with sonographic gel, then put the sheathed transducer in it. Apply additional lubrication to the outside of the condom before insertion. A small rubber hose can be attached to the transducer pathway to introduce or aspirate water from the sheath to adjust for any air bubbles that might occur and cause artifacts.
  - (b) Apply gel to the end of the transducer, then cover it with a condom. Secure the condom with a rubber band and make sure there are no air bubbles at the tip. Apply additional lubrication to the outside of the condom before insertion. Use an inner balloon filled with 30 to 50 ml of nonionized water as a water path.
  - (c) Cover a transducer with a condom and secure it with a rubber band. Lubricate the outside of the condom, then insert the transducer into the rectum. Fill the condom with 30 to 50 ml of nonionized water for a water path.

ORIENTATION

- Sagittal and transverse views of the prostate are obtained.

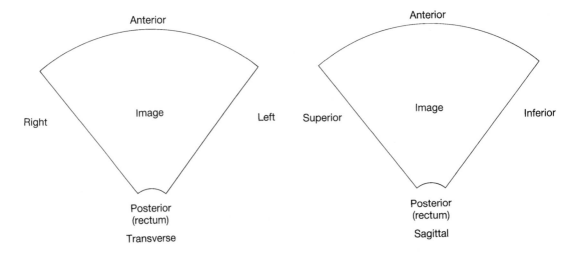

PROSTATE SURVEY

N O T E :   While surveying the prostate evaluate the periprostatic fat and vessels for asymmetry and disruption in echogenicity. Also evaluate the perirectal space for pathology.

☰ TRANSVERSE SURVEY

Transverse Plane • Rectal Approach

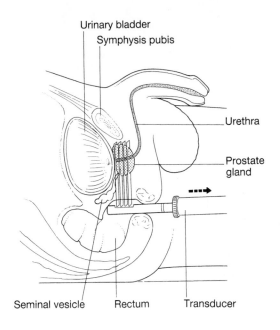

Urinary bladder
Symphysis pubis
Urethra
Prostate gland
Seminal vesicle   Rectum   Transducer

N O T E :   To survey the prostate transversely, the transducer is inserted into the rectum and then withdrawn sequentially to examine the prostate superiorly (base) to inferiorly (apex).

1. With the transducer inserted, the survey begins at the level of the seminal vesicles.

2. After the seminal vesicles and vas deferens have been evaluated, slowly withdraw the transducer to scan through the prostate from its superior to inferior margins. The lateral margins should be well defined.

Note the size, shape, and symmetry of the prostate.

☰ LONGITUDINAL SURVEY

Sagittal Plane • Rectal Approach

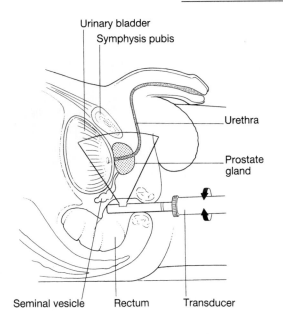

Urinary bladder
Symphysis pubis
Urethra
Prostate gland
Seminal vesicle   Rectum   Transducer

N O T E :   To survey the prostate longitudinally the transducer is rotated clockwise, and counterclockwise to examine the prostate from one lateral edge to the other.

1. Begin at the midline of the prostate. The superior and inferior margins should be well defined and the prostatic urethra visualized.

2. To examine the lateral aspects of the prostate, seminal vesicles, and vas deferens, rotate the transducer clockwise and counterclockwise.

REQUIRED IMAGES*

≡ TRANSVERSE IMAGES

Transverse Plane • Rectal Approach

1. Transverse image of the seminal vesicles.

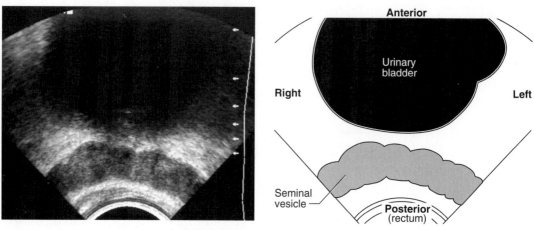

L A B E L E D :   ER TRV SEM V
("ER" INDICATES ENDORECTAL)

N O T E :   Because of the limited field of view, both seminal vesicles may not be entirely visible on a single view. If so, take these additional images:

2. Transverse image of the right seminal vesicle to include its right lateral margin.

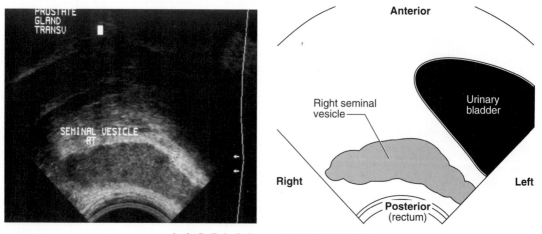

L A B E L E D :   ER TRV SEM V RT

3. Transverse image of the left seminal vesicle to include its left lateral margin.

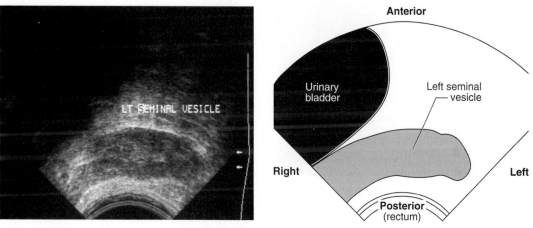

L A B E L E D :   ER TRV SEM V LT

4. Transverse image of the base of the prostate.

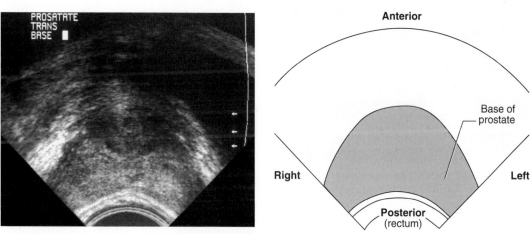

L A B E L E D :   ER TRV BASE

5. Transverse image of the mid prostate.

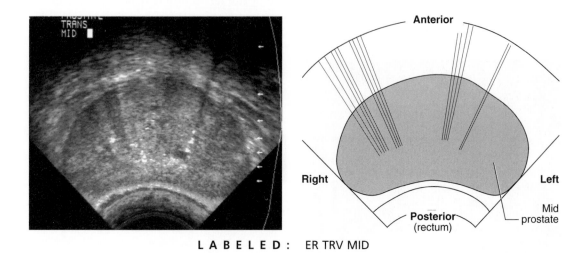

L A B E L E D :   ER TRV MID

6. Transverse image of the apex of the prostate.

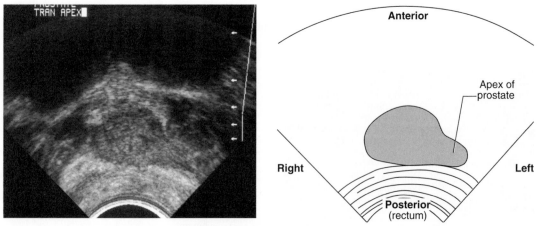

L A B E L E D :   ER TRV APEX

☰ LONGITUDINAL IMAGES

Sagittal Plane • Rectal Approach

7. Longitudinal midline image of the prostate.

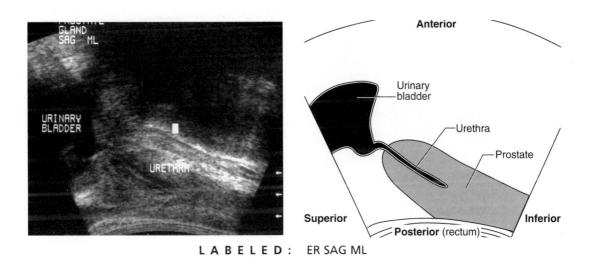

L A B E L E D :   ER SAG ML

8. Longitudinal image of the right lateral portion of the prostate gland and seminal vesicle.

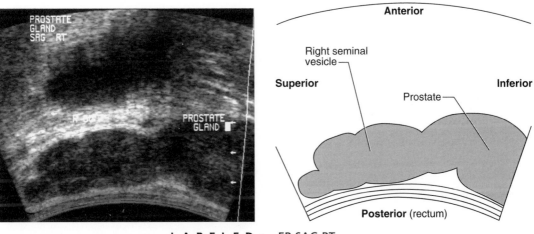

L A B E L E D :   ER SAG RT

9. Longitudinal image of the left lateral portion of the prostate gland and seminal vesicle.

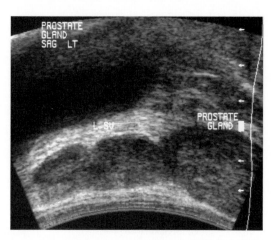

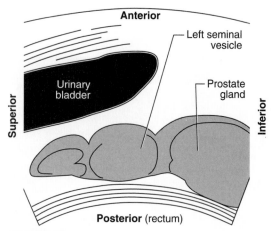

L A B E L E D :   ER SAG LT

---

*Images in this section are by courtesy of the Ultrasound Department of the Methodist Hospital, Houston, Texas.

Small Parts Scanning Protocols

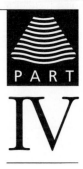

PART

IV

Overview

- "Small part" indicates a structure that is superficial or close to the surface of the skin. In most cases, it requires a real time, high-frequency transducer.

- Protocols provide specific survey steps with "how-to" illustrations.

- Protocols provide image specifications.

- Patient care and safety are always a priority.

- Use good clinical skills and always practice professional behavior.

- **Only physicians can give a legal diagnostic impression.**

- **Only physicians can give a diagnosis.**

275

SURVEYS

- The small part and structures or areas immediately adjacent are completely evaluated in at least two scanning planes.

- Surveys are used to set correct imaging techniques, to rule out pathologies, and recognize any normal variants.

- If an abnormality is identified, it is surveyed in at least two scanning planes *following* the completed survey of the small part. Refer to Chapter 2 for specifics on how to survey pathology.

- Images are not taken during a survey.

IMAGE DOCUMENTATION

- Images are taken following the completed survey.

- As with the survey, documented areas of interest must be represented in at least two scanning planes. Single-plane representation is not enough confirmation.

- Documented areas of interest must be done so in a logical sequence. Follow imaging protocol examples.

- After an abnormality is identified and surveyed, it must be documented in at least two scanning planes *following* the completed survey and completed images of the small part even if the abnormality is demonstrated on the standard set of required images. Refer to Chapter 2 for specifics on how to document pathology.

OTHER CONSIDERATIONS

- Patient comfort and the amount of transducer pressure on the skin surface is always an important consideration when scanning any structure, but the significance is more acute with small part structures. Protocols elaborate on specific techniques but generally a lighter approach is recommended.

- Sonographic appearance for superficial structures is discussed in each small part scanning protocol chapter.

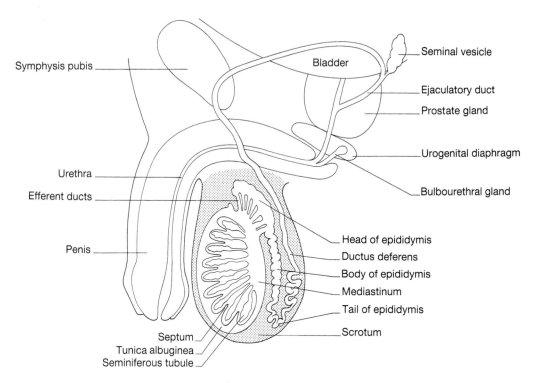

Symphysis pubis

Bladder

Seminal vesicle

Ejaculatory duct

Prostate gland

Urogenital diaphragm

Urethra

Efferent ducts

Bulbourethral gland

Head of epididymis

Ductus deferens

Body of epididymis

Mediastinum

Penis

Tail of epididymis

Scrotum

Septum

Tunica albuginea

Seminiferous tubule

Scrotum anatomy

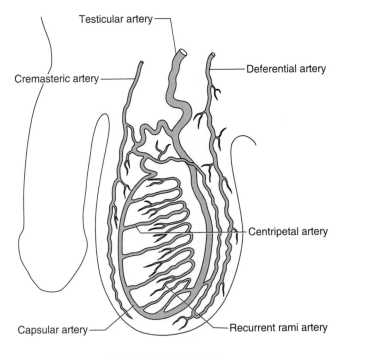

Testicular artery

Deferential artery

Cremasteric artery

Centripetal artery

Capsular artery

Recurrent rami artery

Scrotal blood supply

Scrotum Scanning Protocol

CHAPTER

14

B.B. Tempkin and Wayne C. Leonhardt

ANATOMY

- A two-compartment sac divides the median raphe, a fibrous septum.
- Each compartment contains a testis, epididymis, and a portion of the ductus deferens (spermatic cord).
- The ductus deferens (spermatic cord) is composed of arteries, veins, nerves, lymphatics, and the seminal duct.
- Normal spermatic cord veins are approximately 2 mm in diameter.
- Most of the blood supply to the scrotum is from the internal spermatic (testicular), cremasteric, and deferential arteries.
- The testicular artery provides the major blood supply to the testis. At the posterosuperior aspect of the testis it pierces the tunica albuginea and branches into several capsular arteries. Capsular arteries course along the periphery of the testis in a layer called the tunica vasculosa. They branch into centripetal arteries that penetrate the testicular parenchyma and run toward the mediastinum. Near the mediastinum, centripetal arteries branch into recurrent rami arteries that course back toward the periphery of the testis. In 10-20% of men, a large branch of the testicular artery enters the mediastinum testis and courses through the testis in a direction opposite the centripetal arteries.
- The deferential artery supplies the epididymis and the vas deferens.
- The cremasteric artery supplies the peritesticular tissues.
- Venous outflow from the scrotum is via the pompiniform plexus which empties into the internal spermatis or testicular veins.
- The mediastinum testis is an invagination of the tunica albuginea into the posterior aspect of the testis. It functions as a support system for the ducts and vessels.

279

- The epididymis is bilateral and divided anatomically into three parts: the head (globus major), body (corpus), and tail (globus minor). The head lies superior to the testis. The body and tail are posteroinferior to the testis.
- The epididymal head diameter is approximately 10-12 mm. The body and tail are approximately 2-5 mm in diameter. With increasing age, the epididymis decreases in size.
- Testes are ovoid with the superior pole lying more anterior. A peritoneal layer called the tunica vaginalis surrounds the testis except posteriorly in the region of the epididymis. It contains an inner or visceral layer and an outer or parietal layer, a potential space for fluid to collect.
- Testes are approximately 3-5 cm long and 2-3 cm wide.
- Scrotal wall thickness measures approximately 2-8 mm.

PHYSIOLOGY

- Functions as an endocrine gland by synthesizing and secreting testosterone, the male hormone.
- Functions as an endocrine gland by producing spermatozoa which drain into the epididymis.

SONOGRAPHIC APPEARANCE

- Testes are midgray or medium-level echoes with even texture. Testicular parenchyma is similar to that of the normal thyroid gland.
- The epididymis is midgray or medium-level echoes that are equal to or slightly more echogenic than the normal testes. The head is easier to visualize than the body or tail.
- The mediastinum testis is highly reflective or very echogenic. Longitudinally it appears as a line extending craniocaudally or parallel to the epididymis. Transversely it appears as an ovoid structure in a 3 or 9 o'clock position.
- The appendix testis and appendix epididymis are hyperechoic protuberances superior to the testis and epididymis.
- The spermatic cord appears as multiple hypoechoic linear structures in the longitudinal plane and circular hypoechoic structures in the transverse plane.

NORMAL VARIANTS

- In 10-20% of men, a large branch of the testicular artery (transtesticular artery) enters the mediastinum testis and courses through the testis in a direction opposite the centripetal arteries.

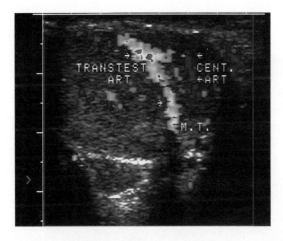

Color flow image of a normal variant. See Color Plate 17 at the back of this book.

COLOR DOPPLER ARTERIAL/VENOUS FLOW CHARACTERISTICS

- The testis has low vascular resistance. Testicular, capsular, centripetal, and recurrent rami arteries have low resistance flow. Their waveforms are characterized by broad systolic peaks and high levels of diastolic flow similar to the internal carotid artery. Cremasteric and deferential arteries have high systolic peaks and lower levels of diastolic flow similar to the external carotid artery.

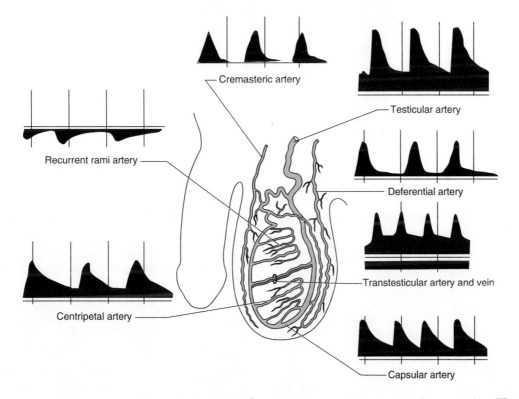

- Intratesticular veins accompany companion arteries. Their waveform signature is continuous or phasic.

- Spermatic cord/Pampiniform plexus: minimal to moderate flow. See Color Plate 18 at the back of this book.

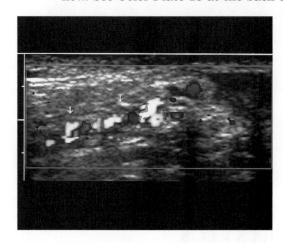

- Epididymis: very slight flicker or dashes of flow. See Color Plate 19 at the back of this book.

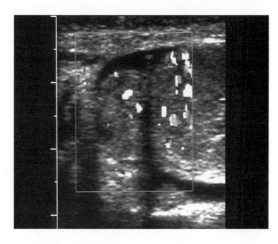

- Testicular, deferential cremasteric, centripetal, and capsular arteries: moderate flow. See Color Plates 20 and 21 at the back of this book.

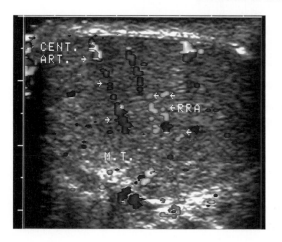
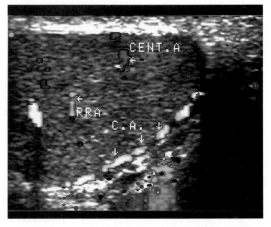

COLOR DOPPLER TECHNICAL CONSIDERATIONS

- Use color Doppler to differentiate vascular from nonvascular structures.
- Confirm intratesticular and epididymal flow using both color and conventional waveform analysis.

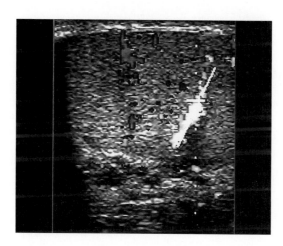

Color flow image and waveform of intratesticular arteries. See Color Plate 22 at the back of this book.

- Use the mediastinum testis as a point of reference when demonstrating intratesticular flow.
- With acute torsion less than 6 hours or chronic torsion more than 24 hours, there is absent intratesticular flow and increased peritesticular flow.
- Color Doppler cannot differentiate malignant hypervascularity from inflammatory hypervascularity.

PATIENT PREP

- The scrotum should be supported on a rolled towel placed between the patient's thighs to isolate and immobilize the scrotum for scanning. Cover the penis with a towel and tape the towel to the abdominal wall.
- Use warm gel as a scanning couplant.

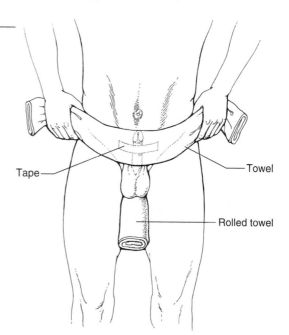

Tape

Towel

Rolled towel

- To scan the scrotum the sonographer's gloved fingers should be placed underneath the scrotum and the thumb over the top of the scrotum. This hand position further stabilizes the scrotum and has the advantage of allowing correlation between a palpable lesion and its sonographic findings. Also, the sonographer's fingers are easily identified as highly reflective or very echogenic and are used as reference points for localizing lesions.

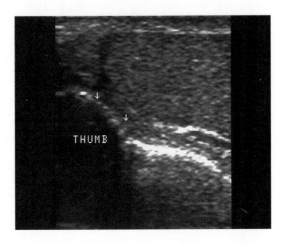

PATIENT POSITION

- **Supine with the legs slightly spread or in a semi-frog-legged position.**
- Upright.

TRANSDUCER

- **5MHz, high resolution, real-time, linear.**
- 7.5MHz, 10MHz.
- Conventional Doppler with color flow imaging (low flow filter, scale, and optimized color gain).
- Gel stand-off pad. Often used for better evaluation of anterior lesions.

BREATHING TECHNIQUE

- **Normal respiration.**
- Perform the valsalva maneuver in the supine or upright position to detect varioceles.

SCROTUM SURVEY

N O T E :   Use the following survey steps for both testes.

≡ LONGITUDINAL SURVEY

Sagittal Plane • Anterior Approach

N O T E :   Evaluation of the testis begins with a survey of the spermatic cord with the patient in normal respiration and valsalva to rule out varicoceles.

1. Begin with the transducer perpendicular at the superior midline portion of the testis at the level of the spermatic cord. Patient should be at normal respiration.

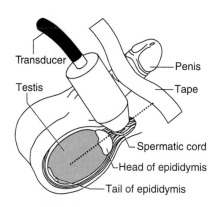

2. Keep the transducer perpendicular at the level of the spermatic cord and slowly slide the transducer medially through the cord until you are beyond it.

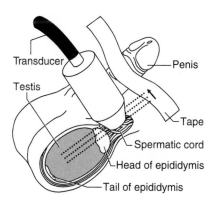

3. Scan back through the medial portion of the spermatic cord to mid testis. Keeping the transducer perpendicular, slowly slide the transducer laterally through the cord until you are beyond it.

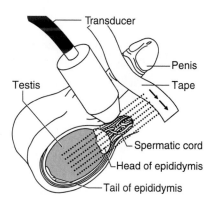

4.-6. Repeat the above survey steps of the spermatic cord with the patient in valsalva.

7. Keep the transducer perpendicular and return to the mid portion of the testis.

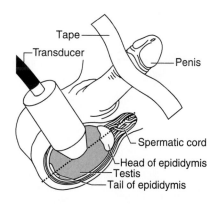

N O T E :   The spermatic cord, epididymal head, and the superior and inferior borders of the testis should be visible on longitudinal views. If not, move the transducer superior and inferior as necessary to evaluate all of the anatomy.

8. Slowly slide the transducer medially through and beyond the testis and scrotal sac.

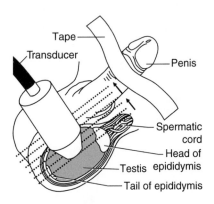

9. Scan back to mid testis and—keeping the transducer perpendicular—slowly move the transducer laterally through and beyond the testis and scrotal sac.

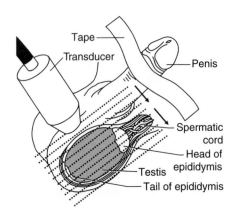

≡ TRANSVERSE SURVEY

Transverse Plane • Anterior Approach

N O T E :   Evaluation of the testis begins with a survey of the spermatic cord with the patient in normal respiration and valsalva to rule out varicoceles.

1. Begin with the transducer perpendicular at the superior portion of the testis at the level of the spermatic cord. Patient should be at normal respiration.

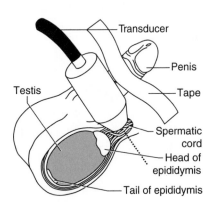

2. Keep the transducer perpendicular at the level of the spermatic cord and slowly slide the transducer superiorly through the cord until you are beyond it.

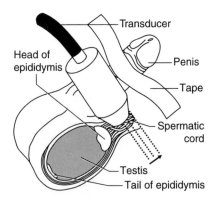

3. Scan back through the superior portion of the spermatic cord to mid cord. Keeping the transducer perpendicular, slowly slide the transducer inferiorly through the cord until you are beyond it.

N O T E : The medial and lateral borders of the testis should be visible on transverse views. If not, move the transducer medial and lateral as necessary to evaluate all of the anatomy.

8. Slowly slide the transducer superiorly through the superior portion of the testis to the head of the epididymis.

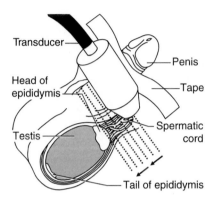

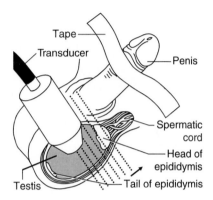

4.-6. Repeat the above survey steps of the spermatic cord with the patient in valsalva.

7. Keep the transducer perpendicular and return to the mid portion of the testis.

9. Keep the transducer perpendicular and continue to move the transducer superiorly through the head of the epididymis, spermatic cord, and scrotal sac until you are beyond it.

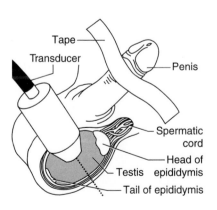

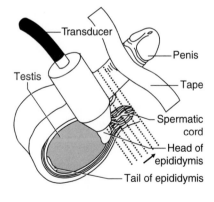

10. Scan back to mid testis and—keeping the transducer perpendicular—slowly move the transducer inferiorly through the inferior portion of the testis to the tail of the epididymis.

11. Continue to move the transducer inferiorly through the tail of the epididymis and scrotal sac until you are beyond it.

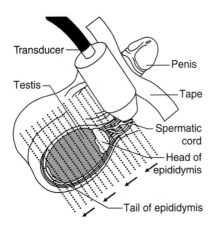

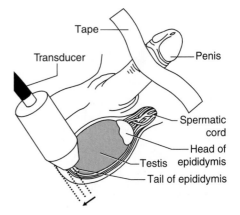

REQUIRED IMAGES

Right Hemiscrotum

≡ LONGITUDINAL IMAGES

Sagittal Plane • Anterior Approach

1. Long axis image of the spermatic cord at normal respiration or rest with *anterior to posterior measurement*.

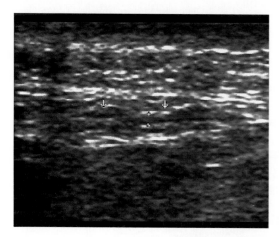 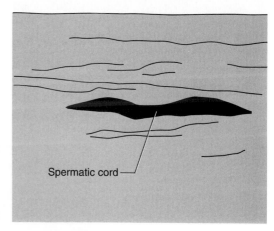

Spermatic cord

L A B E L E D : RT CORD SAG REST

2. Same image as number 1 without calipers.

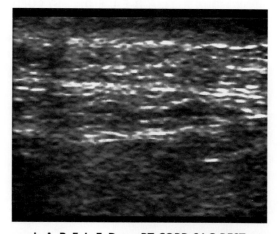

L A B E L E D : RT CORD SAG REST

3. Long axis image of the spermatic cord at valsalva with *anterior to posterior measurement*.

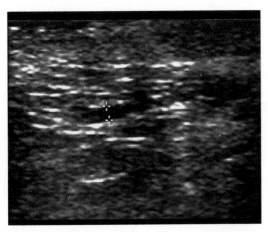 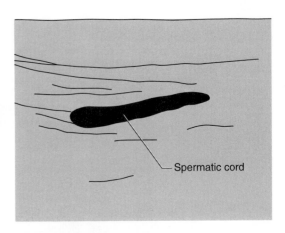

Spermatic cord

L A B E L E D :   RT CORD SAG VAL

4. Same image as number 3 without calipers.

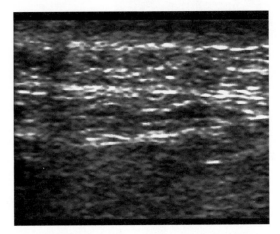

L A B E L E D :   RT CORD SAG VAL

5. Longitudinal image of the head of the epididymis.

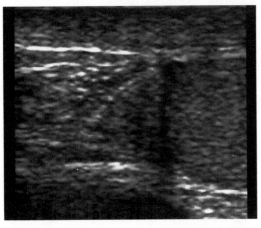 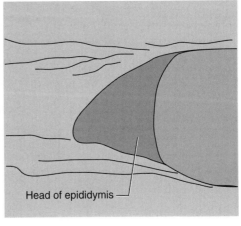

Head of epididymis

L A B E L E D :   RT EPI HEAD SAG

6. Longitudinal image of the right testis at its most superior border.

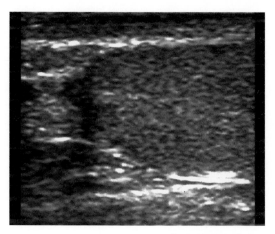 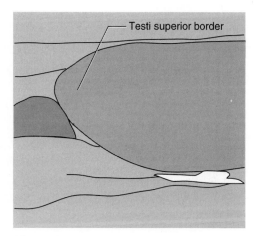

Testi superior border

L A B E L E D :   RT TESTIS SAG SUP

7. Longitudinal image of the mid portion of the right testis.

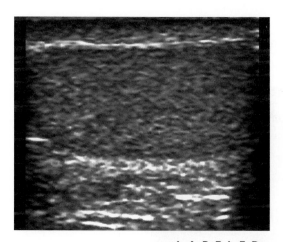 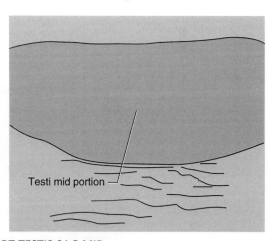

Testi mid portion

L A B E L E D :   RT TESTIS SAG MID

8. Long axis image of the right testis with *superior to inferior measurement.*

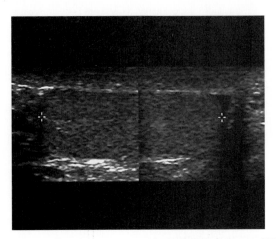 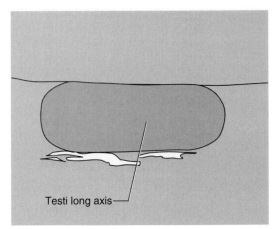

Testi long axis

L A B E L E D :   RT TESTIS SAG LONG AXIS

N O T E :   If necessary, use dual imaging to obtain entire long axis of testis on image.

9. Same image as number 8 without calipers.

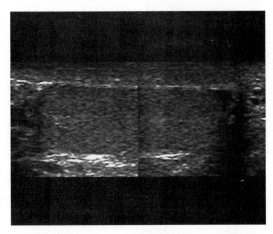

L A B E L E D :   RT TESTIS SAG LONG AXIS

10. Longitudinal image of the medial portion of the right testis.

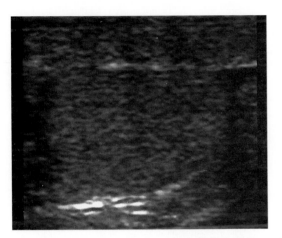 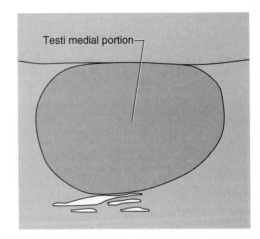

L A B E L E D :   RT TESTIS SAG MED

11. Longitudinal image of the lateral portion of the right testis.

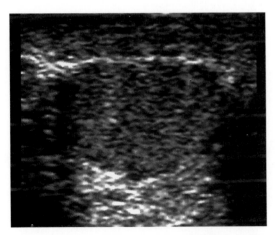 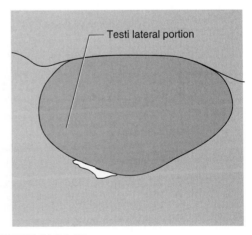

L A B E L E D :   RT TESTIS SAG LAT

12. Longitudinal image of the right testis at its most inferior border.

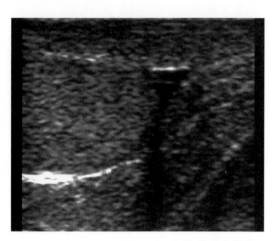 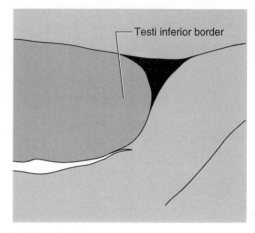

L A B E L E D :   RT TESTIS SAG INF

13. Longitudinal image of the tail of the epididymis.

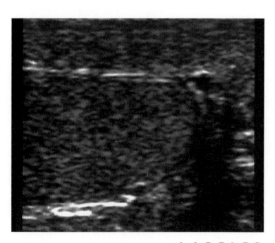 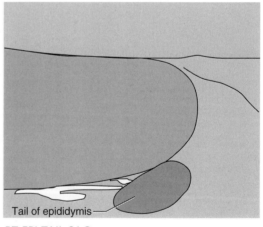

L A B E L E D :   RT EPI TAIL SAG

≡ TRANSVERSE IMAGES

Transverse Plane • Anterior Approach

14. Transverse image of the spermatic cord at normal respiration or rest with *anterior to posterior measurement.*

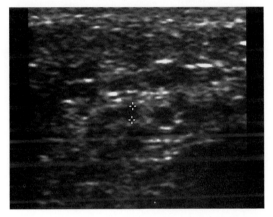 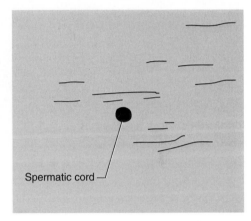

Spermatic cord

L A B E L E D :   RT CORD TRV REST

15. Same image as number 14 without calipers.

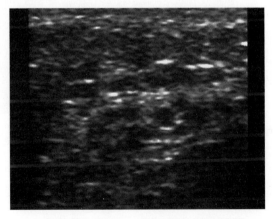

L A B E L E D :   RT CORD TRV REST

16. Transverse image of the spermatic cord at valsalva with *anterior to posterior measurement.*

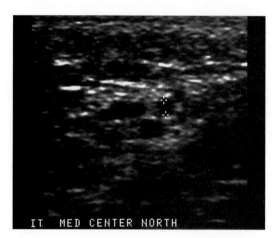 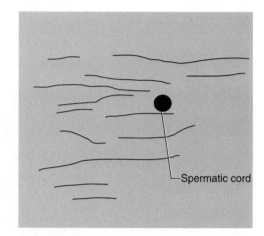

L A B E L E D :   RT CORD TRV VAL

17. Same image as number 16 without calipers.

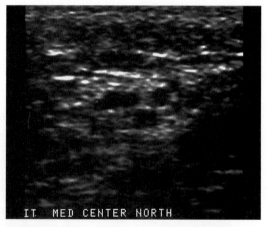

L A B E L E D :   RT CORD TRV VAL

18. Transverse image of the epididymal head.

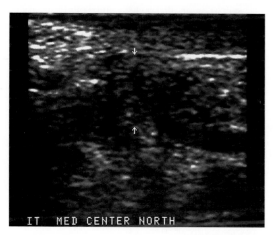 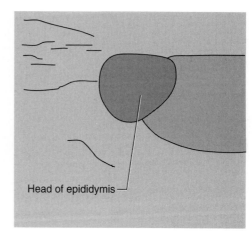

Head of epididymis

L A B E L E D :   RT EPI HEAD TRV

19. Transverse image of the superior portion of the right testis.

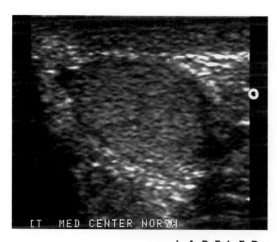 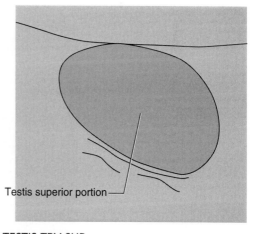

Testis superior portion

L A B E L E D :   RT TESTIS TRV SUP

20. Transverse image of the mid portion of the right testis with *medial to lateral measurement.*

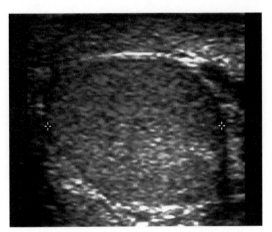 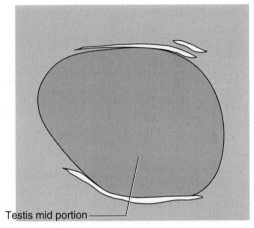

Testis mid portion

L A B E L E D :   RT TESTIS TRV MID

21. Same image as number 20 without calipers.

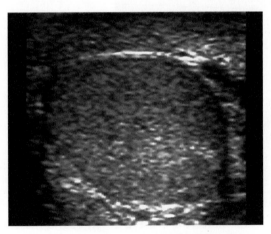

L A B E L E D :   RT TESTIS TRV MID

22. Transverse image of the inferior portion of the right testis.

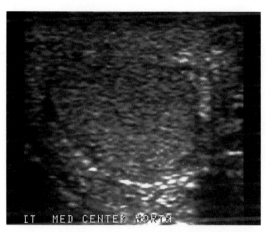 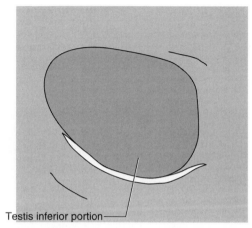

L A B E L E D :   RT TESTIS TRV INF

23. Transverse image of the tail of the epididymis.

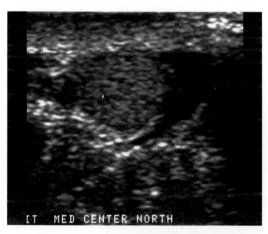 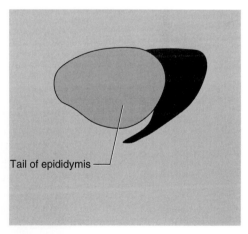

L A B E L E D :   RT TESTIS TRV INF/EPI TAIL

Left Hemiscrotum

☰ LONGITUDINAL IMAGES

Sagittal Plane • Anterior Approach

1. Long axis image of the spermatic cord at normal respiration or rest with *anterior to posterior measurement.*

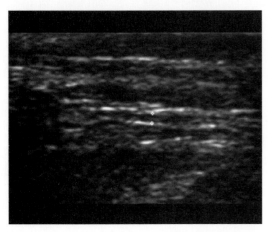

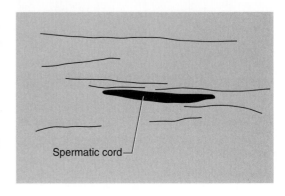

Spermatic cord

L A B E L E D :   LT CORD SAG REST

2. Same image as number 1 without calipers.

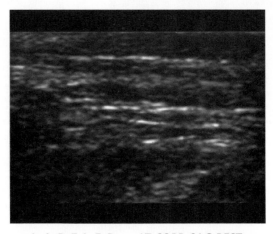

L A B E L E D :   LT CORD SAG REST

3. Long axis image of the spermatic cord at valsalva with *anterior to posterior measurement.*

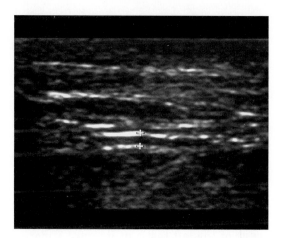 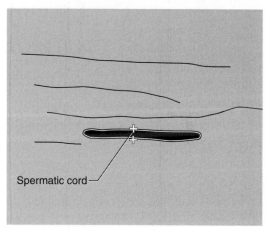

Spermatic cord

L A B E L E D :   LT CORD SAG VAL

4. Same image as number 3 without calipers.

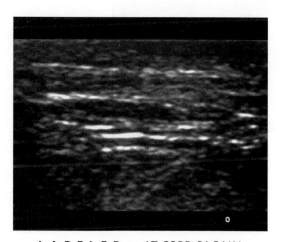

L A B E L E D :   LT CORD SAG VAL

5. Longitudinal image of the head of the epididymis.

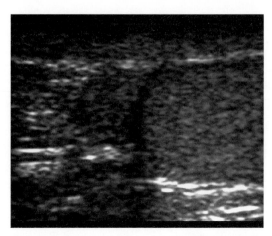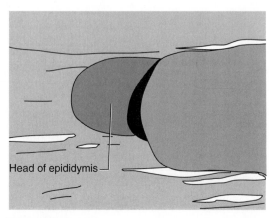

L A B E L E D :   LT EPI HEAD SAG

6. Longitudinal image of the left testis at its most superior border.

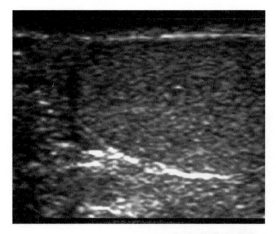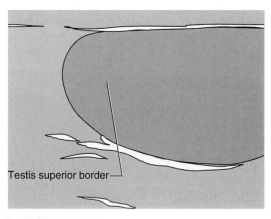

L A B E L E D :   LT TESTIS SAG SUP

7. Longitudinal image of the mid portion of the left testis.

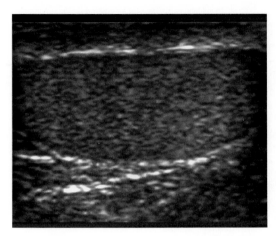 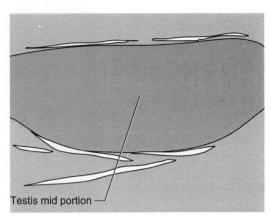

Testis mid portion

L A B E L E D :   LT TESTIS SAG MID

8. Long axis image of the left testis with *superior to inferior measurement.*

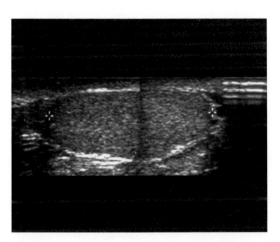 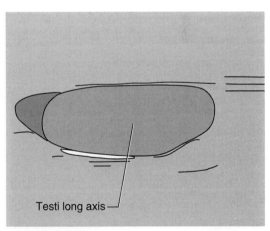

Testi long axis

L A B E L E D :   LT TESTIS SAG LONG AXIS

N O T E :   If necessary, use dual imaging to obtain entire long axis of testis on image.

9. Same image as number 8 without calipers.

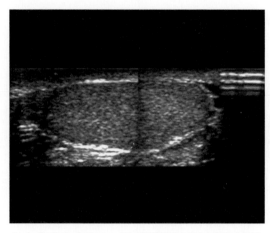

L A B E L E D : LT TESTIS SAG LONG AXIS

10. Longitudinal image of the medial portion of the left testis.

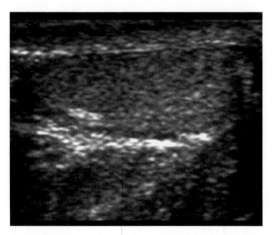 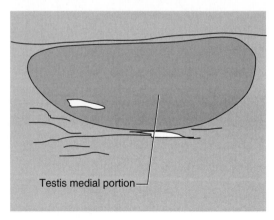

Testis medial portion

L A B E L E D : LT TESTIS SAG MED

11. Longitudinal image of the lateral portion of the left testis.

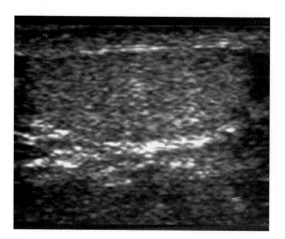 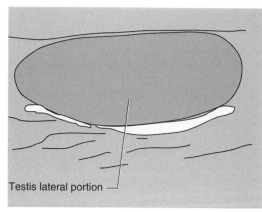

Testis lateral portion

L A B E L E D :   LT TESTIS SAG LAT

12. Longitudinal image of the left testis at its most inferior border.

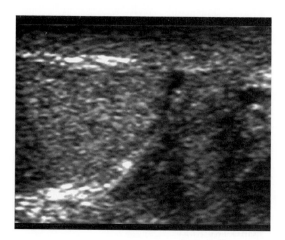 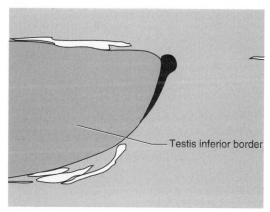

Testis inferior border

L A B E L E D :   LT TESTIS SAG INF

13. Longitudinal image of the tail of the epididymis.

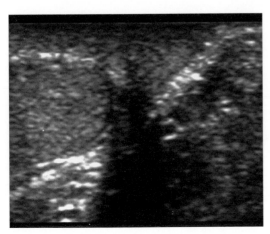 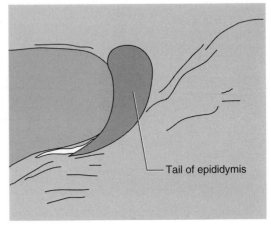

LABELED: LT EPI TAIL SAG

≡ TRANSVERSE IMAGES

Transverse Plane • Anterior Approach

14. Transverse image of the spermatic cord at normal respiration or rest with *anterior to posterior measurement*.

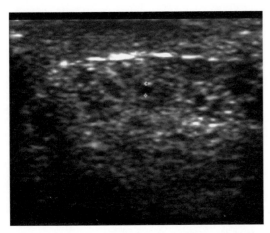 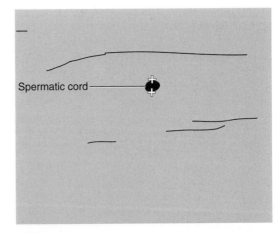

LABELED: LT CORD TRV REST

15. Same image as number 14 without calipers.

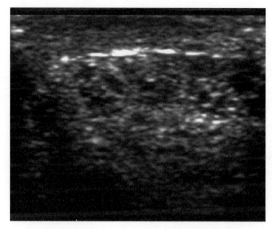

L A B E L E D : LT CORD TRV REST

16. Transverse image of the spermatic cord at valsalva with *anterior to posterior measurement.*

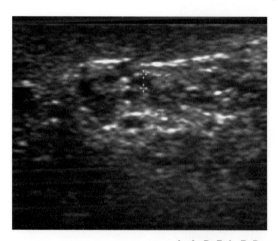
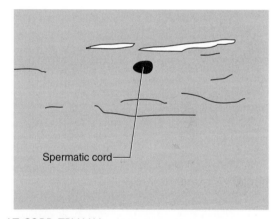

Spermatic cord

L A B E L E D : LT CORD TRV VAL

17. Same image as number 16 without calipers.

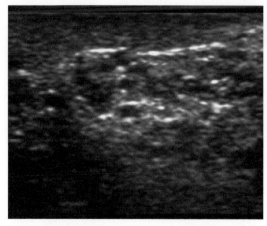

L A B E L E D : LT CORD TRV VAL

18. Transverse image of the epididymal head.

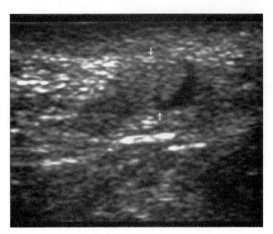 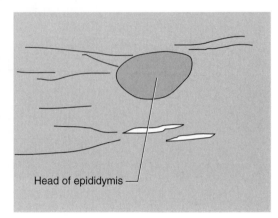

Head of epididymis

L A B E L E D :   LT EPI HEAD TRV

19. Transverse image of the superior portion of the left testis.

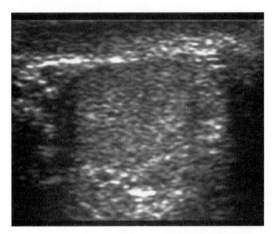 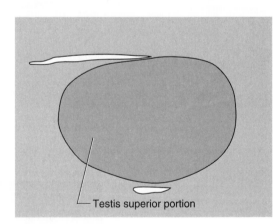

Testis superior portion

L A B E L E D :   LT TESTIS TRV SUP

20. Transverse image of the mid portion of the left testis with *medial to lateral measurement.*

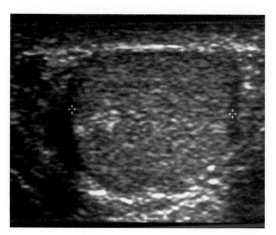 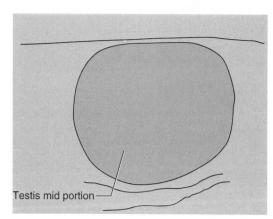

Testis mid portion

L A B E L E D :   LT TESTIS TRV MID

21. Same image as number 20 without calipers.

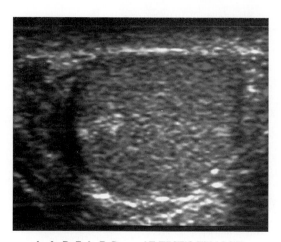

L A B E L E D :   LT TESTIS TRV MID

22. Transverse image of the inferior portion of the left testis.

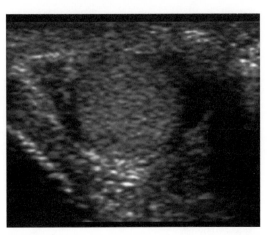 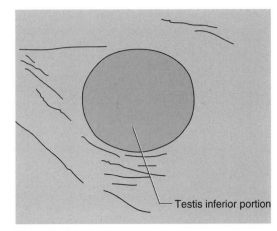

L A B E L E D :   LT TESTIS TRV INF

23. Transverse image of the tail of the epididymis.

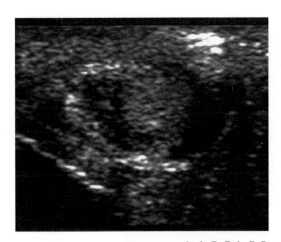 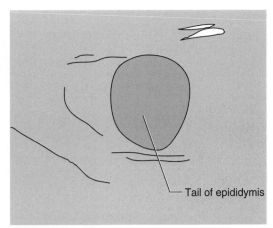

L A B E L E D :   LT EPI TAIL TRV

24. Transverse image of the mid portion of both testes.

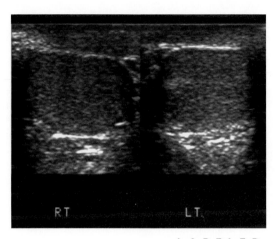
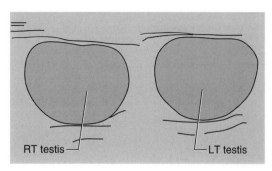

L A B E L E D :   BILAT TESTES TRV

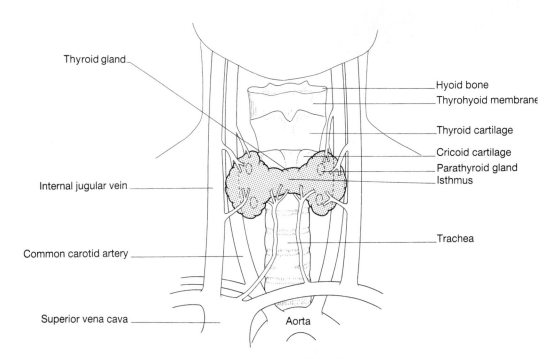

Thyroid gland

Hyoid bone
Thyrohyoid membrane
Thyroid cartilage
Cricoid cartilage
Parathyroid gland
Isthmus

Internal jugular vein

Common carotid artery

Trachea

Superior vena cava

Aorta

Location and anatomy of thyroid gland

Thyroid and Parathyroid Glands Scanning Protocols

CHAPTER 15

B.B. Tempkin and Wayne C. Leonhardt

LOCATION

- Lower, anterior portion of the neck.
- Lies anterior to the trachea and inferior to the larynx.
- The lateral borders of the lobes are the common carotid artery and internal jugular vein.
- The medial border of the lobes is the trachea.
- The isthmus of the gland unites the lower third of the lobes at the level of the second, third, and fourth tracheal rings.
- The sternocleidomastoid, sternothyroid, and sternohyoid muscles are anterior to the thyroid.
- The longus colli muscle and minor neurovascular bundle (consisting of the inferior thyroid artery and recurrent laryneal nerve) are posterior to the thyroid.
- The four parathyroid glands lie between the posterior aspect of the thyroid gland and the longus colli muscle.
- While the parathyroid glands are typically symmetric in position, the two superior glands are situated slightly more medial than the two inferior glands.

ANATOMY

- Superficial, butterfly-shaped gland with right and left lobes.
- The right and left lobes are connected at the midline by a narrow portion of the gland called the isthmus.
- The thyroid is variable in size but weighs approximately 25-35 grams. It is larger in women and becomes enlarged during pregnancy.
- Each lobe is approximately 4-6 cm long, 2-3 cm anterior to posterior, and 3 cm at its greatest width. The isthmus measures approximately 2-6 cm anterior to posterior.
- The thyroid is a highly vascular gland. Its blood supply consists of paired superior and inferior arteries and veins, and often, middle thyroid veins.
- The parathyroid glands are oval or bean shaped.

313

- Each parathyroid gland is approximately 5–7 mm long, 1–2 mm thick, and 3–4 mm wide.
- Blood is supplied to the parathyroids by separate small branches of the inferior and superior thyroid arteries. Venous drainage is via the superior, inferior, and middle thyroid veins.

PHYSIOLOGY

- Endocrine gland that synthesizes, stores, and secretes thyroid hormones.
- Maintains body metabolism.
- The thyroid produces three hormones, triiodothyronine (T3), thyroxine (T4), and calcitonin.
- The parathyroid glands secrete parathormone (PTH) which controls the calcium level in the blood.

SONOGRAPHIC APPEARANCE

- Lobes are midgray or medium-level echoes with even texture which is similar to normal testis and liver parenchyma.
- Lobes appear more echogenic or hyperechoic to adjacent muscles.
- Branches of intrathyroidal veins and arteries appear as 1-2 mm anechoic tubular structures.
- The esophagus appears hypoechoic with an echogenic center representing mucosa.
- Normal parathyroid glands are not usually seen by ultrasound but occasionally a single gland may be identified as a flat hypoechoic structure posterior to the thyroid and anterior to the longus colli muscle.

NORMAL VARIANTS

- Pyramidal lobe:
  Triangular-shaped, superior extension of the isthmus. Present in 15% to 30% of thyroid glands. Variable in size and extends more often to the left side. Parenchyma appears the same as the normal thyroid.
- Dilated follicles:
  Interspersed throughout the thyroid, they appear as 1- to 3-mm cystic areas.
- Ectopic thyroid:
  Lingual thyroids account for 90% of ectopic thyroids.
- Ectopic parathyroid glands:
  Represent approximately 15–20% of the total.

- Variant parathyroid gland shapes:
  Elongated (11%), bi-lobed (5%), or multi-lobed (1%).

COLOR DOPPLER FLOW CHARACTERISTICS

- Utilize color Doppler to differentiate vascular from non-vascular structures.
- Adjust color Doppler parameters to detect normal, or increased flow in the thyroid gland.
- Color Doppler shows increased vascularity within and in the periphery of autonomous functioning adenomas and thyroid cancer.
- Utilize color Doppler to follow the superior or inferior thyroid arteries to locate parathyroid adenomas.

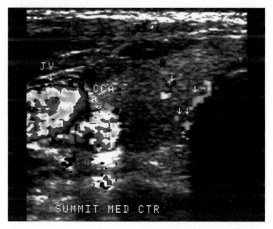

PATIENT PREP

- None.

PATIENT POSITION

- Supine with the patient's neck mildly hyperextended and the head turned slightly away from the side of interest.
- Place a sponge, pillow, or rolled towel under the patient's shoulders to maintain hyperextension of the neck.

TRANSDUCER

- High resolution, real-time, linear transducer. **7.5–10 MHz.**
- 5.0 MHz recommended for a very muscular or fat neck.
- According to the transducer and machine used, a water path or standoff pad may be necessary.
- Doppler color flow imaging (low-flow filter, scale, and optimized color gain).

BREATHING TECHNIQUE

- **Normal respiration.**

THYROID SURVEY

> **N O T E :**   The thyroid gland is small and can be seen in its entirety by some transducers, but it is still evaluated by viewing the lobes individually.

☰ TRANSVERSE STUDY

Transverse Plane • Anterior Approach

1. Begin with the transducer perpendicular at the sternal notch.

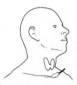

2. Move the transducer slightly superior and toward the patient's right, lateral enough to view the right lobe from its medial to lateral margins.

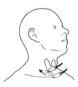

3. Keep the transducer perpendicular and scan superiorly through and beyond the right lobe to the level of the mandible. Note the isthmus medially.

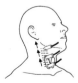

4. Move the transducer inferiorly from the mandible back through and beyond the inferior margin of the right lobe to the level of the sternal notch.

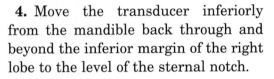

5. Move the transducer slightly superior and toward the patient's left, lateral enough to view the left lobe from its medial to lateral margins.

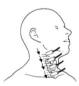

6. Keep the transducer perpendicular and scan superiorly through and beyond the right lobe to the level of the mandible. Note the isthmus medially.

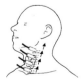

7. Move the transducer inferiorly from the mandible back through and beyond the inferior margin of the left lobe to the level of the sternal notch.

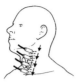

8. Move to the midline of the sternal notch and scan superiorly until you scan through and beyond the isthmus.

≡ LONGITUDINAL SURVEY

Sagittal Plane • Anterior Approach

9. Begin with the transducer perpendicular at the midline of the sternal notch.

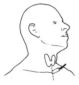

10. Move the transducer slightly superior and toward the patient's right, enough to view the right lobe from its superior to inferior margins.

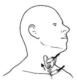

11. Keep the transducer perpendicular and scan toward the patient's right, laterally through and beyond the right lobe.

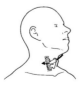

12. Move back onto the lobe and scan through to the midline and the isthmus.

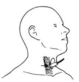

13. From the midline move the transducer slightly toward the patient's left, enough to view the left lobe from its superior to inferior margins.

14. Keep the transducer perpendicular and scan toward the patient's left, laterally through and beyond the left lobe.

15. Move back onto the lobe and scan through to the midline and the isthmus.

N O T E : Imaging the inferior portion of the lobes can be improved by having the patient swallow. This raises the gland superiorly.

REQUIRED IMAGES

Right Lobe

≡ TRANSVERSE IMAGES

Transverse Plane • Anterior Approach

1. Transverse image of the inferior portion of the right lobe.

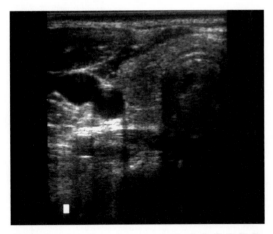
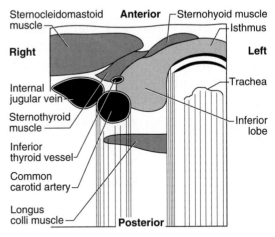

Sternocleidomastoid muscle
Anterior
Sternohyoid muscle
Isthmus
Right
Left
Internal jugular vein
Trachea
Sternothyroid muscle
Inferior lobe
Inferior thyroid vessel
Common carotid artery
Longus colli muscle
Posterior

L A B E L E D :   RT LOBE TRV INF

2. Transverse image of the midportion of the right lobe.

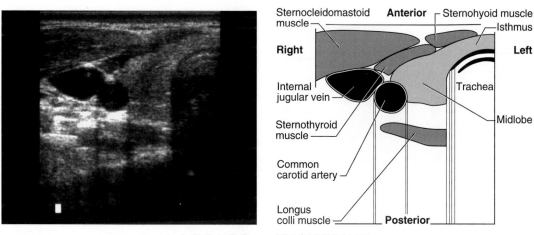

L A B E L E D :   RT LOBE TRV MID

3. Transverse image of the superior portion of the right lobe.

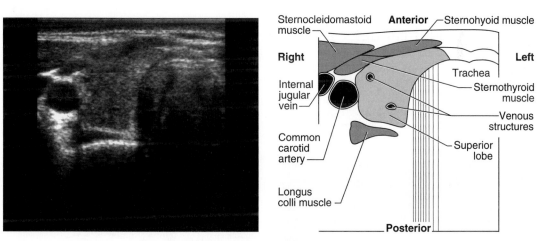

L A B E L E D :   RT LOBE TRV SUP

4. Transverse image of the isthmus to include both the right and left lobe attachments.

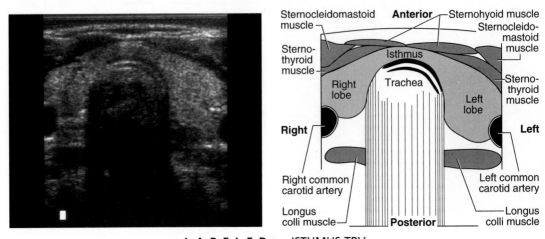

L A B E L E D :   ISTHMUS TRV

≡ LONGITUDINAL IMAGES

Sagittal Plane • Anterior Approach

5. Longitudinal image of the medial portion of the right lobe.

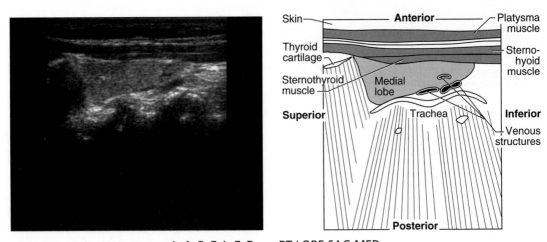

L A B E L E D :   RT LOBE SAG MED

6. Longitudinal image of the lateral portion of the right lobe.

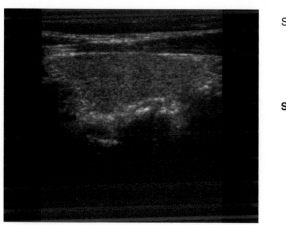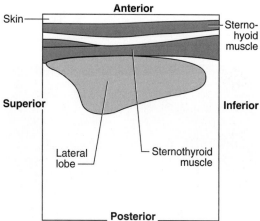

L A B E L E D :   RT LOBE SAG LAT

Left Lobe

≡ TRANSVERSE IMAGES

Transverse Plane • Anterior Approach

7. Transverse image of the inferior portion of the left lobe.

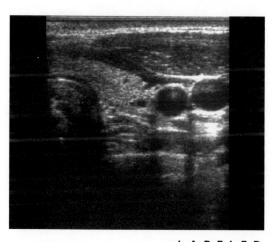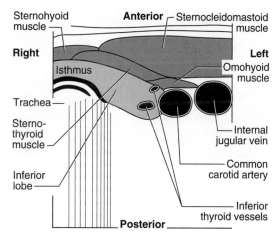

L A B E L E D :   LT LOBE TRV INF

8. Transverse image of the midportion of the left lobe.

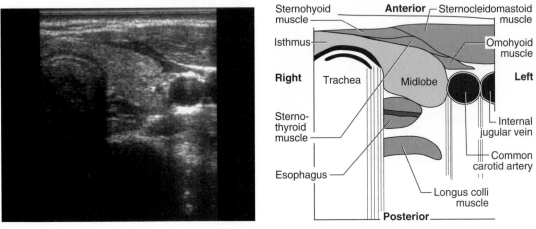

L A B E L E D :   LT LOBE TRV MID

9. Transverse image of the superior portion of the left lobe.

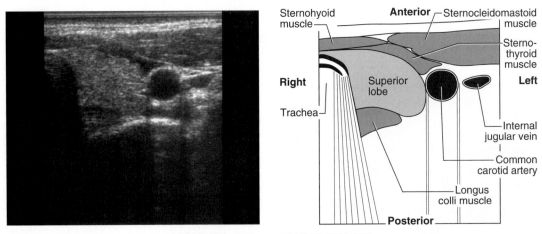

L A B E L E D :   LT LOBE TRV SUP

≡ LONGITUDINAL IMAGES

Sagittal Plane • Anterior Approach

10. Longitudinal image of the medial portion of the left lobe.

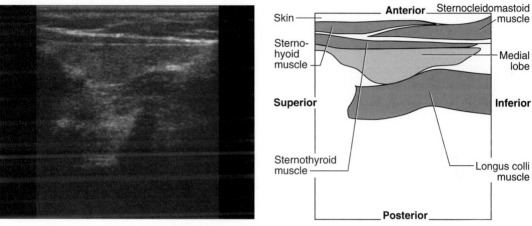

L A B E L E D :   LT LOBE SAG MED

11. Longitudinal image of the lateral portion of the left lobe.

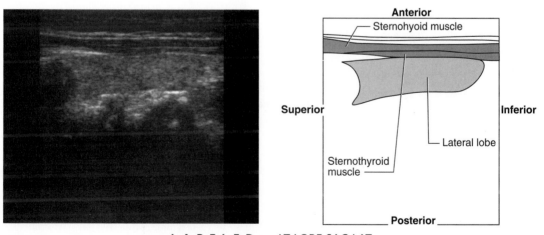

L A B E L E D :   LT LOBE SAG LAT

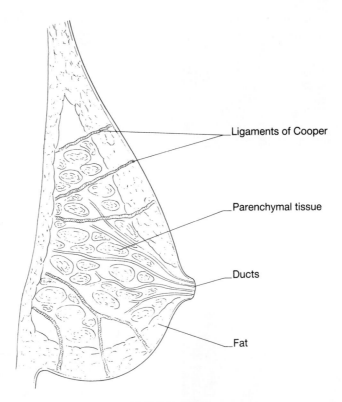

Ligaments of Cooper

Parenchymal tissue

Ducts

Fat

Breast anatomy

Breast Scanning Protocol

B.B. Tempkin and Felicia M. Jones

CHAPTER

16

ANATOMY

- The breast parenchymal elements are lobes, ducts, lobules, and acini.
- Most posterior aspect is connected to the pectoral musculature.
- Most anterior aspect is connected to the skin.

PHYSIOLOGY

- Mammary function is to secrete milk during lactation.

SONOGRAPHIC APPEARANCE

- The skin line, nipple, and the retromammary layer are highly echogenic.
- The areolar area is slightly less echogenic than the nipple and skin.
- Internal nipple appearance is quite variable.
- The mammary layer (active glandular tissue) is the core of the breast and has a mixed parenchymal appearance depending on the amount of fat that is present.

N O T E :   Appearance with the presence of little fat is highly echogenic because of collagen and fibrotic tissue. When fat is present, the appearance is of areas of low-level echoes mixed with areas of high echogenicity.

- Cooper's ligament and other connective tissue can be seen as highly echogenic linear areas within the fat tissue.
- The sonographic appearance of the breast changes with age. Older patients' breasts tend to have more fatty tissue.

PATIENT PREP

- None.

PATIENT POSITION

- **Supine.**
- Sitting erect.

TRANSDUCER

- **5 MHz linear.**
- 7.5 MHz.
- 10 MHz.

CLINICAL REASONING

- Sonography of the breast should be performed only after mammography unless the patient is under 25 years old.
- Breast sonography is generally performed to determine the composition of a localized area(s) that may or may not be palpable.
- Whole breast scanning may be indicated for diffuse diseases such as fibrocystic disease.

BREAST SURVEY

N O T E :   For localized area(s) see pathology scanning protocol, Chapter 2.

≡ WHOLE BREAST SURVEY

1. Begin scanning the breast in question at the 12 o'clock position.

2. Transducer orientation is set up so that the breast is viewed in sections from nipple outward, where the orientation notch is located.

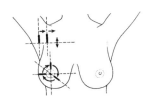

3. Scan around the breast in a clockwise manner, covering all anatomy, including the axillary regions.

N O T E :   If it is necessary to scan the entire breast for diffuse disease, you must scan both breasts.

REQUIRED IMAGES

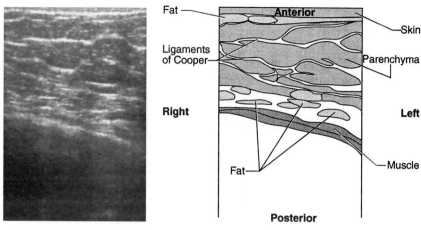

Fat — Anterior
— Skin
Ligaments of Cooper —
Parenchyma
Right   **Left**
Fat —
— Muscle
Posterior

Breast image reference

1. 12 o'clock image of breast tissue with the base of the transducer toward the nipple and the end of the transducer facing outward so that the nipple area is closest to the top of the imaging screen.

L A B E L E D :   12 O'CLOCK RT or LT

2. 3 o'clock image (same orientation as number 1).

L A B E L E D :   3 O'CLOCK RT or LT

3. 6 o'clock image.

L A B E L E D :   6 O'CLOCK RT or LT

4. 9 o'clock image.

L A B E L E D :   9 O'CLOCK RT or LT

5. Transverse image through the nipple.

L A B E L E D :   NIP TRV RT or LT

6. Longitudinal image through the nipple.

L A B E L E D :   NIP SAG RT or LT

7. Longitudinal image of the axillary region.

L A B E L E D :   AXILLARY SAG RT or LT

8. Transverse image of the axillary region.

L A B E L E D :   AXILLARY TRV RT or LT

9. to 16. Will be the same corresponding images of the other breast.

N O T E :   In some cases, whole breast scanning includes images from 12 o'clock, 1 o'clock, 2 o'clock, 3 o'clock, etc. If so, label accordingly and include nipple and axillary images.

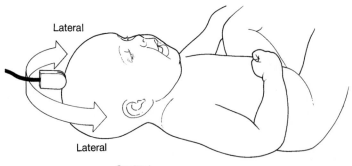

Lateral

Lateral

Sagittal

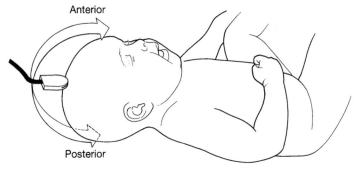

Anterior

Posterior

Coronal

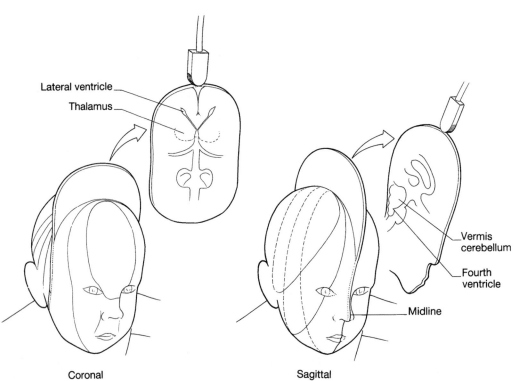

Lateral ventricle

Thalamus

Vermis cerebellum

Fourth ventricle

Midline

Coronal

Sagittal

Neonatal Brain Scanning Protocol

Kristin Dykstra-Downey

CRANIAL VAULT ANATOMY AND SONOGRAPHIC APPEARANCE

- Four ventricles:
  - (a) Two lateral ventricles:

    Each ventricle is divided segmentally into a frontal horn, body, occipital horn, and temporal horn. The atrium or trigone is the junction of the body and occipital and temporal horns. The ventricle walls appear echogenic and curvilinear. These slit-like structures lie the same distance from the interhemispheric fissure. The cavities contain cerebrospinal fluid (CSF) and appear anechoic.

  - (b) Third ventricle:

    The third ventricle is a small, teardrop-shaped, midline cavity that lies between the thalami and is connected to the lateral ventricles via the foramen of Monro. The walls appear echogenic. The cavity contains CSF and appears anechoic.

  - (c) Fourth ventricle:

    The fourth ventricle is a small, thin, arrowhead-shaped, midline cavity that appears to project into the cerebellum. It is vaguely seen except with massive ventricular dilatation. The walls appear echogenic. The cavity contains CSF and appears anechoic when seen.

- Corpus callosum:

  The corpus callosum is a midline structure that bridges horizontally to the roof of the lateral ventricles. It has an echogenic "double-walled" -like appearance. The parenchyma appears midgray or as medium- to low-level echoes.

- Cavum septum pellucidum and vergae:

  The cavum septum pellucidum (anterior portion) and vergae (posterior portion) appear comma-shaped sagitally or triangular-shaped coronally. This is a midline, anechoic,

329

fluid-filled structure projecting superoanterior to the third ventricle and lies between the frontal horns and bodies of the two lateral ventricles.

- Thalamus:

  The two egg-shaped thalami lie on each side of the third ventricle. They appear midgray or as medium- to low-level echoes.

- Cerebellum:

  The cerebellum lies immediately posterior to the fourth ventricle and occupies the majority of the posterior fossae of the skull. The vermis is the central echogenic portion of the cerebellum, whereas the surrounding parenchyma appears midgray or as medium-level echoes.

- The cisterna magna:

  The cisterna magna is a small, anechoic, fluid-filled space, immediately posteroinferior to the cerebellum.

- Choroid plexus:

  The choroid plexus consists of two curvilinear, echogenic structures that arch around the thalami anteriorly from the floor of the body of the lateral ventricle and posteriorly to the tip of the temporal horn. Note that the choroid plexus does not extend into the frontal or occipital horns.

- Aqueduct of Sylvius:

  The aqueduct of Sylvius is a midline channel that connects the third and fourth ventricles. It is rarely seen sonographically unless dilated.

- Foramen of Monro:

  The foramen of Monro consists of anechoic, midline channels that connect the third ventricle with each lateral ventricle.

- Brain stem:

  The brain stem is a columnar-appearing structure that connects the forebrain and the spinal cord. Consists of the midbrain, pons, and the medulla oblongata. It appears midgray or as medium- to low-level echoes.

- Interhemispheric fissure:

  The interhemispheric fissure is a linear, echogenic area in which the midline falx (fold of dura mater) lies separating the two cerebral hemispheres.

- Massa intermedia:

  The massa intermedia is a pea-shaped, soft tissue structure that is suspended within the third ventricle. It appears midgray or as medium-level echoes and is best seen with ventricular dilatation.

- Hippocampal gyrus (choroidal fissure):

  The hippocampal gyrus is an echogenic, spiral-like fold embodying each temporal horn.

- Cerebral peduncle:

  The cerebral peduncle is a medium- to low-level echo, Y-shaped structure inferior to the thalami and fused at the level of the pons.

- Sulci:

  The sulci are echogenic, spider-like fissures separating the gyri or folds of the brain. They appear fewer in number in the premature neonate.

- Tentorium:

  The tentorium is an echogenic structure (tent-shaped coronally) that separates the cerebrum from the inferior cerebellum and resembles a pine tree.

- Sylvian fissure:

  The sylvian fissure resembles an echogenic "Y" turned on its side and is located bilaterally between the temporal and frontal lobes of the brain. The middle cerebral artery can be seen pulsating here.

- Caudate nucleus:

  The caudate nucleus is located within the concavity of the lateral angles of each lateral ventricle and appears midgray or as medium-level echoes.

- Germinal matrix/caudothalamic groove:

  The germinal matrix is a vascular network located in the region of the caudate nucleus and thalamus called the caudothalamic groove. When visualized, it appears small and echogenic. Note that this is the most common site for a subependymal hemorrhage.

- Quadrigeminal plate:

  The quadrigeminal plate is an echogenic structure immediately superior to the apex of the tentorium resembling the top of a pine tree.

PATIENT PREP

- Keeping the infant warm is of utmost importance.
- The infant should be disturbed as little as possible, preferably left in the isolette.
- Gowns and gloves are recommended.
- The portable ultrasound system should be wiped down with a cleaning agent.
- Coupling gel should be body temperature.

PATIENT POSITION

- Supine with the head face up.
- Prone with the head lying on either side.

TRANSDUCER

- **7.5 MHz** for premature infants less than 32 weeks' gestation or less than 1500 g.
- 5.0 to 3.0 MHz for term and older infants with open anterior fontanelle.

NEONATAL BRAIN SURVEY

N O T E :   Use the anterior fontanelle as a window through which to angle or pivot the transducer. The diameter of the fontanelle may restrict the amount of angulation and anatomy seen.

N O T E :   While surveying the brain, close attention should be paid to all intracranial anatomy and its symmetry.

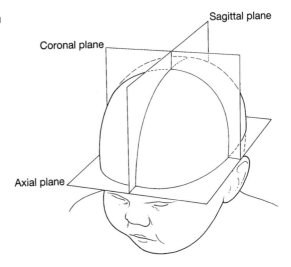

≡ CORONAL SURVEY

Coronal Plane • Anterior Fontanelle Approach

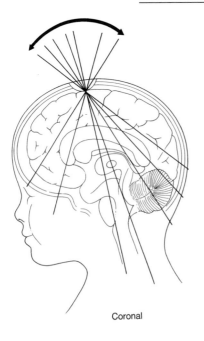

Coronal

1. Begin with the transducer perpendicular at the anterior fontanelle.

2. Slowly angle the transducer toward the face. Scan through the frontal horns into the frontal lobes of the brain.

3. Slowly angle the transducer back to perpendicular.

4. Slowly angle the transducer posteriorly. Scan through the occipital horns into the occipital lobes of the brain.

5. Slowly angle the transducer back to perpendicular.

☰ SAGITTAL SURVEY

Sagittal Plane • Anterior Fontanelle Approach

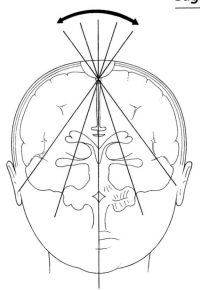

1. Begin with the transducer perpendicular at the anterior fontanelle.

2. Slowly angle the transducer laterally toward the right lateral ventricle. Scan through the temporal lobe of the brain to the level of the sylvian fissure.

3. Slowly angle the transducer back to perpendicular.

4. Repeat the first, second, and third steps, but angle the transducer through the left hemisphere.

REQUIRED IMAGES

☰ CORONAL IMAGES

Coronal Plane • Anterior Fontanelle Approach

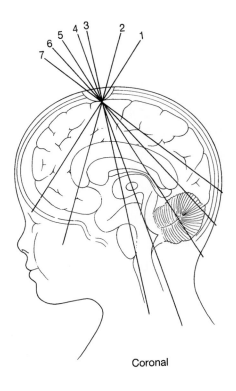

Coronal

1. Coronal image of the frontal lobes of the brain with the interhemispheric fissure. Include the orbital cones and ethmoid sinus.

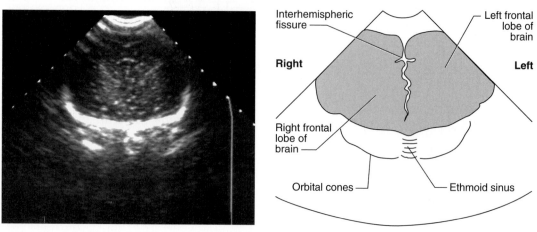

L A B E L E D : CORONAL

2. Coronal image of the frontal horns of the ventricles encompassing the caudate nucleus. Include the germinal matrix adjacent to the ventricles and corpus callosum.

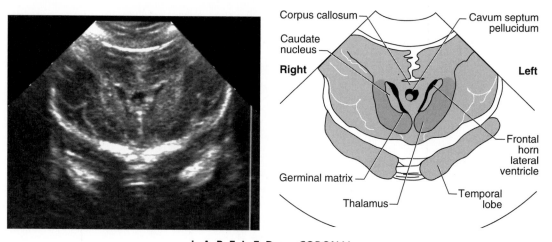

L A B E L E D : CORONAL

3. Coronal image of the frontal horns and thalami. Include the sylvian fissures, septum pellucidum, third ventricle, and foramen of Monro.

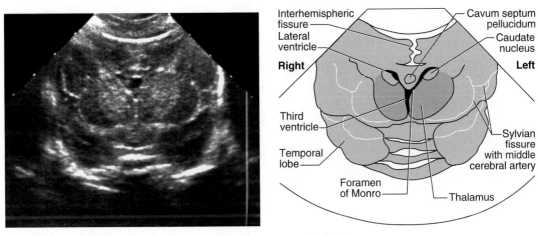

L A B E L E D :   CORONAL

4. Coronal image of the bodies of the lateral ventricles, thalami, sylvian fissures, choroidal fissures, and temporal horns.

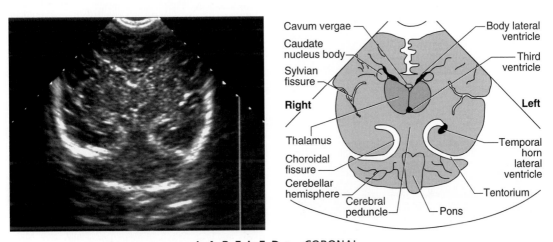

L A B E L E D :   CORONAL

5. Coronal image of the tentorium cerebelli. Include the sylvian fissures and the cisterna magna.

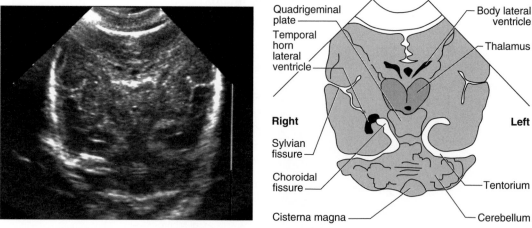

LABELED: CORONAL

6. Coronal image of the choroid plexus in the atrium or trigone region.

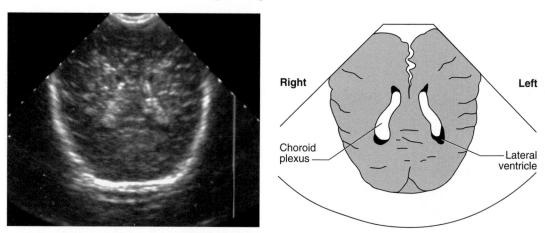

LABELED: CORONAL

7. Coronal image of the occipital lobes of the brain.

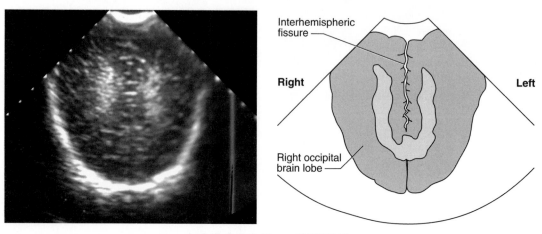

LABELED: CORONAL

☰ SAGITTAL IMAGES

Sagittal Plane • Anterior Fontanelle Approach

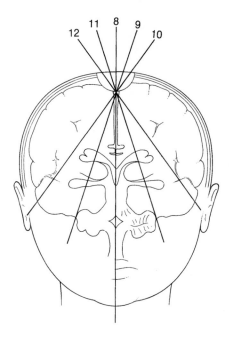

Midline Image

8. Sagittal midline image of the cavum septum pellucidum, corpus callosum, third ventricle, fourth ventricle, and cerebellum, including the massa intermedia (seen in two thirds of infants).

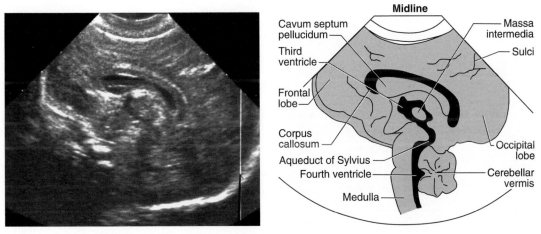

L A B E L E D :   SAG ML

N O T E :   This image should be perpendicular at the midline.

Right Hemisphere Images

9. Sagittal image of the right ventricle, germinal matrix, caudate nucleus, thalamus, and choroid plexus.

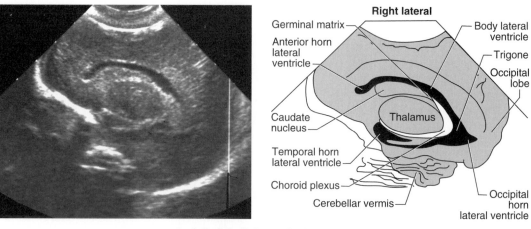

Right lateral

Germinal matrix

Anterior horn lateral ventricle

Caudate nucleus

Temporal horn lateral ventricle

Choroid plexus

Cerebellar vermis

Body lateral ventricle

Trigone

Occipital lobe

Thalamus

Occipital horn lateral ventricle

L A B E L E D :   SAG RT LAT

N O T E :   In some cases the frontal horn, body, temporal horn, and occipital horn cannot be imaged in the same plane. Therefore an additional image(s) may be necessary.

L A B E L E D :   SAG RT LAT

10. Sagittal image of the right temporal lobe of the brain at the level of the sylvian fissure.

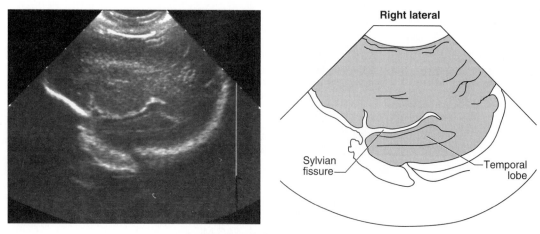

Right lateral

Sylvian fissure

Temporal lobe

L A B E L E D :   SAG RT LAT

Left Hemisphere Images

11. Sagittal image of the left ventricle, germinal matrix, caudate nucleus, thalamus, and choroid plexus.

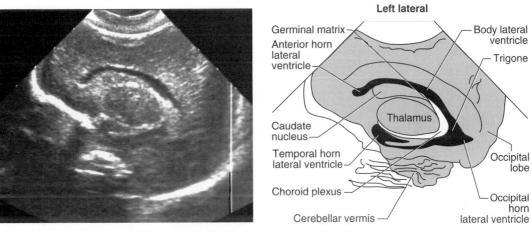

L A B E L E D :   SAG LT LAT

N O T E :   In some cases the frontal horn, body, temporal horn, and occipital horn cannot be imaged in the same plane. Therefore an additional image(s) may be necessary.

L A B E L E D :   SAG LT LAT

12. Sagittal image of the left temporal lobe of the brain at the level of the sylvian fissure.

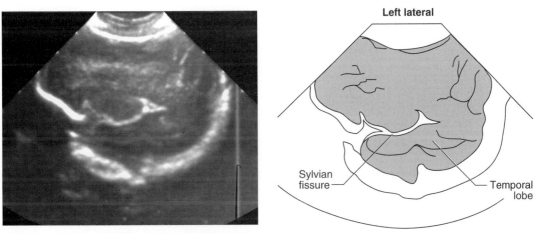

L A B E L E D :   SAG LT LAT

N O T E :   Alternative axial views through the temporal recess or posterior fontanelle are options to further evaluate the lateral ventricular walls and/or the occipital horns, respectively.

Vascular Scanning Protocols

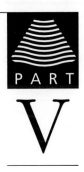

PART

V

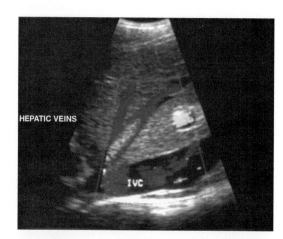

Example of color flow Doppler in hepatic veins. See Color Plate 4 at the back of this book.

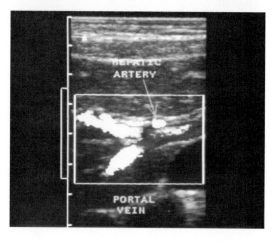

Example of color Doppler image of flow in the portal vein. See Color Plate 5 at the back of this book.

Abdominal Doppler and Color Flow

Marsha Neumyer

BASIC PRINCIPLES

≡ THE DOPPLER EQUATION

$$Fd = \frac{2\ Fo\ V\ Cos\ \theta}{C}$$

Fd = Doppler shifted frequency
Fo = Carrier (operating) Doppler frequency
C = Speed of sound in soft tissue
Cos θ = The Doppler beam angle relevant to the path of blood flow

- As the sound beam is sent out into the body, any motion detected in the path of the beam is depicted as a change or shift in frequency.
  - (a) This is referred to as the Doppler shift frequency.
  - (b) The Doppler shift frequency (Fd) increases as the operating frequency (Fo) increases.
  - (c) The Doppler shift frequency usually falls within the audible frequency range.

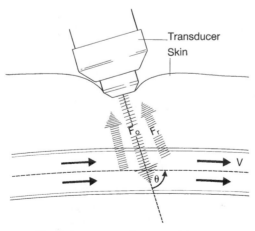

Obtaining a Doppler signal from a moving target.

≡ GENERAL INFORMATION

Frequency Range

- The diagnostic frequency range for ultrasound is 1 to 20 MHz.
- The frequency chosen must depend on the depth of penetration required and the resolution necessary to achieve diagnostic information.
- As you increase the frequency you decrease depth of penetration, increase resolution, and increase blood flow detection.

Angle Detection

- If quantitative information is needed, the angle of the Doppler beam relevant to the path of blood flow must be known.
- The Doppler shift decreases as the Doppler angle increases. The angle of insonation is usually controlled by the operator.
- It must be remembered that if Doppler shifted signals are collected at an angle of O°, the cosine of zero is 1.0 and, therefore, a very accurate representation of velocity is possible.
- This is usually operator-controllable and should be set between 45 and 60 degrees to ensure maximum signal return.
- If the angle select is set at 90 degrees or perpendicular to flow, the computer will be unable to detect forward from reverse flow.

Doppler angle correction

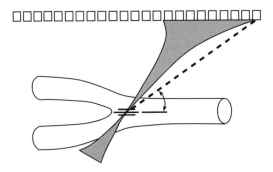

True angle corrected peak velocity

Image demonstrating proper Doppler angle correction. (Courtesy of Diasonics, Inc., Milpitas, California.)

☰ SAMPLE VOLUME

- When examining very small abdominal vessels, sample volume size may be initially enlarged to ensure that all returning Doppler shift signals are detected.
- When examining larger vessels, the sample volume size should be kept smaller.
  - (a) Sampling should be complete throughout the entire vessel as peak systolic and end-diastolic velocities may be encountered not only at mid-vessel, but may be adjacent to the wall dependent on the amount and surface contour of vessel pathology.

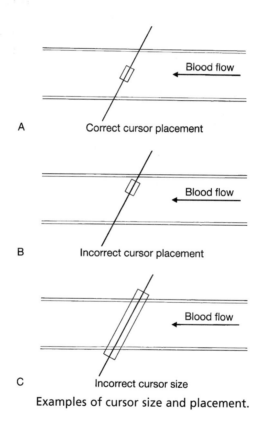

A   Correct cursor placement

B   Incorrect cursor placement

C   Incorrect cursor size

Examples of cursor size and placement.

Doppler Gain

- Doppler spectral gain should be optimized to ensure display of the full range of velocity information without aliasing.

Most Frequently Used Doppler Controls

- Doppler gain: will increase or decrease the total gain applied to the Doppler spectral information.
- Wall filter: will increase or decrease the low amplitude echoes present because of vessel wall "thumping." Different from the "Thump filter." Must be careful not to set too high or you will delete useful information.
- Angle Control: as discussed previously.
- Zero Baseline: may be adjusted to allow display of high velocities.
- Scale size: if operator-controllable, may be used with pulsed Doppler to help eliminate aliasing and to optimize the spectral display.

≡ DOPPLER INSTRUMENTATION

Continuous Wave Doppler (CW)

- Cheaper.
- Generally a small pencil probe.
- Lacks axial resolution.

  (a) Cannot determine vessel depth.

  (b) Filters may be used to help decrease noise interference.

- An area of overlap between the outgoing and incoming beams is used as a basis for comparison to determine Doppler shift frequency.

  (a) A demodulator (often a quadrature phase detector) is used to determine the Doppler shift frequency.

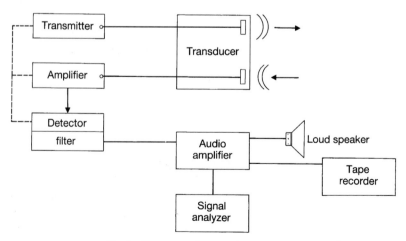

Block diagram of a continuous-wave Doppler system.

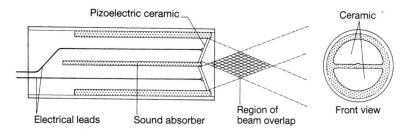

Diagram of a continuous-wave Doppler transducer.

Pulsed Wave Doppler (PW)

- Often duplex instrumentation. A combination of real-time Doppler velocity spectral display and B-Mode image instrumentation.
  - (a) The Doppler velocity information may be collected from discrete sample sites within the gray-scale image.
  - (b) The Doppler crystals are located within the imaging transducer.
- Allows Doppler velocity spectral analysis (temporal display) from a small, specific operator-controllable region (sample volume).
- Is able to examine only a limited frequency range.
  - (a) Will alias because the Doppler shift frequencies are determined by sampling multiple times along the same pulse line. Due to time and depth limitations (PRF), the internal computer may not be able to sample often enough within a given time frame to display the full range of frequencies.
- Has poor signal to noise ratios (it may be difficult to detect low flow signals because of noise interference).
  - (a) Hard to remove noise without removing real information.
- May use high power levels:
  - (a) SPTA levels may reach 1 W/cm^2
- The use of an operator-set Doppler angle correction allows easy calculation of flow velocities by the internal computer using the Doppler equation.

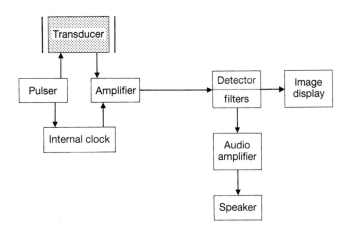

Block diagram of a duplex Doppler instrument.

Color Doppler

- Offers a display of mean flow velocities (spatially) by sampling multiple points at a very fast rate.
- Multiple sampling often causes noise from tissue movement as well as from moving blood signals. Filters must be used to eliminate all but the continuously moving signals.
- Frequency shifts are detected through autocorrelation.

Power Doppler

- Newest technology.
  - (a) Color encodement is based on the relative intensity of the Doppler signal rather than the Doppler shift. Because of this feature, direction of blood flow cannot be determined.

≡ DOPPLER ANALYSIS

Audible Sound

- The Doppler shift frequency falls within the audible range of 200 Hz to 15 kHz.

Spectral Analysis

- The Doppler signal is displayed such that the power or intensity of each velocity is displayed as a shade of gray.

Color Doppler Analysis

- The color used for display is based on three characteristics of color.
  - (a) Hue: the three primary colors are used to create color maps (red, blue, and green).
  - (b) Saturation: the amount of white present in a color. This creates color shades.
  - (c) Luminosity: the brightness of a color.
- Color Doppler systems MAY use two monitors. One color and one gray scale. There is better gray scale resolution available on a dedicated gray scale monitor because of increased spatial resolution.
  Larger color monitors allow better spatial resolution.
- Red hue generally represents flow toward the transducer.
- Blue hue generally represents flow away from the transducer.
- Mosaic color patterns or "desaturation" of a primary color represent high velocity or complex flow. Choice of color maps is controlled by the operator.

- With color imaging, spectral broadening may be viewed as "variance."
  - (a) One color is arbitrarily chosen to display a wide range of velocities present.
  - (b) The color green is frequently chosen to "tag" a threshold velocity to facilitate recognition of increased velocity.
- These patterns are operator-controllable.
- Other color Doppler controls:
  - (a) The number of cycles per color line (often referred to as dwell time, ensemble length, or packet size).

    If this is increased, flow sensitivity increases, but frame rate decreases.
  - (b) Gray scale/color priority: This determines whether gray scale or color Doppler information will be emphasized in display.

    Increasing this increases the color saturation.

    Decreasing this helps to decrease the color present from wall and tissue motion.

    This acts as a filter by suppressing color information above a certain operator-set level.

≡ DOPPLER PITFALLS

Aliasing

- Does not occur with CW Doppler.
- Occurs in PW and color Doppler when the Nyquist limit (1/2 PRF) is exceeded.
- Appearance: An aliased signal will wrap around the baseline.

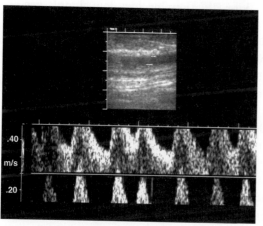

Example of Doppler mirroring.

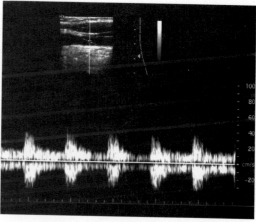

Example of Doppler aliasing. (Courtesy of Mary Washington Hospital, Fredericksburg, Virginia.)

- This phenomenon occurs because the pulsed Doppler system cannot sample often enough.
- Aliasing may also occur in color Doppler systems.

  It will appear as an abrupt color change within the same vessel that is not caused by flow reversal.

  It is often seen as a change in high-frequency color codes (i.e., light red to light blue).
- Flow reversal will be seen as adjacent deep shades separated by black (zero baseline) on the color image.
- The Doppler signal is backscattered from the moving red blood cells (Rayleigh scattering). As frequency increases, Rayleigh scattering increases. As in gray-scale imaging, the operator must choose the incident Doppler frequency for adequate penetration that will allow acceptable resolution and signal amplitude without aliasing.

Doppler Mirror Image

- An artifactual display of the Doppler spectral waveform appearing on the opposite side of the zero baseline from the waveform corresponding to the appropriate direction of flow.
- Results from inappropriate angle of insonation or PRF.

Color Imaging Pitfalls

N O T E :   Like PW Doppler, color Doppler is limited by the frame rate, tissue depth, and PRF of the system.

- Color Doppler systems tend to have poorer resolution.
- Color Doppler systems are unable to detect flow less than approximately 0.05 meters per second.
  - (a) If there is a low-flow color map available, color may well be the best way to visualize low-velocity flow because with CW or PW Doppler, low-flow signals are often covered up by noise or eliminated by the wall filter (set too high).
  - (b) Color Doppler systems use frame rates of 4 to 32 frames per second.
  - (c) This may be operator-controllable. Increase for better resolution.
  - (d) To better detect low-velocity flow, use a higher frequency transducer.
  - (e) To decrease tissue or vessel wall vibrations, decrease the color wall filter.
- Mirror image artifacts:
  - (a) To correct range ambiguity artifacts:
    Decrease PRF.

Increase frequency of the transducer.

Decrease far gain.

(b) Grating lobes:

Result from decreased lateral resolution because the beam is not perpendicular to the target.

To correct, adjust the transducer angle and/or Doppler steering angle.

≡ BIOLOGICAL EFFECTS

- The American Institute of Ultrasound in Medicine states that for imaging transducers, no known bioeffects have been proved below scanning intensity levels of 100 mW/cm^2 SPTA.
- No known bioeffects have been documented at currently used diagnostic intensity levels.
- All sonographers should be familiar with their equipment and the intensity levels stated by the manufacturer's owner's manual.
- Sonographers should scan conscientiously at all times using the ALARA (as low as reasonably acceptable) principle to adjust power, or intensity.
- The AIUM recommends using high power for as brief a period as possible to allow diagnostic studies. This practice ensures that the valuable diagnostic information will still be obtained without introducing any remote risk of harmful biological effects.
- The AIUM has approved fetal Doppler for the examination of the fetal heart and umbilical cord.

PURPOSE OF ABDOMINAL DOPPLER AND/OR COLOR FLOW IMAGING

- To assess patency of vessels.
- To rule out arterial stenosis.
- To rule out venous thrombosis.
- To determine flow direction.
- To determine volume flow.
- To assess hepatic shunts.
- To quantitate vascular resistance.
  (a) Cirrhotic liver disease.
  (b) Renal transplants.
  (c) Assessment of high-risk pregnancy.

(d) Formulae used:

Resistance Index:

$$\frac{\text{Peak Systolic Velocity} - \text{End Diastolic Velocity}}{\text{Peak Systolic Velocity}}$$

Pulsatility Index:

$$\frac{\text{Peak Systolic Velocity} - \text{End Diastolic Velocity}}{\text{Mean Velocity}}$$

Diastolic to Systolic Ratio:

$$\frac{\text{End Diastolic Velocity}}{\text{Peak Systolic Velocity}}$$

(e) To differentiate vascular from avascular abdominal masses.

(f) To assess anomalous vessels.

(g) To confirm normal anatomy.

CLINICAL NOTES

≡ EXAMINATION PROTOCOL

- Abdominal duplex and color flow imaging are performed only to confirm patency of vessels, detect the presence and severity of disease, and to define the location of disease processes.

≡ PATIENT PREP

- Patients should be fasted for 8 to 12 hours to decrease abdominal gas which may interfere with acquisition of image and Doppler flow information.

≡ PATIENT POSITION

- The examination will generally begin with the patient in the supine position with the head of the bed slightly elevated.
- Lateral decubitus and prone positions may be used as necessary to obtain adequate "windows" for interrogation of organs and blood vessels.

≡ TRANSDUCERS

- A range of transducers from 2.25 MHz to 5.0 MHz phased or curved linear array probes will be necessary to penetrate to the depth of the abdominal aorta and distal renal arteries.

≡ ARTERIAL FLOW

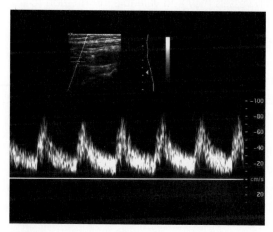

Example of a low-resistance arterial signal. (Courtesy of Milton S. Hershey Medical Center, Hershey, Pennsylvania.)

- Pulsates with cardiac cycle.
- Most arterial flow within the abdomen has fairly low resistance (Celiac, hepatic, splenic, and renal arteries).
- This typically means that the signal will not cross the baseline.
- Low flow vessels or abdominal masses often have a spectral appearance with lower systolic peaks and a more pronounced diastolic component.
- In contrast, the Doppler spectral waveform recorded from the fasting superior and inferior mesenteric arteries will demonstrate low diastolic flow consistent with high resistance arterial flow.
- Examples of abdominal arterial flow:

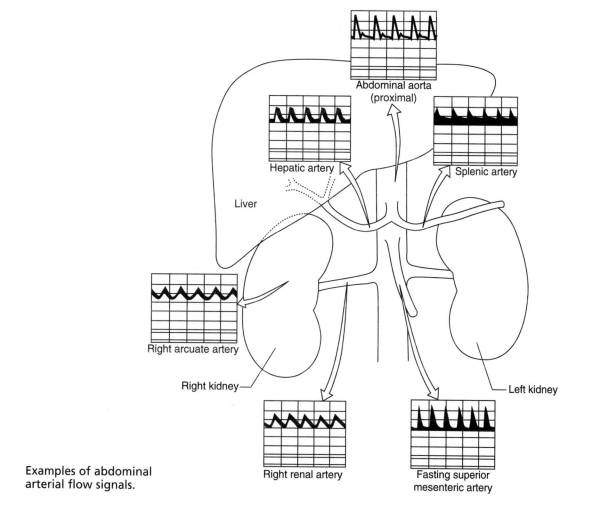

Examples of abdominal arterial flow signals.

N O T E :   Each vessel has a characteristic appearance. The investigation of certain vessels may add valuable information to the clinical question concerning the presence of pathology.

(a) Hepatic arteries:

Tend to have low impedance flow pattern characterized by forward diastolic flow.

Flow-reducing stenosis is suggested by peak systolic velocity greater than 220 cm/sec with post-stenotic turbulence.

Increased flow, in the absence of stenosis, may suggest portal hypertension or portal vein thrombosis.

Must confirm the presence of hepatic artery flow in liver transplants.

(b) Splenic artery:

Low resistance vascular flow pattern characterized by constant forward diastolic flow.

Frequently tortuous; may, therefore, demonstrate minimal spectral broadening due to flow disturbance.

Flow-reducing stenosis is suggested by peak systolic velocity greater than 220 cm/sec with post-stenotic turbulence.

(c) Mesenteric arteries:

The normal fasting celiac artery has low resistance Doppler velocity signals with constant forward diastolic flow consistent with the common hepatic and splenic arteries.

There is no significant change in the normal celiac peak systolic or diastolic velocities post-prandially.

With greater than 70% diameter reducing celiac artery stenosis, there will be at least 220 cm/sec peak systolic velocity with post-stenotic turbulence apparent.

The normal fasting superior mesenteric artery (SMA) signal should show low diastolic flow.

The normal post-prandial superior mesenteric arterial signal will demonstrate increased systolic flow, at least a 50% increase in diastolic flow and loss of the reverse flow component. Exceptions: Patients with diabetic gastroparesis and those with gastric "dumping" syndrome.

With greater than 70% diameter-reducing SMA stenosis, there will be a peak systolic velocity greater than 275 cm/sec with post-stenotic turbulence.

With critical stenosis or occlusion of the SMA and celiac arteries, the inferior mesenteric artery may enlarge and course antegrade along the mid- to lateral abdomen to reconstitute the more proximal mesenteric arteries.

Retrograde flow may be noted in the splenic and superior mesenteric veins if the SMA and celiac arteries are critically stenosed or occluded.

(d) Renal arteries:

Assess renal artery stenosis associated with hypertension or decreased renal function.

Normal spectral pattern: low vascular resistance; constant forward diastolic flow.

Mild to moderate stenosis: peak systolic velocities less than 180 cm/sec. Renal-aortic peak systolic velocity ratio less than 3.5.

Flow-reducing stenosis: peak systolic velocity greater than 180 cm/sec; post-stenotic turbulence; renal-aortic peak systolic velocity ratio greater than 3.5.

Occlusion: no flow in renal artery; Doppler signal in the renal parenchyma may show delayed systolic upstroke and deceleration (tardus-parvus signal).

(e) Renal transplants:

Rejection: often see decreased blood flow due to decreased renal function and increased capillary resistance (often due to external compression or narrowing of smaller blood vessels). There will be decreased diastolic flow.

Infarction: must optimize color flow display and Doppler to rule out possibility of very low flow.

Renal artery stenosis: as discussed previously.

Spectral waveform from a renal transplant at the level of the renal artery. (Courtesy of Mary Washington Hospital, Fredericksburg, Virginia.)

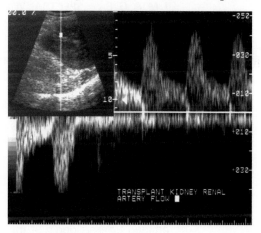

(f) Miscellaneous:

Blood supply to any area of interest.

- Exam protocol and required images

(a) Select images:

Renal arteries.

Renal perfusion.

Hepatic artery at porta hepatis.

N O T E :   Examination of the abdominal arteries and veins may be performed concurrently for each organ system, e.g., renal, mesenteric.

Mesenteric Arterial Images

1. Scan the abdominal aorta in longitudinal and transverse planes from the level of the diaphragm to the bifurcation (see Chapter 3).

   Return to the proximal aorta. Locate the celiac trunk as it arises from the anterior abdominal aortic wall just inferior to the diaphragm.

2. Sample with Doppler throughout the celiac trunk.

3. Return to a transverse image of the aorta at the level of the celiac origin. Locate the artery and its bifurcation into the common hepatic and splenic arteries. The celiac and splenic arteries may be tortuous.

I M A G E :   LONGITUDINAL VIEW CELIAC ARTERY, COMMON HEPATIC AND SPLENIC ARTERIES AT THE BIFURCATION

L A B E L E D :   CELIAC BIFURCATION

4. Sample with Doppler throughout the length of the celiac trunk and the proximal common hepatic and splenic arteries.

I M A G E :   SPECTRAL WAVEFORMS FROM THE CELIAC, COMMON HEPATIC AND SPLENIC ARTERIES

L A B E L E D :   CELIAC ART or COMMON HEP ART or SPLENIC ART

N O T E :   The hepatic artery may be followed from the celiac bifurcation to the level of its entry into the liver at the porta hepatis. Images and Doppler spectral waveforms should be documented throughout the proximal, mid and distal segments of the vessel.

N O T E :   In a similar manner, the splenic artery may be examined from its origin at the celiac bifurcation to the level of the splenic hilum. Images and Doppler spectral waveforms are documented throughout the proximal, mid and distal segments of the vessel. The splenic artery is frequently quite tortuous and color flow imaging may facilitate examination of this vessel.

I M A G E :   DOPPLER SPECTRAL WAVEFORM FROM THE DIS-TAL CELIAC TRUNK

Color Doppler image demonstrating flow in the region of the porta hepatis. See Color Plate 3 at the back of this book. (Courtesy of ATL, Bothell, Washington.)

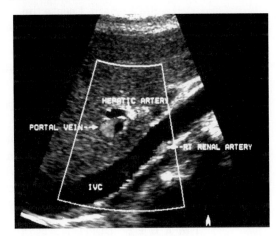

L A B E L E D :   CELIAC DIST

5. Return to the longitudinal image of the aorta just inferior to the origin of the celiac artery. Locate the origin of the superior mesenteric artery, which is usually 1-2 cm inferior to the celiac. The celiac and SMA may share a common origin.

I M A G E :   LONGITUDINAL VIEW OF THE SMA FROM ITS ORIGIN TO THE MID-SECTION OF THE VESSEL

L A B E L E D :   PROX-MID SMA

6. Sample with Doppler throughout the visualized segments of the SMA beginning at its origin.

I M A G E :   SPECTRAL WAVEFORMS FROM THE PROXIMAL TO THE MID SMA

L A B E L E D :   PROX SMA or MID SMA

N O T E :   The inferior mesenteric artery (IMA) is not routinely examined. If the celiac and/or SMA are critically stenosed or occluded, the IMA would be evaluated in a manner similar to the study of the SMA.

Renal Arterial Examination

1. Scan the abdominal aorta in longitudinal and transverse planes from the level of the diaphragm to the bifurcation (see Chapter 5). Return to the longitudinal view.

I M A G E :   LONGITUDINAL VIEW OF THE AORTA

L A B E L E D :   LONG AO

2. Return to the transverse view of the aorta. Locate the left renal vein as it crosses anterior to the aorta just inferior to the SMA origin. Locate the right and left renal arteries immediately posterior to the renal veins.

I M A G E :   TRANSVERSE VIEW OF THE AORTA AT THE LEVEL OF THE LEFT RENAL VEIN AND ORIGIN OF THE RIGHT OR LEFT RENAL ARTERY

L A B E L E D :   ORIGIN RT or LT REN ART

3. Continuously sample with Doppler from within the lumen of the aorta through the renal artery orifice by moving the Doppler sample volume slowly along this course. This will allow the examiner to detect the presence of stenosis at the origin of the renal artery.

I M A G E :   DOPPLER SPECTRAL WAVEFORMS FROM THE ORIGIN OF THE RIGHT or LEFT RENAL ARTERY

L A B E L E D : ORIGIN RT or LT REN ART

4. Using gray-scale or color flow imaging, follow the course of the renal artery from the proximal to the mid-segment of the vessel.

I M A G E :   LONGITUDINAL AORTA-CELIAC ORIGIN

Color Doppler image demonstrating renal artery origins. See Color Plate 1 at the back of this book. (Courtesy of Diasonics, Inc., Milpitas, California.)

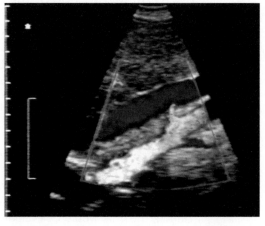

L A B E L E D :   AORTA-CELIAC ORIGIN

5. Sample continuously with Doppler throughout the visualized length of the renal artery.

I M A G E :   DOPPLER SPECTRAL WAVEFORMS FROM THE PROXIMAL THROUGH THE MID SEGMENTS OF THE RENAL ARTERY

L A B E L E D :   PROX or MID RT/LT REN ART

6. Move the patient to a lateral decubitus or other position

which allows adequate visualization of the kidney and distal to mid-renal artery. Image the renal artery from the hilum of the kidney as far proximal as possible.

I M A G E :   TRANSVERSE VIEW OF THE KIDNEY AND THE DISTAL TO MID RENAL ARTERY FROM THE LEVEL OF THE HILUM

L A B E L E D :   DIST RT/LT REN ART

7. Sample continuously with Doppler from the level of the renal hilum throughout the distal to mid renal artery.

I M A G E :   DOPPLER SPECTRAL WAVEFORMS FROM THE DISTAL TO MID RENAL ARTERY

L A B E L E D :   DIST RT/LT REN ART

8. Obtain a longitudinal view of the kidney. Measure the pole-to-pole length. You may use color flow imaging to demonstrate the arterial and venous perfusion of the organs.

I M A G E :   DOPPLER SPECTRAL WAVEFORM FROM THE ORIGIN OF THE CELIAC

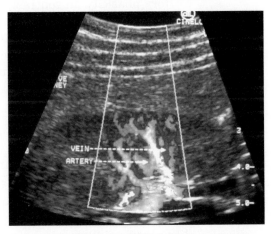

Color Doppler image demonstrating renal perfusion. See Color Plate 2 at the back of this book. (Courtesy of ATL, Bothell, Washington.)

L A B E L E D :   AORTA—CELIAC ORIGIN

9. Sample with Doppler throughout the intersegmental arteries of the renal medulla and the arcuate arteries of the renal cortex. You will obtain both arterial and venous signals at the cortical level due to the small size of the vessels and the arterio-venous shunting that occurs at this level.

I M A G E :   DOPPLER SPECTRAL WAVEFORMS FROM THE RENAL MEDULLA AND CORTEX

L A B E L E D :   RT or LT REN MED COR

N O T E : Approximately 20% of patients will have more than one renal artery on each side. These accessory or multiple renal arteries may be detected using several strategies:

- Power Doppler (Doppler power angio) may be useful as this technique relies on the intensity of the signal and is less affected by the angle of insonation than color Doppler imaging.
- Accessory renal arteries usually course to the surface of the lower pole of the kidney. As a consequence, the Doppler signals from the renal pole with the additional artery may have higher amplitude than the signal from the other region of the organ.
- Enlarge the Doppler sample volume and listen along the wall of the aorta for additional low resistance renal artery signals. Multiple renal arteries may arise anywhere along the aortic wall to the level of the common iliac arteries.

≡ VENOUS FLOW

- Respiratory phasicity varies throughout the abdominal venous system.
    - (a) Portal veins and splenic veins show little or no respiratory phasicity. In contrast, the hepatic venous and inferior vena caval Doppler waveforms show both respiratory phasicity and cardiac influences.
    - (b) In venous hypertension, the splanchnic vessels will dilate to diameters greater than 1.5 cm.
- Clinical examples:
- Clinical Notes:
    - (a) Inferior vena cava:
      Demonstrate impedance to outflow due to thrombus.
      Assess for thrombus surrounding IVC clips or filters.
      Must document patency in all liver transplants.
      Rule out propagation of tumor thrombus from renal masses.
    - (b) Splenic vein: see section on mesenteric ischemia; confirm patency and flow direction.
    - (c) Superior mesenteric vein: see section on mesenteric ischemia; confirm patency and flow direction.
    - (d) Portal vein:
      Normally has steady, minimally phasic flow.
      Assess for thrombus; if thrombosed, assess for recanalization.
      Confirm hepatopetal flow direction.
      The presence of marked respiratory variations (biphasic signals) suggest portal hypertension. Such signals are due to the increase in hepatic vascular resistance.

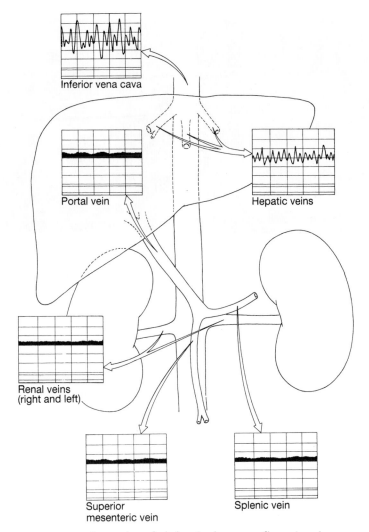

Examples of abdominal venous flow signals.

Portal vein branches should be differentiated from dilated biliary ducts.

(e) Renal veins:

Normally have steady, minimally phasic flow.

Assess for patency and propagation of renal tumor thrombus.

(f) Venous color Doppler of the abdomen:

Hepatic veins.

Portal vein.

IVC.

Mesenteric veins.

Renal veins.

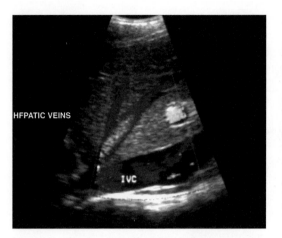

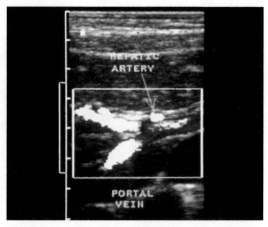

Example of color flow Doppler in hepatic veins. See Color Plate 4 at the back of this book. (Courtesy of ATL, Bothell, Washington.)

Example of color Doppler image of flow in the portal vein. See Color Plate 5 at the back of this book. (Courtesy of Diasonics, Inc., Milpitas, California.)

≡ MISCELLANEOUS

- Vascular tumors: often have three primary characteristics:
  (a) High-amplitude signals.
  (b) Increased peak systolic velocities.
  (c) A "roaring" sound due to edge motion and interference from the increased vascularity.
- Hepatomata: demonstrate high pitched signals due to arteriovenous communications.
- Pseudoaneurysms: contained hematomas that may have disorganized, pulsatile, or circular flow with low velocity signals within the hypo- or anechoic blood-filled mass.
  (a) Are located most often near a vessel branch or surgical anastomosis.
  (b) A characteristic "to-fro" flow pattern is noted within the tract, or pedicle, which connects the pseudoaneurysm to the artery.
  (c) If thrombosed, no Doppler signal should be obtained within the pedicle or the pseudoaneurysm.
- A/V fistulae (arteriovenous fistulae).
  (a) The arterial component will show increased velocity and a decreased resistive index proximal to the arteriovenous communication.
  (b) The outflow vein will show pulsatile flow.
- Gallbladder cancer versus sludge.
  (a) A cancer will show some low flow.
  (b) Sludge shows no flow.

≡ GYNECOLOGICAL STUDIES

- An active ovary shows increased peak systolic flow and a diastolic flow component.

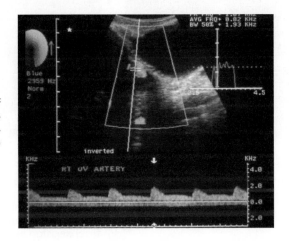

Doppler spectral display of blood flow in an active ovary. (Courtesy of Diasonics, Inc., Milpitas, California.)

- An inactive ovary shows no diastolic flow component.
  (a) Diastolic flow decreases normally during the follicular phase of ovulation.
- Ectopic pregnancies: spectral or color Doppler may help to show trophoblastic flow with high diastolic flow components.
- Infertility: may help to demonstrate the presence of ovarian flow associated with ovulation.

≡ OBSTETRICAL STUDIES

N O T E :   Remember to scan prudently.

- The flow resistance within the umbilical artery may be directly related to the presence of intrauterine growth retardation.

  The umbilical artery may show the following changes when IUGR is present due to increased placental pressure:
  (a) Increased resistance.
  (b) Decreased diastolic flow in the umbilical artery.
- Doppler of the umbilical cord:
  (a) To identify a three-vessel cord.
  (b) To assess cord insertions.
  (c) To rule out nuchal cord.
- Doppler of the fetal heart: will help to identify cardiac chambers and flow patterns.
- Doppler of the placenta.
  (a) Rule out chorioangiomata versus placental lakes.

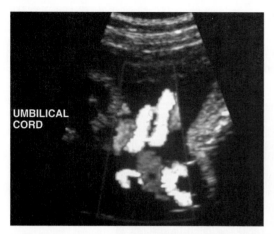

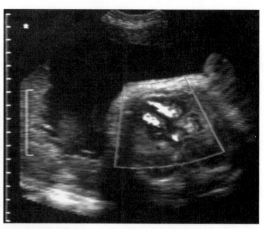

Color Doppler image of a three-vessel umbilical cord. See Color Plate 6 at the back of this book. (Courtesy of ATL, Bothell, Washington.)

Color Doppler image of a fetal four-chamber heart. See Color Plate 7 at the back of this book. (Courtesy of Diasonics, Inc., Milpitas, California. Diasonics does not have the Food and Drug Administration approval to market their probes for this fetal Doppler application. However, the final decision as to how a medical device will be used is the prerogative of the medical practitioner. Please check FDA approval for all manufacturers' probes used in any examination.)

≡ BREAST SONOGRAPHY

- Current studies are showing an increase in detection of Doppler signals in malignant lesions versus nonmalignant lesions.

≡ SCROTAL ULTRASOUND

- The testicular artery has low peripheral resistance with broad systolic peaks and high diastolic flow.

Color Doppler image demonstrating arterial flow in a testicular artery. See Color Plate 8 at the back of this book. (Courtesy of Diasonics, Inc., Milpitas, California.)

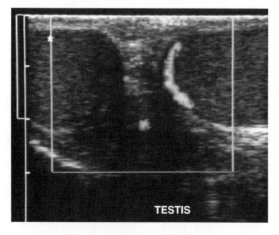

- The deferential artery has high resistance with narrow systolic peaks and low diastolic flow.

- Pathology:
  - (a) Inflammatory conditions:
    Epididymitis.
    Orchitis.
  - (b) Abscesses:
    Demonstrate hypervascularity.
    Have decreased Resistive Indices (RI).
    Gray scale shows decreased echogenicity due to edema.
  - (c) Torsion/ischemia:
    Complete or near complete absence of flow.
    Nuclear medicine is still the study of choice.
  - (d) Neoplasms:
    Gray-scale images remain most helpful in defining masses.
    Doppler or color Doppler may help define vascular tumors.
  - (e) Varicoceles:
    These are often easily visible.
    A vein greater than 3 mm during a Valsalva maneuver is considered a varicocele.

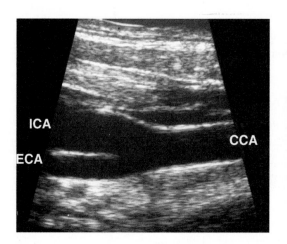

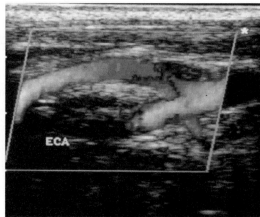

Color Doppler image of the carotid artery bifurcation: See Color Plate 9 at the back of this
book.

Cerebrovascular Duplex Scanning Protocol

CHAPTER
19

Marsha M. Neumyer

LOCATION

- Medial to internal jugular vein.
- Lateral to thyroid gland.
- Posteromedial to the sternocleidomastoid muscle.

ANATOMY

- Right common carotid artery originates from the innominate artery.
- Left common carotid artery originates from the aortic arch.
- At approximately the level of the superior border of the thyroid cartilage, the common carotid artery bifurcates into a more anteromedial external carotid artery and a more posterolateral internal carotid artery.
- The external carotid artery can be differentiated from the internal carotid artery by looking for branches within the neck.
- The internal carotid artery tends to be larger than the external, although size is variable.

PHYSIOLOGY

- The external carotid artery provides vascular flow to the face and facial muscles.
- The internal carotid artery provides blood flow to the brain and the eyes.

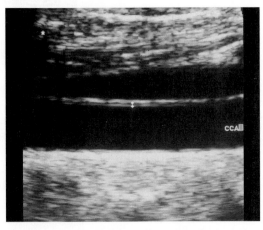

Common carotid artery. (Courtesy of Diasonics, Inc., Milpitas, California.)

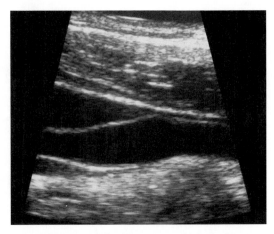

Carotid artery bulb. (Courtesy of Diasonics, Inc., Milpitas, California.)

SONOGRAPHIC APPEARANCE

- The normal vessel lumen should be echo-free.
- If viewing the vessel at a perpendicular angle, you may be able to appreciate the intimal lining.
- Using multiple scan planes, you should be able to image the common, external, and internal carotid arteries as separate vessels.

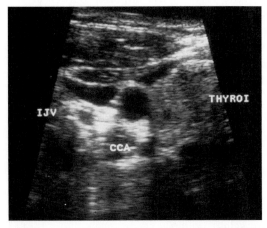

Common carotid artery. Note the sternocleido-mastoid muscle. (Courtesy of Diasonics, Inc., Milpitas, California.)

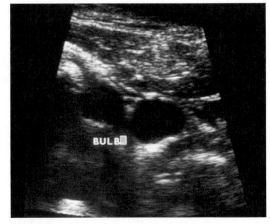

Carotid artery bulb. (Courtesy of Diasonics, Inc., Milpitas, California.)

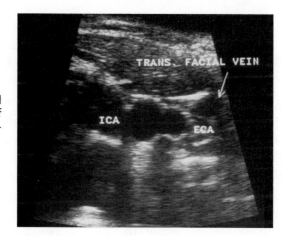

Internal and external carotid artery origins. (Courtesy of Diasonics, Inc., Milpitas, California.)

PATIENT PREP

- None.

PATIENT POSITION

- Supine with the head resting flat and turned slightly away from the side to be scanned. Hyperextension of the neck must be avoided as this will make it difficult to maintain full transducer contact with the skin and may cause the vessels to lie in an inappropriate anatomical plane.
- As the examiner, you should sit at the head of the table with the patient's head directly in front of you. You should be able to rest your elbow on the corner of the table. You must then scan ambidextrously to be easily able to reach the machine.
- Or you may stand next to the patient table and lean one arm across the patient's chest in order to reach the neck. A pillow may be placed over the patient's chest in order to ensure patient comfort.
- The examination may be performed with the patient in an erect position if he or she is unable to lie down.

PULSED DOPPLER TRANSDUCERS

- 10 MHz—better resolution, may not be able to visualize all anatomy if vessels lie deep within the neck.
- 7.5 MHz—allows slightly better penetration.
- 5.0 MHz—may require use of a standoff pad due to decreased resolution unless using a broadband transducer with auto focusing.

SURVEY

1. Begin in anterior, coronal (lateral), or posterior scanning plane.

2. Start on the right side immediately superior to the clavicle. Move laterally and identify the jugular vein. Move medially through the common carotid artery and identify the thyroid gland.

3. Return to a longitudinal view of the common carotid artery and angle as inferiorly as possible in order to view as much of the origin as possible.

4. Move superiorly, continuously rocking through the vessel medial to lateral in order to view as much of the vessel walls as possible.

5. While at the level of the middle common carotid artery, angle the probe in a posterolateral manner and look for the vertebral bodies. Running in between the vertebral bodies you should see the vertebral artery, which often lies posterior to the vertebral vein. Angle the probe in a very slightly medial/lateral manner to ensure the best visualization of the artery. Follow the course of the vertebral artery inferiorly to its origin from the subclavian artery.

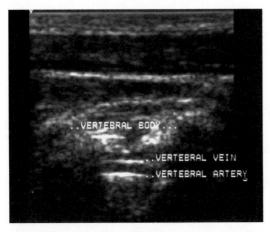

Vertebral artery. (Courtesy of Mary Washington Hospital, Fredericksburg, Virginia.)

6. Angle the probe anteromedially and return to the common carotid survey.

7. Continue superiorly to the level of the bifurcation, then rock in an anteromedial/posterolateral motion and identify both the internal and external cartoid arteries.

8. Continue to move superiorly with a slight posteromedial angle to view the internal carotid artery. Continue to rock lateral to medial to view the vessel walls completely. Follow the vessel as superiorly as possible to the mandible.

N O T E :   As you move superiorly, it may be easier to view a greater length of the internal carotid artery by moving from a more anterior or lateral approach to a more posterior approach.

9. Return inferiorly to the level of the bulb and rock anteromedially to identify the external carotid artery. Move superiorly along the length of the external carotid artery rocking laterally and medially through the vessel to fully visualize walls.

N O T E :   Follow each vessel as superiorly as possible until the mandible makes it impossible to go further.

10. Once you have viewed both the internal and external carotid arteries in a longitudinal plane, move inferiorly again back to the level immediately superior to the clavicle.

11. Rotate the transducer 90 degrees and begin the transverse survey on the right common carotid artery.

12. Angle as inferiorly as possible noting as much of the origin as possible. It may be possible to view the subclavian artery at this level.

13. Move superiorly noting vessel walls and internal components.

14. Make special note of the bifurcation and view the internal and external carotid arteries superiorly to the bifurcation.

15. Follow as superiorly as possible to the mandible.

16. Move inferiorly again to the level of the clavicle. Rotate the probe 90 degrees and begin the spectral survey by turning on the Doppler sample volume (refer to owner's manual for equipment specifications). Follow the vessel longitudinally, adjusting the sample volume to maintain a midvessel location.

17. Be sure to sample adequately throughout the common carotid, bulb, internal and external carotid arteries. Use the smallest sample volume size available. Listen for evidence of disturbed flow.

18. With the sample volume still on, move inferiorly back to a level immediately superior to the clavicle. This acts as a second sampling and ensures a complete Doppler investigation. Now move toward the level of the middle common carotid, and angling the probe posterolateral, sample the vertebral artery.

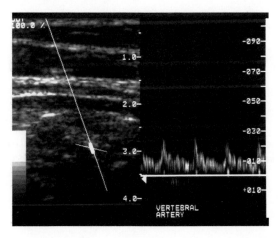

N O T E :   If plaque is present, sample at sites proximal, within, and distal to determine the presence of disturbed flow and significant stenosis.

19. Once flow has been assessed thoroughly in all vessels, you may return to the common carotid artery and begin to obtain the required images.

N O T E :   Deep vessel bifurcation may make it very hard to differentiate vessels by appearance alone. Always use Doppler signals.

N O T E :   Long-standing occlusions of the internal carotid artery may cause an enlargement of the external carotid artery and its branches, which may cause erroneous vessel identification.

N O T E :   Normal flow disturbance is possible and should not be mistaken for pathology. Look for vessel bends or kinks.

N O T E :   When scanning with color Doppler, it is easiest to turn the color Doppler on after the longitudinal and transverse gray scale survey.

20. Once the transverse survey has been completed, return to the level of the clavicle and turn on the color Doppler. Set color gains and other controls.

21. Then perform a transverse survey in the same manner as you would a gray scale survey pass. You may need to scan more slowly to allow proper color filling of the vessel lumen.

22. When you have scanned as superiorly as possible, again return to the level of the clavicle. Rotate the probe 90 degrees and adjust the color

Spectral display of vertebral artery blood flow. (Courtesy of Mary Washington Hospital, Fredericksburg, Virginia.)

Doppler steering angle according to the course of the vessel. Follow the vessel superiorly. It is often necessary to change the steering angle at least once as the vessel changes lie. The steering angle should remain as close to parallel to the angle of flow as possible.

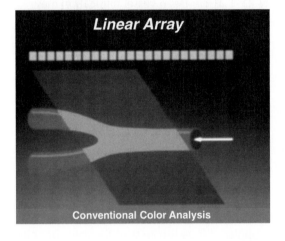

Color Doppler angle adjustment. (Courtesy of Diasonics, Inc., Milpitas, California.)

23. Once the common, internal, and external carotid vessels have been thoroughly investigated, you may return to the level of the middle common carotid artery, locate the vertebral artery, and confirm flow.

24. You may then return to the level of the clavicle and begin to obtain your spectral tracings.

25. Color Doppler may be left on for the remainder of the examination, although color Doppler cannot replace the spectral analysis throughout the vessel. It may, however, help you to identify high-velocity jets through which you may want to sample more carefully.

REQUIRED IMAGES

1. Longitudinal image of the right proximal common carotid artery.

LABELED: SAG RT PCCA

2. Spectral waveform from the right proximal common carotid artery with peak systolic and end diastolic velocities measured.

LABELED: RT PCCA

3. Longitudinal image of the right distal common carotid artery.

LABELED: SAG RT DCCA

4. Spectral waveform from the right distal common carotid artery with peak systolic and end diastolic velocities measured.

LABELED: RT DCCA

5. Longitudinal image of the right proximal internal carotid artery showing its origin from the bulb.

L A B E L E D : SAG RT PICA

6. Spectral waveform from the proximal internal carotid artery with peak systolic and end diastolic velocities measured.

L A B E L E D : DIST RT ICA

7. Longitudinal image of the right middle internal carotid artery.

L A B E L E D : SAG RT MICA

8. Spectral waveform from the middle internal carotid artery with peak systolic and end diastolic velocities measured.

L A B E L E D : RT MICA

9. Longitudinal image of the right distal internal carotid artery.

L A B E L E D : SAG RT DICA

10. Spectral waveform from the distal internal carotid artery with peak systolic and end diastolic velocities measured.

L A B E L E D : RT DICA

11. Longitudinal image of the right external carotid artery.

L A B E L E D : SAG RT ECA

12. Spectral waveform from the external carotid artery with peak systolic and end diastolic velocities measured.

L A B E L E D : RT ECA

13. Optional longitudinal image of the right vertebral artery.

L A B E L E D : SAG RT VERT

N O T E : The spectral image of this vessel is often not satisfactory because of the depth of the vertebral vessels.

14. Spectral waveform from the right vertebral artery with peak systolic and end diastolic velocities measured.

L A B E L E D : RT VERT

15. Transverse image of the carotid bulb just prior to vessel bifurcation.

L A B E L E D :   TRV RT BULB

N O T E :   Repeat the required images on the left side beginning with a thorough survey.

N O T E :   The image and spectral data from the vertebral arteries and the subclavian are required for billing a *complete* carotid examination and for vascular laboratory accreditation.

N O T E :   Even in the absence of pathology, it is important to carefully image the bulb. It is thought that this area is most prone to atherosclerosis due to the shear forces imposed on the vessel wall by the blood flow patterns and the vessel geometry. Stenotic lesions are often asymptomatic until they reduce the diameter of the vessel lumen by more than 60%. Lesser lesions may occasionally be detected only with careful, thorough scanning in the transverse plane.

N O T E :   Stenotic plaque may be measured in the transverse plane to ensure accuracy.

N O T E :   Additional images of plaque may be necessary. It is important to look for irregularities along the borders of the plaque, which may indicate ulcerations.

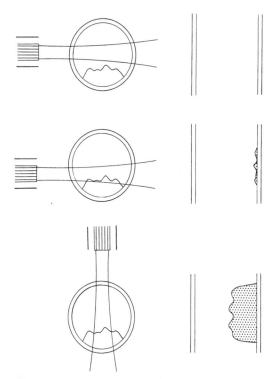

The importance of thoroughly examining the vessel is shown here. With an improper survey, this plaque might be missed.

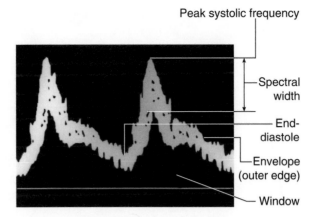

Example of a spectral display from the carotid arteries.

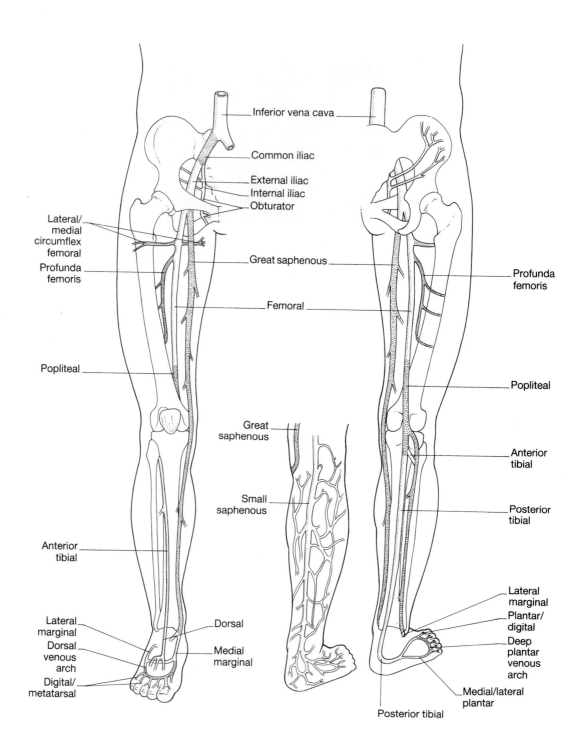

Inferior vena cava

Common iliac

External iliac
Internal iliac
Obturator

Lateral/
medial
circumflex
femoral

Profunda
femoris

Great saphenous

Profunda
femoris

Femoral

Popliteal

Popliteal

Great
saphenous

Anterior
tibial

Small
saphenous

Posterior
tibial

Anterior
tibial

Lateral
marginal
Plantar/
digital

Lateral
marginal
Dorsal
venous
arch

Dorsal

Deep
plantar
venous
arch

Medial
marginal

Digital/
metatarsal

Medial/lateral
plantar

Posterior tibial

**VENOUS SYSTEM OF
THE LOWER LIMB**

Normal deep and superficial venous anatomy of the legs.

Peripheral Arterial and Venous Duplex Scanning Protocols

CHAPTER

20

Marsha M. Neumyer

LOWER EXTREMITY VENOUS DUPLEX ULTRASONOGRAPHY

- Purpose: to noninvasively determine the presence of venous thrombosis.

≡ ANATOMY

- The common femoral vein (CFV) lies medial to the common femoral artery (CFA).
- The superficial vein (SFV) lies posterior to the superficial femoral artery (SFA) superiorly.
- The SFV follows a medial course along the inner curve of the thigh and at its inferior aspect, just superior to the knee, lies posterior to the SFA.
- The popliteal vein lies posterior and lateral to the popliteal artery.
- The saphenous vein is located medial to the SFV and CFV at the level of the SFV insertion.
- Valves are located in the larger veins to prevent the back flow of blood. These are commonly seen in the CFV, SFV, and popliteal veins.
- The deep femoral vein or profunda vein is found posterior to the SFV with its insertion at approximately the same level.
- All veins are thin-walled and collapse easily with a minimum of pressure.

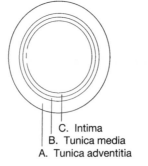
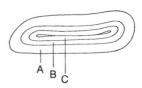

Noncompressed and compressed images of a vein.

C. Intima
B. Tunica media
A. Tunica adventitia

A B C

≡ PATIENT PREP

- None.

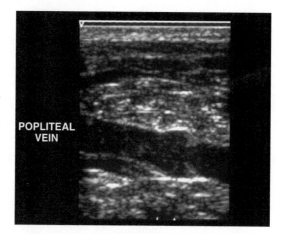

Gray-scale image demonstrating a venous valve. (Courtesy of ATL, Bothell, Washington.)

POPLITEAL VEIN

≡ PATIENT POSITION

- Supine with the examination table in the reversed Trendelenberg position to promote venous pooling.

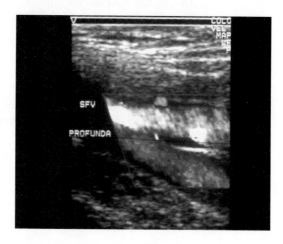

Color flow Doppler image at the level of the SFV and profunda vein insertions. See Color Plate 10 at the back of this book. (Courtesy of ATL, Bothell, Washington.)

SFV

PROFUNDA

☰ TRANSDUCER

- 5.0 or 7.0 MHz linear array with Doppler and/or color Doppler capabilities.

☰ NORMAL SONOGRAPHIC FINDINGS

- There are five normal findings in duplex sonography of the lower extremity venous system.
  - (a) Spontaneous flow: Doppler interrogation of the vessel should demonstrate flow without necessity to augment manually or with Valsalva maneuver. A lack of flow may suggest thrombosis or extrinsic compression of the vessel.
  - (b) Phasicity: Doppler flow patterns vary because of the patient's respiratory changes:

    There will be a decrease in flow during inspiration due to increased intraabdominal pressure.

    Flow will increase with expiration. Continuous flow with no noticeable respiratory changes suggest a proximal obstruction.
  - (c) Augmentation: with distal compression there should be a sudden rush of venous flow superiorly. This indicates no complete thrombosis between the transducer and the point of compression.

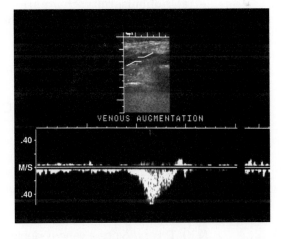

Doppler spectral display demonstrating venous augmentation. (Courtesy of Mary Washington Hospital, Fredericksburg, Virginia.)

N O T E :   If you need to compress a vein a second time to assess augmentation, you will need to wait a few seconds between compressions to allow the vein to refill distally.

  - (d) Competence of venous valves: with proximal compression of the veins the presence of competent valves should prevent remarkable retrograde (inferior) flow.

    If retrograde flow is noted with firm, extended proximal compression or release of distal compression of the limb, valvular incompetence is suggested. Incompetence may be caused by varicose veins or the presence of old clot which has left the valve leaflets stiff and nonpliable.

A minimal amount of retrograde flow may be noted if quick, hard compressions are applied to the limb. Such compressions do not allow enough time for the valve leaflets to close adequately.

A Valsalva maneuver may also be used to assess valvular competence.

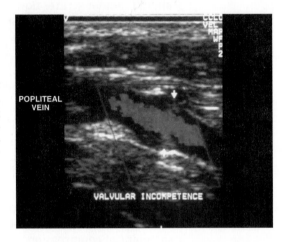

Color Doppler image demonstrating valvular incompetence. See Color Plate 11 at the back of this book. (Courtesy of ATL, Bothell, Washington.)

(e) Nonpulsatility: there are flow variations with respiratory cycles, not with each heartbeat.

N O T E :   Pulsatile venous flow suggests congestive heart failure, fluid overload, or tricuspid insufficiency.

≡ EXAM PROTOCOL AND REQUIRED IMAGES

N O T E :   Examination of veins is easiest in a transverse plane, but longitudinal imaging should also be performed to help ensure adequate venous mapping (so that no small thrombosis is missed) and assessment of the venous valves especially with color flow Doppler.

N O T E :   Since a venous duplex examination requires a thorough mapping of the veins, it is unnecessary to perform a "survey" and then a more detailed exam to obtain images. Images may be obtained as you go. A diagnosis is rarely made from hard copy alone in this exam.

N O T E :   Always examine both legs for comparative purposes. It may be helpful to examine the asymptomatic leg first.

- Begin transversely high on the thigh at or above the level of the groin crease. Locate the CFV and CFA.

To confirm that you are in the CFV, identify the insertion of the saphenous vein and the bifurcation into the SFV and the profunda femoris vein (PFV).

- Assess the entire length of the CFV for compressibility by compressing every 1 to 2 cm. The walls of the CFA should not deform with adequate compression of the vein.

1. Images of noncompressed and compressed common femoral vein (on split screen if available).

L A B E L E D :   LT or RT CFV

N O T E :   For split screen imaging use the left side for non-compressed views and the right side for compressed.

- Still at the level of the CFV turn on the Doppler placing the cursor toward flow.

  Spontaneous, phasic flow should be present throughout the CFV.

2. Duplex image of Doppler spectral CFV waveform demonstrating respiratory changes and augmentation.

L A B E L E D :   RT or LT CFV

- Return to a gray scale image. Move inferiorly and locate the insertion of the saphenous vein medially.

  Assess the proximal portion of the saphenous vein for compressibility.

N O T E :   A complete exam requires assessment of the entire length of the greater saphenous vein.

3. Images of noncompressed and compressed saphenous vein (split screen).

L A B E L E D :   RT or LT SAPH V

- Investigate the saphenous vein with Doppler to confirm normal flow characteristics.

4. Duplex image of a Doppler spectral waveform from the saphenous vein demonstrating augmentation and respiratory changes.

L A B E L E D :   RT or LT SAPH V

- Return to gray scale imaging and return to the level of the CFV. Move inferiorly to locate the insertion of the profunda vein. This lies posterior and lateral to the SFV. Follow this vein as inferiorly as possible assessing compressibility.

N O T E :   Compressibility may be difficult to assess in vessels lying deep or tangent to the skin.

5. Images of noncompressed and compressed profunda vein (split screen).

L A B E L E D :   RT or LT PROF V

- Return superiorly to the deep vein insertion and begin sampling with Doppler. Assess for normal characteristics. Follow as inferiorly as possible.

6. Duplex image of a Doppler spectral waveform from the profunda vein demonstrating augmentation and respiratory changes.

L A B E L E D :   RT or LT PROF V

- Return to a gray scale image and move superior to the level of the SFV insertion. Begin following that vein inferiorly compressing every 1 to 2 cm at a level near its insertion.

7. Images of noncompressed and compressed superficial femoral vein near its insertion (split screen).

L A B E L E D :   RT or LT SFV SUP

- Sample the same segment of vein with Doppler. Assess for normal characteristics.

8. Duplex image of a Doppler spectral waveform from the SFV near its insertion demonstrating augmentation and respiratory changes.

L A B E L E D :   RT or LT SFV

- Return to a gray scale image and continue to follow the SFV inferiorly assessing for compressibility.

N O T E :   Make very careful note of vein compressibility because that is the most important indicator of venous thrombosis.

9. Images of noncompressed and compressed superficial femoral vein at approximately midthigh (split screen).

L A B E L E D :   RT or LT SFV MID

- Sample SFV at a midthigh level with Doppler. Assess for normal characteristics.

10. Duplex image of a Doppler spectral waveform from the SFV at midthigh level demonstrating augmentation and respiratory changes.

L A B E L E D :   RT or LT SFV MID

- Return to a gray scale image and investigate the remaining segment of SFV, compressing at regular intervals.

N O T E :   As you approach Hunter's canal just superior to the knee, compression is often very difficult if possible at all. This is due to the tendons present here.

11. Images of noncompressed and compressed superficial femoral vein as inferiorly as possible (split screen).

L A B E L E D :   RT or LT SFV INF

- Doppler in the SFV just superior to the knee. The vein will have passed medially and now lies posterior to the artery.
  Augmentation is especially important here because compression is often less than adequate.

12. Duplex image of a Doppler spectral waveform from the SFV just superior to the knee demonstrating augmentation.

L A B E L E D :   RT or LT SFV INF

- The popliteal veins can be examined either with the patient prone or with the knee bent and relaxed away from the patient to the side.

N O T E :   Document any vessel duplication, which is fairly common at this level. If there is more than one popliteal vessel they must both be carefully examined.

- Locate the popliteal vein posterior to the artery and assess for normal characteristics.
  Follow the vein as far superiorly behind the thigh as possible. Continue to assess compression.
  Begin to move inferiorly, following the popliteal vein to the level of its bifurcation into the anterior tibial trunk and the tibio-peroneal trunk. Follow the tibio-peroneal trunk to the level where it bifurcates into the posterior tibial and peroneal trunks.
  Once the entire length of the popliteal vein has been adequately assessed for compressibility, return to a mid-popliteal level.

13. Images of noncompressed and compressed popliteal vein at its midpoint (split screen).

L A B E L E D :   RT or LT POP V MID

- Sample with Doppler throughout the entire length of the popliteal vessels. At mid-popliteal level:

14. Duplex image of a Doppler spectral waveform from the midpopliteal vein demonstrating augmentation.

L A B E L E D :   RT or LT POP V MID

N O T E :   It may be awkward to squeeze a patient's thigh and maintain transducer location at the same time. Having the patient quickly flex the ipsilateral foot will have a similar effect.

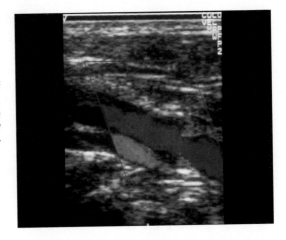

Color Doppler image of popliteal vein and artery. See Color Plate 12 at the back of this book. (Courtesy of ATL, Bothell, Washington.)

- Color Doppler may be used to rescan the entire leg in a longitudinal plane.

  Color Doppler provides a visual means of assessing spontaneous flow, augmentation, and valve competence.

- To assess valve competence we rescan quickly to locate a venous valve (this may be done within the scanning protocol of that particular venous segment) and scan to a level just inferior to the valve.

  While observing color flow Doppler (or a spectral waveform), squeeze the patient's leg superior to the valve. If the valve is too superior to the scanning site, have the patient take in a deep breath, hold it, bear down hard, and release (Valsalva maneuver).

  There should be no remarkable amount of retrograde (inferior) venous blood flow through the valve. Significant retrograde flow indicates the presence of an incompetent valve.

  Any valve can be examined in this manner.

- Examine only the deep veins of the thigh.

  It has been shown that the majority of life-threatening pulmonary emboli originate in the proximal deep veins of the leg. Although pulmonary emboli may originate from the smaller veins of the calf, these emboli are usually not clinically significant. Controversy regarding the importance of detecting and treating isolated calf vein thrombi still exists.

- Repeat on the affected leg.

≡ PATHOLOGY

Noncompressible Veins

- Clot: With acute thrombosis of the vein, the vein lumen may be enlarged when compared with the same vein at that level in the opposite leg and usually contains some internal low to medium echoes.

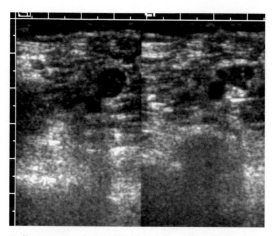

Split screen of clot-filled vein. Note small residual or recanalized lumen. (Courtesy of Mary Washington Hospital, Fredericksburg, Virginia.)

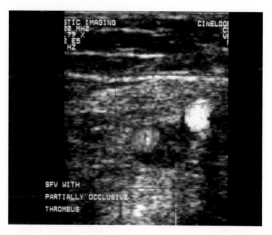

Color Doppler image demonstrating thrombus in the SFV. See Color Plate 13 at the back of this book. (Courtesy of ATL, Bothell, Washington.)

Flow may be present if recanalization (reopening of the lumen) has begun.

- Proximal obstruction: venous flow may be decreased and/or continuous. There are often no respiratory changes seen.

    The size of the vein may increase.

- Some veins are normally noncompressible due to

    (a) Depth within the tissues

    (b) Angle or course relevant to the transducer plane of compression

    (c) Position relevant to boney processes

- Chronic thrombosis: the vessel walls may be scarred after an episode of venous thrombosis. The vein walls may be thickened, preventing complete compressibility. Be aware of the patient's history. Prior phlebitic episodes may have resulted in valvular incompetence. Assess carefully.

Baker's Cyst

- A loculated fluid collection behind the knee (usually laterally) may cause leg swelling resulting from compression of the popliteal vein and associated poor venous drainage.

Cellulitis

- General inflammation of the skin and interstitial tissues of the leg. This most often affects the ankle and calf.

    The legs are often red and shiny.

    The deep veins may be more difficult to visualize because of the inflammation present.

    There is often increased echogenicity of the inflamed tissues, which may obscure vein visualization.

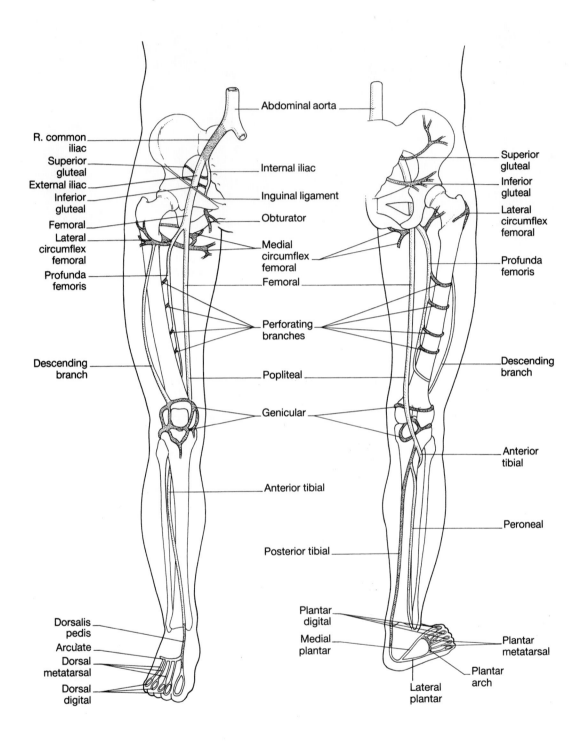

R. common iliac

Superior gluteal

External iliac

Inferior gluteal

Femoral

Lateral circumflex femoral

Profunda femoris

Descending branch

Dorsalis pedis

Arcuate

Dorsal metatarsal

Dorsal digital

Abdominal aorta

Internal iliac

Inguinal ligament

Obturator

Medial circumflex femoral

Femoral

Perforating branches

Popliteal

Genicular

Anterior tibial

Posterior tibial

Plantar digital

Medial plantar

Lateral plantar

Plantar arch

Plantar metatarsal

Superior gluteal

Inferior gluteal

Lateral circumflex femoral

Profunda femoris

Descending branch

Anterior tibial

Peroneal

**ARTERIAL SYSTEM OF
THE LOWER LIMB**

LOWER EXTREMITY PERIPHERAL ARTERIAL DUPLEX ULTRASONOGRAPHY

- Purpose: to noninvasively determine the presence, amount, and location of arterial disease and plaque accumulation in the legs.
  - (a) To assess claudication (pain in the leg associated with exercise and relieved by rest). The pain occurs because there is an increased need for blood flow to the large muscle groups in the leg following exercise, but an inadequate blood supply because of arterial blockage due to disease.
  - (b) To assess graft patency (no blood pressures should be taken over or very close to a graft site. This could cause a leakage of blood at an anastomosis).

≡ PATIENT PREP

- You may need to fast the patient for 8 to 12 hours prior to an examination of the abdominal aorta and iliac arteries.

≡ TRANSDUCER

- 5.0- or 7.0-MHz linear probe with Doppler and/or color Doppler capabilities. A 3.0-MHz probe is also helpful to examine the distal aorta and proximal iliac arteries.

≡ NECESSARY EQUIPMENT

- Arm blood pressure cuff.
- Adult thigh blood pressure cuffs.

≡ EXAM PROTOCOL AND REQUIRED IMAGES

- Beginning with the patient in a supine position, obtain bilateral brachial blood pressures. Record on worksheet (see section on blood pressures).
- With the patient in supine position, palpate the following pulses:
  Groin (iliac/common femoral artery)
  Popliteal
  Posterior tibial
  Dorsalis pedis
- Using a low frequency probe (2.25 to 3.0 MHz), the distal aorta and proximal iliac arteries may be examined in both longitudinal and transverse planes.

  1. Longitudinal view of the distal aorta.

  L A B E L E D :   SAG AORTA DIS

  2. Longitudinal view of the right iliac artery.

  L A B E L E D :   SAG RT ILIAC

3. Longitudinal view of the left iliac artery.

L A B E L E D :   SAG LT ILIAC

N O T E :   The iliac arteries may be examined simultaneously from a coronal plane with the patient in a right lateral decubitus position.

4. Transverse view of the distal aorta.

L A B E L E D :   TRV AORTA DIS

5. Transverse view of the right and left iliac arteries.

L A B E L E D :   TRV RT/LT ILIAC

N O T E :   If one leg is significantly more symptomatic than the other, begin with the less symptomatic leg.

- Begin scanning with a 5.0- or 7.0-MHz transducer. You will need to start superior to the groin crease in a sagittal plane. Locate the common femoral artery (CFA).
- Sample with Doppler thoroughly to assess blood flow velocity and waveform morphology throughout the length of the CFA.
  Use simultaneous imaging for duplex studies if available. Although this may slightly decrease image resolution on some ultrasound systems, it will make scanning much quicker.

N O T E :   If simultaneous imaging is not available, you will have to B-scan for a short segment, freeze an image, then move a Doppler cursor thoroughly over that frozen image, and continue on to the next segment through the entire vessel.

Normal triphasic arterial signal from a high-resistance system.

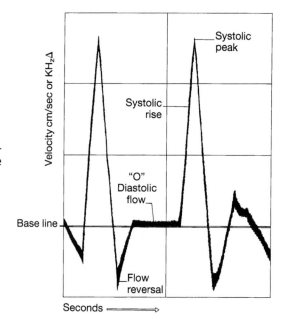

6. Longitudinal gray scale view of the common femoral artery.

L A B E L E D :   SAG RT or LT CFA

7. Dopper spectral waveform of the CFA.

L A B E L E D :   RT or LT CFA

- The CFA will bifurcate into the superficial femoral artery (SFA) and the deep femoral or profunda femoris artery.
- Follow the profunda femoris artery as inferiorly as possible with duplex sampling.

8. Longitudinal view of the profunda femoris artery origin.

L A B E L E D :   SAG RT or LT PROF ART

9. Doppler spectral waveform of the profunda femoris artery near its insertion.

L A B E L E D :   SAG RT or LT PROF ART

N O T E :   It may be difficult to follow the profunda for more than a few centimeters because the vessel usually courses deep into the leg. If you are able to follow the profunda artery for a longer length, another set of images should be documented more inferiorly along the vessel.

- Return superiorly to the level of the bifurcation and locate the SFA. Follow this artery inferiorly to just above the knee.

10. Longitudinal view of the superficial femoral artery origin.

L A B E L E D :   SAG RT or LT PROX SFA

11. Doppler spectral waveform of the SFA near its origin.

L A B E L E D :   SAG RT or LT PROX SFA

12. Longitudinal view of the SFA at approximately midthigh.

L A B E L E D :   SAG RT or LT MID SFA

13. Duplex spectral waveform at midthigh.

L A B E L E D :   SAG RT or LT MID SFA

14. Longitudinal view of the SFA just superior to the knee.

L A B E L E D :   SAG RT or LT DIST SFA

15. Duplex spectral waveform just superior to knee SFA.

L A B E L E D :   SAG RT or LT DIST SFA

• Next the popliteal artery is to be examined. This may be done in a number of ways. The patient may be placed in a prone position with the knee slightly flexed, the leg may be bent slightly and positioned out to the side away from the patient, or the patient may be placed in a lateral decubitus position with the knee slightly flexed.

Placing the patient in a prone position will allow for a more direct, easier approach, but it may be difficult or time-consuming to have the patient roll over.

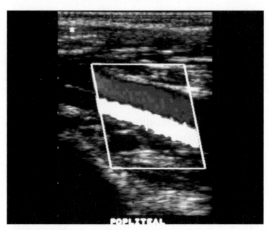

Color Doppler image of the popliteal artery. See Color Plate 14 at the back of this book. (Courtesy of Diasonics, Inc., Milpitas, California.)

• Locate the popliteal artery posterior and slightly lateral to the vein.

Follow the artery as superiorly as possible into the thigh while gray scale imaging.

Begin duplex scanning and follow the artery inferiorly to the superior aspect of the calf to the level of the vessel trifurcation into the anterior tibial, posterior tibial, and peroneal arteries.

16. Longitudinal view of the popliteal artery.

L A B E L E D :   SAG RT or LT POP ART

17. Doppler spectral waveform of the popliteal artery.

L A B E L E D :   SAG RT or LT POP ART

• The tibial arteries may be evaluated using color Doppler.
It may be helpful to follow the arteries up the left from the ankle if there is any difficulty following them down the calf.

• After examining the popliteal artery, move down to the patient's ankle to examine the posterior tibial artery (PT) and dorsalis pedis artery (DP).

All three tibial arteries should be sampled with Doppler using a high frequency transducer.

N O T E :   Gray scale images may be taken to demonstrate pathology.

18. Doppler spectral waveform of the posterior tibial artery.

L A B E L E D :   SAG RT or LT PT

19. Doppler spectral waveform of the dosalis pedis artery.

L A B E L E D :   SAG RT or LT DP

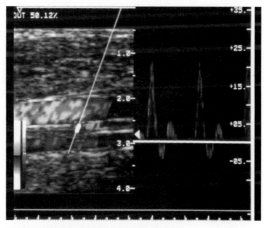

Spectral analysis of the posterior artery demonstrating normal triphasic flow. See Color Plate 15 at the back of this book. (Courtesy of ATL, Bothell, Washington.)

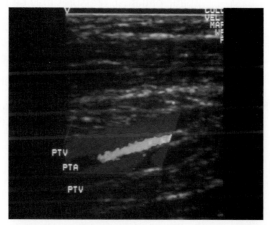

Color flow Doppler image of the posterior tibial artery and vein. See Color Plate 16 at the back of this book. (Courtesy of ATL, Bothell, Washington.)

N O T E :   Determine the strongest and most easily accessible artery to use for pressure monitoring.

Duplex ultrasonography is used to complement arterial assessment using indirect noninvasive physiologic studies. Ankle brachial indices, segmental systolic pressure measurements, pulse volume recording photoplethysmography, and constant-load exercise testing are among the more common procedures employed for primary evaluation. The scope of this chapter does not permit detailed discussion of each of these physiologic test modalities. A brief description of the protocol for segmental systolic pressure measurements follows. The reader is referred to the references listed at the end of this section for additional information.

- Cuff placement depends on whether a 3-cuff or 4-cuff method is to be used. If the 4-cuff procedure is used, appropriately-sized cuffs are to be placed as follows:
  (a) As high as possible on the thigh.
  (b) Just above the knee.
  (c) Just below the knee.
  (d) Just above the ankle.

  If the 3-cuff technique is used, a wide thigh cuff is placed snugly over the thigh and below knee and above ankle cuffs are used.

  Inaccurate blood pressures will be measured if inappropriate cuff sizes are used. It is necessary to use only cuffs that are at least 20% wider than the diameter of the limb at that segment.

- Start at ankle level and measure the pressure at each cuff level, moving superiorly. The popliteal artery signal may be used, if necessary, to measure the thigh pressures.

- Repeat on the contralateral leg.

N O T E :   It may be difficult to obtain a high thigh pressure on obese patients. When the arterial wall is calcified (i.e., with diabetic patients), pressures may be falsely elevated.

N O T E :   If the high thigh pressure is reduced, the Doppler spectral waveform from the common femoral artery will indicate the likelihood of more proximal disease.

Normally, the waveform will be triphasic.

If the CFA Doppler signal demonstrates loss of the reverse diastolic flow component, occlusive disease of the common or external iliac artery is suggested. If the CFA signal is abnormal bilaterally, aorto-iliac disease is indicated.

≡ DATA DOCUMENTATION

Using Blood Pressures

• The severity of atherosclerotic disease may be assessed by using the ankle/arm index.

A/A INDEX

> 1.13.......Arterial calcifications

\+ 1.0.........Normal

0.9-1.0........Minimal ischemia with minimal
 symptoms

0.5-0.9........Mild to moderate ischemia with mild to
 moderate claudication

0.3-0.5........Moderate to severe ischemia with
 severe claudication or rest pain

< 0.3.........Severe ischemia with rest pain or
 gangrene

N O T E : A pressure drop greater than 20 mmHg between two cuffs suggests the presence of flow-reducing stenosis or occlusion proximal to or beneath the measuring cuff. If a 4-cuff technique is used (narrow high thigh cuff), the high thigh pressure should be 30-40 mmHg higher than the highest brachial systolic pressure. Pressures should be compared both vertically on the limb and horizontally, comparing pressures at each cuff site with the pressure in the cuff at the same level on the contralateral limb.

Without Blood Pressures

• Waveform morphology.
  (a) Triphasic signals: have a strong forward systolic component followed by a brief period of diastolic flow reversal and then an end diastolic forward flow segment. This is due to the high resistance flow present in the legs.
  (b) Biphasic signals: have a strong forward systolic component followed by a period of diastolic flow reversal. There is no end diastolic forward flow component. This is frequently seen in elderly patients due to loss of vessel wall elasticity.

- Study impression.
  - (a) Normal-Triphasic signals: may be biphasic in the elderly. No evidence of spectral broadening.
  - (b) 1–19% diameter-reducing stenosis: normal peak systolic velocity; spectral broadening during the deceleration phase of systole. Reverse diastolic flow component remains.
  - (c) 20–49% diameter-reducing stenosis: more than a 30% increase in peak systolic velocity compared to the proximal normal segment; spectral broadening with loss of systolic window; proximal and distal Doppler waveforms are unchanged.
  - (d) 50–79% diameter-reducing stenosis: may be 100% increase in peak systolic velocity compared to more proximal segment; marked spectral broadening; loss of the diastolic flow reversal; proximal waveform remains unchanged; distal waveform may show post-stenotic turbulence.
  - (e) 80–99% diameter-reducing stenosis: more than 100% increase in peak systolic velocity; monophasic signals; a "thumping" signal just proximal to critical stenosis or occlusion; distal waveform will be dampened.
  - (f) Occluded: no Doppler signal or color flow display in an imaged vessel. Collateral vessels may be imaged at the site of reentry and reconstitution of the artery.

MARY WASHINGTON HOSPITAL
PERIPHERAL ARTERIAL STUDY WORKSHEET

NAME: _____   DATE: _____

X RAY #: _____   DOCTOR: _____

AGE: _____

SYMPTOMS: _____

CLAUDICATION: R   L   DIABETES: Y   N   HYPERTENSION: Y   N

PULSES: RT   LT

RADIAL   _____   _____
ULNAR   _____   _____
FEMORAL   _____   _____
PT   _____   _____
DP   _____   _____

BLOOD PRESSURES: RT   LT

        BRACHIAL: _____   _____

                                        RT CIA   LT CIA

RT A/A INDEX: RT FEM A   LT FEM A

    _____

                                        RT POP BP   LT POP BP

LT A/A INDEX: _____   _____

    _____   RT PT   LT PT

                                        _____   _____

An example of a worksheet for a peripheral arterial examination utilizing blood pressure. (Courtesy of Mary Washington Hospital, Fredericksburg, Virginia.)

Echocardiography

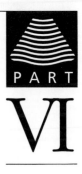

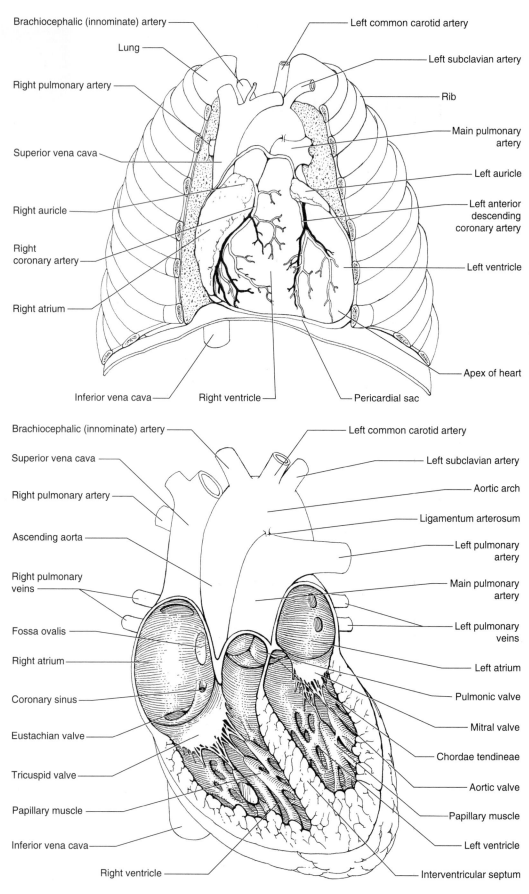

Brachiocephalic (innominate) artery

Lung

Right pulmonary artery

Superior vena cava

Right auricle

Right coronary artery

Right atrium

Left common carotid artery

Left subclavian artery

Rib

Main pulmonary artery

Left auricle

Left anterior descending coronary artery

Left ventricle

Apex of heart

Inferior vena cava

Right ventricle

Pericardial sac

Brachiocephalic (innominate) artery

Superior vena cava

Right pulmonary artery

Ascending aorta

Right pulmonary veins

Fossa ovalis

Right atrium

Coronary sinus

Eustachian valve

Tricuspid valve

Papillary muscle

Inferior vena cava

Right ventricle

Left common carotid artery

Left subclavian artery

Aortic arch

Ligamentum arterosum

Left pulmonary artery

Main pulmonary artery

Left pulmonary veins

Left atrium

Pulmonic valve

Mitral valve

Chordae tendineae

Aortic valve

Papillary muscle

Left ventricle

Interventricular septum

Anatomy of the adult heart

Adult Echocardiography Scanning Protocol

CHAPTER

21

Maureen E. McDonald

LOCATION

- The heart is found within the thoracic cavity in a space called the middle mediastinum.
- Posterior to the ribs and lungs, it is located between the third to fifth intercostal spaces.
- Upper portion, or **base** of the heart, lies closer to the sternum than the lower portion, or **apex,** which lies inferior and to the left of midline.
- Apex is slightly more anterior than the base.

ANATOMY

- The heart is a muscle consisting of three layers:
  - (a) **Epicardium** (smooth, thin outer layer).
  - (b) **Myocardium** (thicker, muscular layer).
  - (c) **Endocardium** (smooth, thin inner surface).
- The heart sits within a sac called the **pericardium** and is surrounded by a small amount of serous fluid to prevent friction as the heart beats.
- The heart has four chambers. The two upper chambers are the right and left **atria.** The two lower chambers are the right and left **ventricles.**
- The upper portion of both atria have a small triangular extension called an **appendage** (a.k.a. auricle) that is tightly lined with muscle called **pectinate muscle.**
- The right atrium's (RA) lining is mostly smooth with some pectinate muscle on the free wall. It receives unoxygenated blood from three major sources:
  - (a) Superior vena cava (SVC) (enters the chamber from above)
  - (b) Inferior vena cava (IVC) (enters from below)
  - (c) Coronary sinus (found between the IVC and the opening to the RV)

- The IVC and coronary sinus have prominent edges that represent remnants of valves that once covered them during fetal days. These are the **eustachian valve** and the **thebesian valve** respectively.
- The Mid-posterior RA wall is also the interatrial septum. It has a thinner area in the mid portion representing the **fossa ovalis.**

N O T E :   During fetal circulation, the fossa ovalis serves as a passage to the left heart, allowing most of the blood to bypass the undeveloped lungs.

- The left atrium (LA) is also smooth walled and receives oxygenated blood from four pulmonary veins. This is the most posterior chamber.
- The right ventricle (RV) is the most anterior chamber whose inner surface is lined with bands of muscle called **trabeculae carneae.** There is a dense band of tissue in the distal part of the chamber that runs perpendicular to the interventricular septum called the **moderator band.**
- The **interventricular septum** (IVS) separates the RV from the LV and consists of mostly muscular tissue with the exception of a small portion of membranous tissue near the insertion of the valves.
- The left ventricle (LV) is more trabeculated than the RV and the walls are also much thicker. The LV makes up the apex of the heart.
- The heart also has four valves that control blood flow in and out of the chambers. There are two atrioventricular (A-V) valves that control the blood flow from the atria to the ventricles and two semilunar valves that control blood flow from the ventricles to the great vessels.
- The mitral and tricuspid valves are the A-V valves. Their leaflets attach to a ring of dense tissue between the chambers called the **annulus fibrosus.** From the free edges of the leaflets are multiple strong, thin fibers called **chordae tendineae.** These chords attach to cone-shaped projections of muscle from the ventricular walls called **papillary muscles.**
- The **mitral valve** is located between the LA and LV and has two leaflets: the anterior leaflet and the posterior leaflet. Also known as the bicuspid valve, its chords attach to the anterolateral and posteromedial papillary muscles.
- The **tricuspid valve** is found between the RA and RV and has three leaflets: the anterior, posterior, and septal. There are three papillary muscles in the RV where the tricuspid chords attach: the anterior, posterior, and septal papillary muscles.
- The semilunar valves are the aortic and pulmonic valves. They are crescent shaped and have no chords or papillary muscles associated with them.

- The **aortic valve** is found in the left heart between the LV and the aortic root and has three cusps: the right coronary cusp, left coronary cusp, and the noncoronary cusp.
- The **pulmonic valve** has three cusps: the anterior, right, and left cusp and is located between the RV and the main pulmonary artery.
- The main pulmonary artery and the aorta comprise the great vessels. These are found at the base or superior aspect of the heart. A short ligament, the **ligamentum arteriosum,** connects the two.

N O T E :   The ligamentum arteriosum was once the ductus arteriosus in the fetus. Blood would flow through the duct from the pulmonary artery to the aorta, bypassing the lungs.

- The **aorta** arises from the ventricle and is divided into three regions: the ascending, arch, and descending aorta. There are three vessels that originate from the arch: the brachiocephalic (a.k.a. innominate), left common carotid, and left subclavian arteries. The brachiocephalic branch is directed rightward and bifurcates into the right common carotid and right subclavian arteries.
- The **main pulmonary artery** (PA) begins at the infundibular region of the RV and moves anteriorly before it bifurcates into the right and left pulmonary arteries. The right PA is directed toward the right lung and moves posterior to the aortic arch. The left PA branches in the direction of the left lung.
- Just beyond the aortic valve are three small crescent-shaped pouches called the **Sinus of Valsalva.** Each is associated with one of the aortic cusps. The right coronary artery originates from the right cusp sinus and the left coronary artery from the left cusp sinus. The remaining sinus has no coronary artery associated with it, hence the name noncoronary cusp.
- The left main coronary artery bifurcates shortly after its origin into the left anterior descending (LAD) and the left circumflex artery. These are found embedded in fat on the exterior surface of the heart. The fat is there to protect the vessels. The LAD runs inferiorly down the anterior interventricular sulcus which is a groove separating the RV from the LV. The left circumflex is located posterolateral to the LAD and runs partly in the atrioventricular groove (a.k.a. coronary sulcus) which is the separation between the RA and RV on the external surface of the heart.
- The right coronary artery (RCA) eventually bifurcates but not so quickly as the left and is also embedded in fat wrapping around the heart in the right atrioventricular groove. The branches of the RCA are the right posterior descending and the marginal artery. The posterior descending artery is found in the posterior interventricular sulcus.

- The cardiac veins drain into the **coronary sinus** which is found in the left atrioventricular groove (coronary sulcus) on the posterior surface of the heart between the LA and LV.

PHYSIOLOGY

- The heart is the center of the circulatory system responsible for directing the flow of deoxygenated blood to the lungs and then distributing the reoxygenated blood to the rest of the body.
- The heart has its own intrinsic conduction system consisting of specialized tissue called **nodes.** These create the impulse that regulates the heart's rate of contraction. The sinoatrial (SA) node, found in the upper portion of the RA near the SVC, is considered the initial pacemaker of the heart. When it fires, an impulse is sent by way of inter-nodal pathways across the atria, causing them to depolarize and contract. The atrioventricular (AV) node, found in the lower portion of the right interatrial septum, is then stimulated and directs the pulse toward the ventricles by way of the **Bundle of His,** which then bifurcates into the right and left bundle branches. These extend towards the apex of the heart by way of the interventricular septum. Multiple small bands called **Perkinjie fibers** branch off the main bundle branches, across the ventricles and into the muscle cells, spreading the impulse through the ventricles and causing them to depolarize and contract simultaneously.
- The conduction system emits an electrical impulse that can be detected on the surface of the body. This is how we get an electrocardiogram (EKG). The EKG consists of three distinct phases. The P wave is a small bump corresponding to atrial contraction and depolarization. The QRS complex, which is a series of downward and upward deflections, relates to ventricular contraction and depolarization. The T wave is a small bump representing ventricular repolarization. Atrial repolarization is not observed on the EKG since it occurs at the same time as the QRS complex.

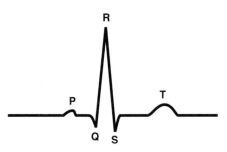

- There are two parts to the cardiac cycle: **systole** (muscular contraction) and **diastole** (muscular relaxation).

SONOGRAPHIC APPEARANCE

- The pericardium is the most reflective structure and appears almost white.
- The papillary muscles and myocardium are medium gray and homogeneous in echotexture.
- The valves are slightly more echogenic than the walls when perpendicular to the ultrasound beam.
- The area within the chambers and great vessels, as well as any other fluid space, is anechoic.

PATIENT PREPARATION

- A basic EKG is attached to the patient to assist with the timing of the cardiac cycle. Leads are attached to the right chest, left chest, and left hip region—avoiding hair, if possible.

PATIENT POSITION

- Left lateral decubitus for most views with the left arm extended above the head and the right arm at the patient's side.
- Subxiphoid: left lateral decubitus or supine. Bend the knees to relax the stomach muscles if needed.
- Suprasternal: the patient is supine with the neck extended. A pillow can also be placed under the shoulders allowing the head to drop back, hyperextending the neck even further.

TRANSDUCER

- **2.5 MHz.**
- 3.5 MHz recommended for smaller, thinner people.
- Use a 5 MHz transducer when structures in the near field need to be further evaluated (e.g., LV apex).

BREATHING TECHNIQUES

- For the majority of patients, normal respiration.
- When ribs or lungs interfere, having the patient either hold their breath or expel all their air and not breathe, may improve the image. You may also need to slide an interspace to follow the movement of the heart. Experiment to find the best possible picture.

TRANSDUCER ORIENTATION

- Images are taken from four routine positions on the chest wall: Parasternal, Apical, Subxiphoid (a.k.a. Subcostal), and Suprasternal.

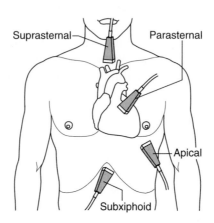

N O T E : Hold the transducer like a pencil, keeping two fingers on the patient at all times. This contact helps to prevent unintentional sliding and allows the sonographer to know how much pressure he or she is applying.

N O T E : To simplify the discussion of transducer orientation, imagine a clock on the patient's chest. The indicator on the transducer, which is some type of mark or indentation, will be directed anywhere from one to twelve o'clock. (To check indicator orientation, put gel on the transducer and touch the face on the indicator side. There should be movement on the left side of the sector. Adjust L/R invert if necessary.)

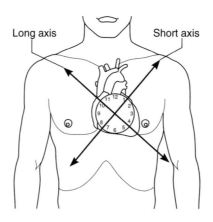

N O T E : Most movements are very slight once the proper interspace is found.

N O T E : Remember, the heart sits on an angle between the right shoulder and the left hip.

HEART SURVEY

≡ 2D EXAMINATION

- The purpose of the 2D examination is to:
  (a) Identify the chambers and walls and valves of the heart, and evaluate their size, thickness, and motion.
  (b) Assess the anatomical relationships of structures to rule out congenital defects.
- Document the presence of any pathology including tumors or fluid surrounding the heart, or thrombi within.

Parasternal Views

1. Begin with parasternal long axis by placing the transducer to the left side of the sternum in the second to third intercostal space with the indicator on the transducer directed towards 10 o'clock. Evaluate the sizes of the LA, LV, aortic root, and the RV. Assess for thickness and motion of the AV, MV, IVS, and posterior wall of the LV.

2. Maintaining the same interspace and 10 o'clock orientation, angle the transducer inferior and medial towards the belly button. This produces the right ventricular inflow view and visualizes the more anterior structure of the heart: the RA, TV, and RV. A remnant of the eustachian valve (a normal variant) may also be observed in the RA.

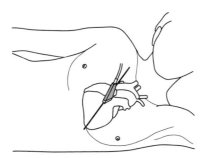

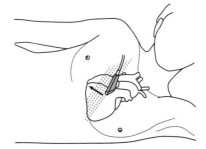

3. To obtain the right ventricular outflow view, the transducer is now angled superior and lateral towards the left shoulder. The indicator is still directed towards 10 o'clock. This will open the pulmonary artery and allow for assessment of the pulmonic valve.

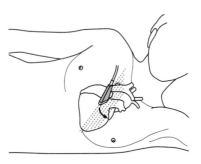

4. Rotate the transducer 90 degrees clockwise towards 1 o'clock, maintaining the same interspace as above and keeping the transducer close to the sternum. The parasternal short axis views are observed here, beginning with the aortic valve level. Tilt the transducer towards the right shoulder. Start by visualizing the area above the aortic valve for the presence of pathology, then slowly sweep towards the level of the aortic valve. The AV should be in the center of the screen with the LA, RA, RV, and PA surrounding it. Evaluate for the presence of three aortic cusps and note the thickness and motion of all the valves.

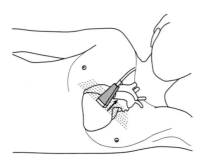

5. Continue to slowly sweep laterally through the left ventricular outflow tract region towards the mitral valve. Only the angle of the transducer has changed and the ultrasound beam is now pointing almost directly anterior to posterior. Both leaflets of the mitral valve should be observed as well as its biphasic motion.

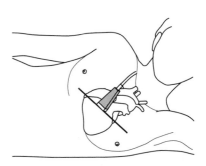

6. Slowly angle the transducer further lateral, towards the left hip. The cross section of the LV appears round with the papillary muscles indenting the inner surface, giving the cavity a mushroom-like appearance. Assess LV function for focal or global abnormalities. Continue to sweep laterally, beyond the papillary muscles as deep into the ventricle as possible allowing for further assessment of LV function.

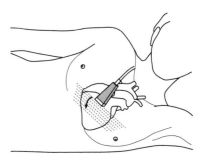

N O T E :   Occasionally, you may need to slide an interspace to obtain the different levels of short axis, though angling is usually sufficient.

Apical Views

1. Place the transducer on the left flank, lateral to the left breast and point upwards, in the direction of the right shoulder. The indicator is oriented to 3 o'clock. The heart is transected from apex to base and the four chambers, MV, TV, interventricular septum, and lateral wall of the LV are seen. In addition, the walls in the apical region are now visualized. Each structure is evaluated in respect to its size, thickness, and motion. This is known as the apical four-chamber view.

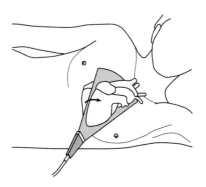

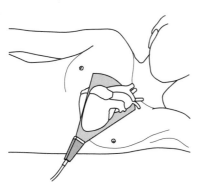

N O T E :   If unable to find the proper apical interspace, locate the PMI (point of maximal impulse) by placing two fingers on the left side of the chest and feeling for the heartbeat. The transducer is placed at this position. This is the apex of the heart.

N O T E :   It is important to visualize the endocardium of the LV in order to assess function. Evaluate the walls to see if they are thickening and if there are any focal or global ischemic abnormalities. When estimating motion it is easiest to segmentalize the ventricle, looking first at the proximal, mid, then distal walls, and then to check overall function.

2. For the apical five-chamber view, angle the transducer slightly superior to open the LVOT and the aortic valve. The MV and TV become obscured. Evaluate for the presence of any obstruction in the outflow tract region.

3. Rotate the transducer counterclockwise towards 12 o'clock while still pointing towards the right shoulder. The MV, LA, and LV are visualized and thus called the apical two-chamber view. The inferior, anterior, and apical walls of the LV can now be assessed.

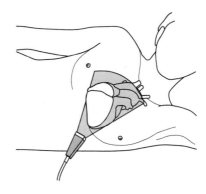

4. Rotate the transducer further counterclockwise towards 11 o'clock, opening up the apical long axis view. The structures seen in the parasternal long axis are visualized again in this view, but due to the different orientation, the apical region of the heart is now observed.

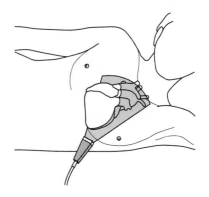

Subxiphoid Views

1. To obtain the subxiphoid long axis, place the transducer below the xiphoid process and slightly to the right of midline away from the stomach on a softer portion of the abdomen. Using the liver as a window, point the transducer toward the left shoulder. Hold the hand above the transducer, rather than like a pencil. This enables the transducer to be angled under the ribs and prevents the hand from interfering with the scan. The indicator is pointed towards 3 o'clock. The four chambers of the heart are visualized and assessed for relative sizes. If the chambers appear foreshortened, the transducer should be rotated accordingly. The area around the heart should also be evaluated for the presence of pericardial fluid, tumors, and masses. The interatrial septum is also best evaluated in this view.

2. For the subxiphoid short axis views, rotate the transducer 90 degrees counterclockwise towards 12 o'clock. Sweeping the transducer from the direction of the left shoulder to the direction of the right shoulder produces the same three levels as the parasternal short axis views (papillary muscles, mitral valve, and aortic valve levels) but with the heart on a slightly different tilt. In addition, the hepatic veins and IVC can be seen to enter the RA by pointing more rightward, beyond the aortic valve level. Make sure the IVC is clear with no thrombi.

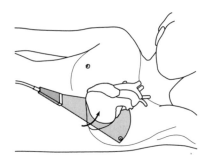

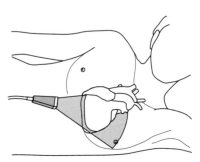

Suprasternal View

1. With the patient in the supine position, neck extended, place the transducer at the sternoclavicular groove and angle inferior towards the heart. This will visualize the aortic arch and its branches, along with a cross section of the right pulmonary artery. The transducer is oriented towards 12 o'clock.

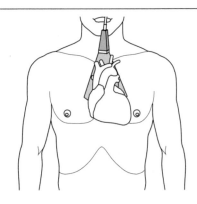

2. For a short axis of the aorta, rotate the transducer 90 degrees clockwise to 3 o'clock. A longitudinal section of the right pulmonary artery may also be seen anterior to the LA.

N O T E : This view should be used when questions involving the aorta arise, such as in dissection or Marfans syndrome.

REQUIRED IMAGES

N O T E : The study is videotaped allowing for real-time assessment of structures. At least 6–10 beats of each view should be recorded with additional images of any pathology.

1. Parasternal long axis.

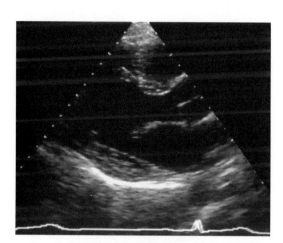 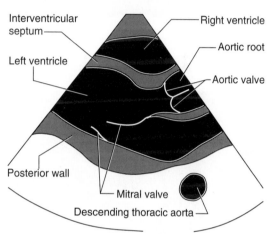

N O T E : The anterior portion of the aortic root and the interventricular septum should be continuous and as perpendicular to the ultrasound beam as possible. The posterior portion of the aortic root runs continuous with the anterior mitral valve leaflet.

2. Right ventricular inflow view.

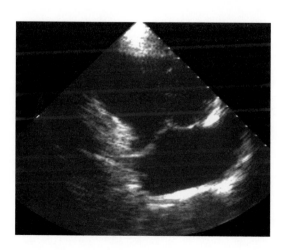 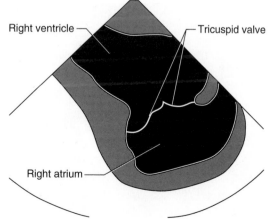

3. Right ventricular outflow view.

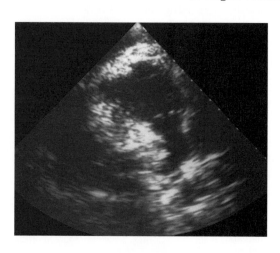
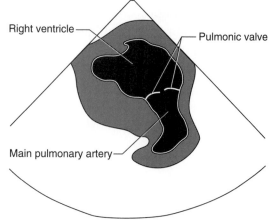

4. Parasternal short axis at the level of the aortic valve.

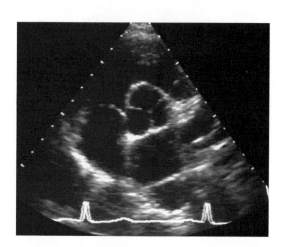
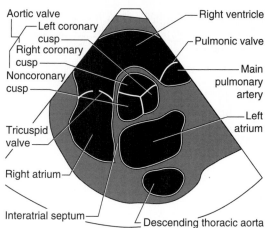

5. Parasternal short axis at the level of the mitral valve.

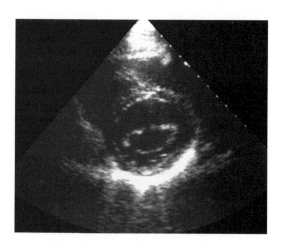
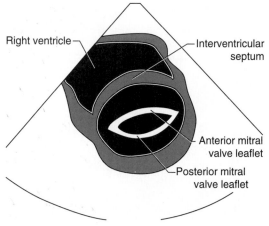

6. Parasternal short axis at the level of the papillary muscles.

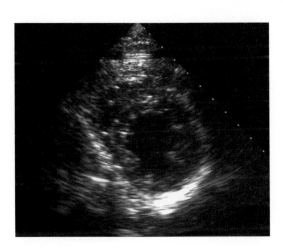 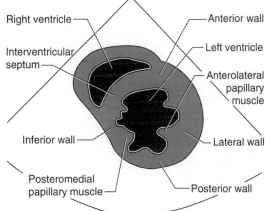

7. Apical four-chamber view.

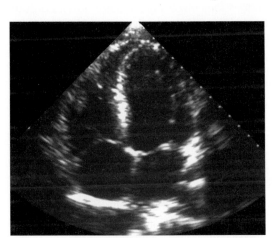 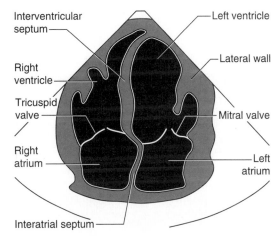

8. Apical five-chamber view.

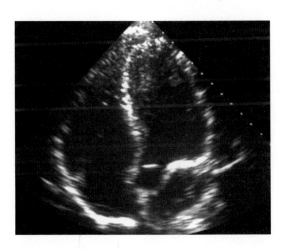 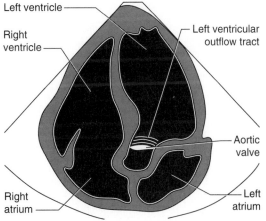

9. Apical two-chamber view.

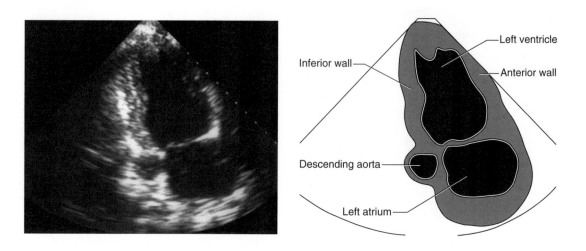

N O T E :   When questions involving the aorta arise, a portion of the descending thoracic aorta can be visualized posterior to the two-chamber view and should be evaluated for pathology.

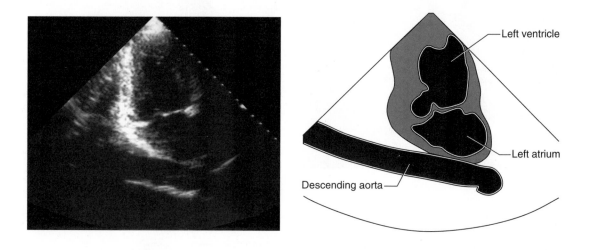

10. Apical long axis.

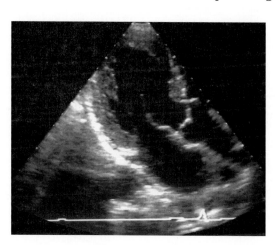

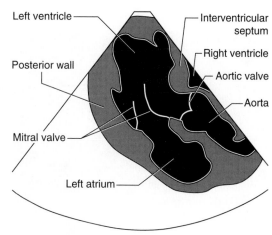

11. Subxiphoid four chamber.

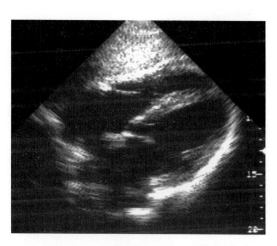

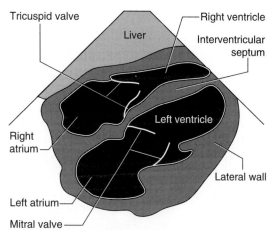

12. Subxiphoid short axis papillary muscle level.

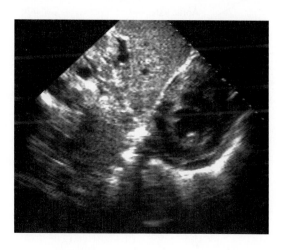

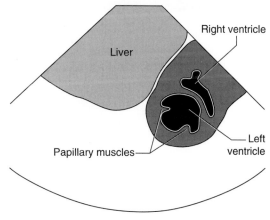

13. Subxiphoid short axis at the level of the mitral valve.

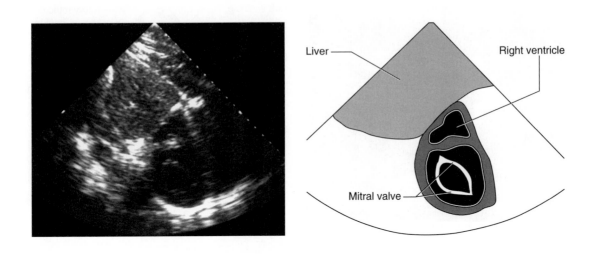

14. Subxiphoid short axis at the level of the aortic valve.

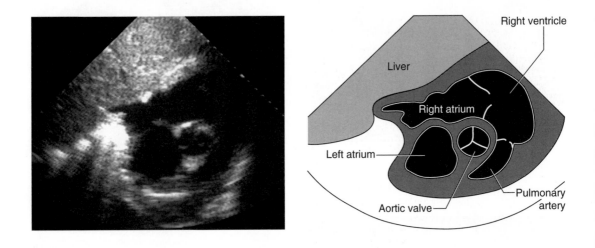

15. Subxiphoid short axis viewing the IVC entering the RA.

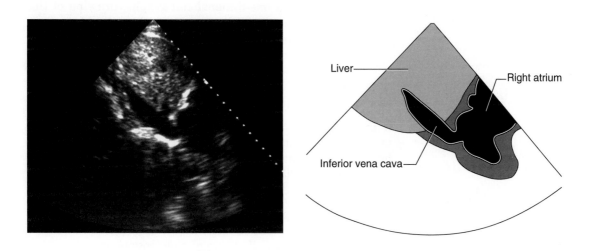

16. Suprasternal notch viewing the long axis of the aorta.

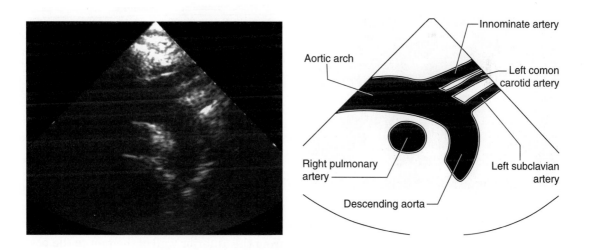

N O T E :   This view should be used when questions involving the aorta arise, such as dissection or Marfans syndrome. A short axis of the aorta should also be evaluated in these cases.

≡ M-MODE EVALUATION

- The M-mode is a one-dimensional graphic drawing of the heart used to measure distance over time. An M-mode is useful for obtaining dimensions of the heart and assessing fine movements too subtle for the eye to see.

N O T E :   A minimum of six beats should be recorded at each level demonstrating both systolic and diastolic motion.

N O T E :   The M-mode may be documented on either video-tape or strip chart recorder. If the strip chart is used, begin with a frozen image of the parasternal long axis view to demonstrate the orientation of the heart.

N O T E :   The 2D image must be as perpendicular to the ul-trasound beam as possible, lessening the chance for inaccurate measurements. (A tipped ventricle will yield exaggerated num-bers.) When measuring, if unsure of a dimension, omit it.

Aortic Valve Level

- The cursor is placed so that it transects the RV, aorta, and LA in either the parasternal long or short axis view.

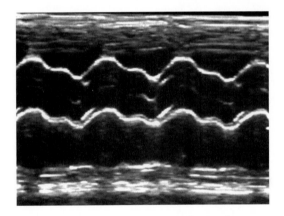
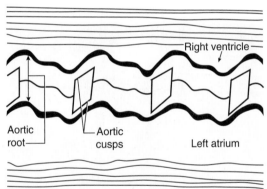

- Measurements taken[1]:
  - (a) Aortic root: from the anterior wall of the root to the pos-terior wall of the root, at the level of the Q wave on the ECG; normally 1.9–4 cm
  - (b) Aortic valve cusp separation: normally has the shape of a box when open with the right coronary cusp more an-terior and the noncoronary cusp posterior. Measured at the onset of systole (when the valve first opens); nor-mally 1.5–2.6 cm.
  - (c) Left atrium: measured at the largest dimension (end systole); normally 1.9–4 cm.

---

[1]Normal values used in the lab at Thomas Jefferson University, Philadel-phia, Pennsylvania.

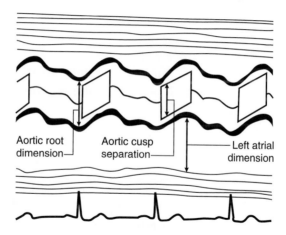

Aortic root dimension — Aortic cusp separation — Left atrial dimension

N O T E :   Always measure structures from leading edge to leading edge.

Mitral Valve Level

- Slowly sweep the cursor through the LVOT region to the tip of the mitral valve leaflets. This sweep will demonstrate structural continuity. The biphasic opening of both mitral leaflets should then be documented.

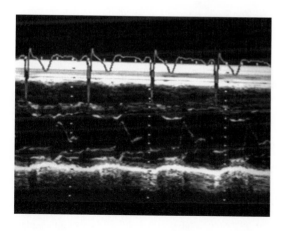

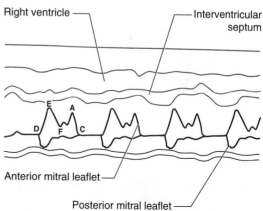

Right ventricle — Interventricular septum

Anterior mitral leaflet — Posterior mitral leaflet —

N O T E :   The mitral valve is labeled to describe the different phases of its motion.

D—beginning of diastole.

E—maximal excursion of the valve.

F—point to which the valve had closed following the passive filling phase.

A—atrial contraction (P wave on the ECG).

B—extra bump between A and C (occurs only when pathology, such as diastolic dysfunction, is present).

C—closure of the valve and the beginning of systole.

- Measurements[2]:
  - (a) D to E excursion; normally greater than 1.6 cm
  - (b) E to F slope over the period of one second (expressed in mm/sec); normally greater than 70 mm/sec.
  - (c) E point to septal separation; normally no greater than 1 cm.

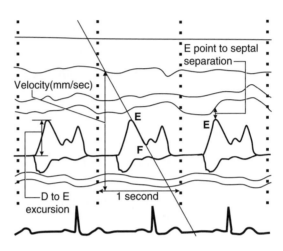

Left Ventricular Level

- Slowly sweep the cursor just beyond the mitral leaflets but stopping before the papillary muscles. Both systolic and diastolic dimensions of the LV should be documented.

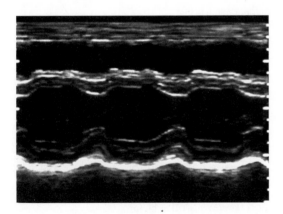 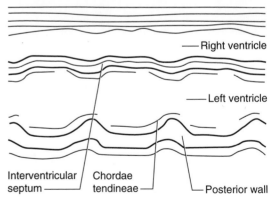

---

[2]Normal values used in the lab at Thomas Jefferson University, Philadelphia, Pennsylvania.

- Measurements[3]:
    - (a) All of the following are measured at the level of the Q wave on the EKG: RV (no greater than 2.7 cm); IVS, posterior LV wall (both normally between .6–1.2 cm); and LV end diastolic dimension (LVEDD) (normal range 3.5–5.7 cm).

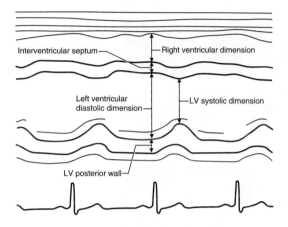

N O T E :   Often the free wall of the RV is not visualized due to its close proximity to the transducer, making it difficult to determine the true size of the chamber. The measurement is therefore taken from the point where motion is first observed, to the leading edge of the interventricular septum. Then subtract .5 cm from the total to compensate for the RV wall thickness.

    - (b) LV end systolic dimension (LVESD): measure at the smallest dimension.

N O T E :   The LVEDD and the LVESD should be measured on the same beat.

N O T E :   Be careful not to include chordae tendinea in the thickness of the LV walls.

Tricuspid and Pulmonic Valves

- An M-mode of the tricuspid or pulmonic valve is used to demonstrate thickness and motion and are not necessarily a routine part of the exam. There are no standard measurements obtained.

---

[3]Normal values used in the lab at Thomas Jefferson University, Philadelphia, Pennsylvania.

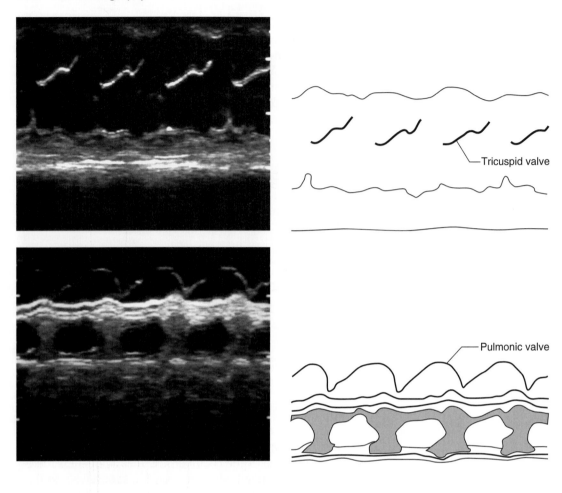

≡ DOPPLER EVALUATION

- Used to assess blood flow through the heart, including increased velocities, stenosis, regurgitation, and shunts.
- Both continuous and pulsed-wave Doppler are used in conjunction with each other. In addition, color Doppler simplifies the mapping process and gives a visual representation of the size and direction of blood flow disturbances.

Normal Valve Profiles

Mitral Valve

- The flow profile is shaped like an M and is best sampled in the apical four-chamber view. Here, blood flow moves towards the transducer during diastole; therefore, the waveform appears above the baseline. Peak velocity should not exceed 1.3 m/sec.[4]

---

[4]Hatle, L., Angelsen, B.: *Doppler Ultrasound in Cardiology,* second edition. Philadelphia: Lea & Febiger, 1985, p. 93.

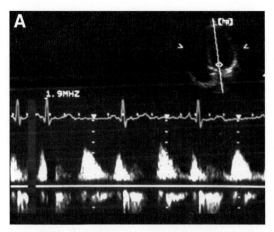

Figure A: Continuous-Wave Mitral
Valve Doppler

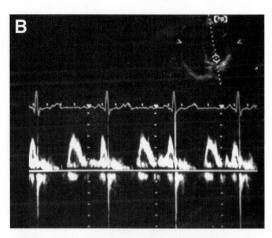

Figure B: Pulsed-Wave Mitral
Valve Doppler

N O T E :   Pulsed-wave Doppler has an envelope (whiter outline) and window (darker interior) versus the filled-in profile of
continuous wave. In cases of turbulent flow, this PW window can
become filled in and is called spectral broadening.

Tricuspid Valve

- The flow profile also looks like an M and occurs during diastole. It is best sampled in either the right ventricular inflow view or the apical four-chamber view. Blood flow
moves towards the transducer; therefore, the profile appears above the baseline. Peak velocity should not exceed
0.7 m/sec.[5]

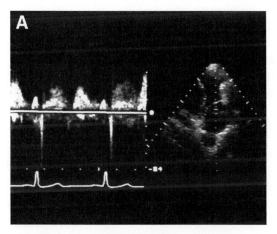

Figure A: Continuous-Wave Tricuspid
Valve Doppler

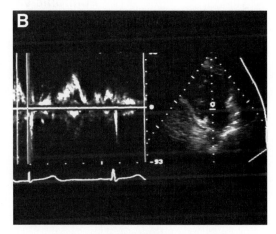

Figure B: Pulsed-Wave Tricuspid
Valve Doppler

[5]ibid.

Aortic Valve

- A sample is best taken from the apical five-chamber view and the profile has the shape of a bullet. In this case, blood flow is moving away from the transducer during systole and therefore appears below the baseline. Peak velocity should not exceed 1.7 m/sec.[6]

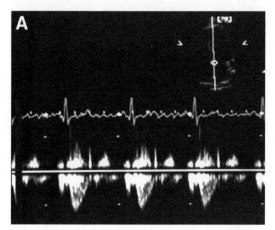

Figure A: Continuous-Wave Aortic
Valve Doppler

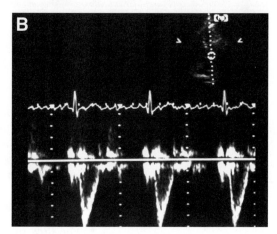

Figure B: Pulsed-Wave Aortic
Valve Doppler

Pulmonic Valve

- The profile is also shaped like a bullet, but is best sampled in parasternal short axis at the level of the aortic valve. Flow moves away from the transducer during systole; therefore, it appears below the baseline. Peak velocity should not exceed 0.9 m/sec.[7]

[6]ibid.
[7]ibid.

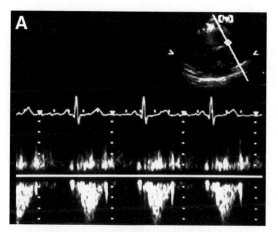

Figure A: Continuous-Wave Pulmonic
Valve Doppler

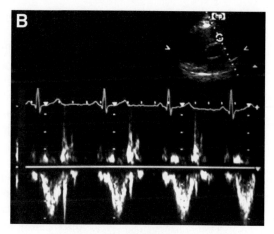

Figure B: Pulsed-Wave Pulmonic
Valve Doppler

Left Ventricular Outflow Tract

* Systolic flow sampled in this region is also shaped like a bullet and appears below the baseline. It is best sampled in the apical five-chamber view and peak velocity should not exceed 1.1 m/sec.[8]

N O T E :   Doppler is best when flow is parallel to the ultrasound beam. In contrast, 2D is best when perpendicular. Therefore, the best Doppler image is not necessarily the best 2D image.

Valve Survey

N O T E :   The following sequence should be used in the evaluation of each valve: color Doppler, continuous-wave (CW) Doppler, then pulse-wave (PW) Doppler. Assess each value separately beginning with the mitral valve. Repeat this process on the aortic, tricuspid, and pulmonic valves, and the left ventricular outflow tract (LVOT) if necessary.

---

[8]ibid.

Color Doppler Survey

N O T E : Flow moving towards the transducer appears as various shades of red. Flow moving away is blue. A lower velocity would be deeper in color and gradually lighten as the velocity increases to almost yellow or white. At times, a variance map is used. This is usually a green color tagged on the end of the color spectrum. The green makes the higher velocities or turbulent flows stand out.

- The color sector should be placed so that the valve or area being assessed is in the center of the sample. Normally, mitral and tricuspid flow appear red, and pulmonic and aortic flow are blue. When the valves are closed, no color (regurgitation) should be seen below them. Mitral and tricuspid regurgitation appear blue; aortic and pulmonic regurgitation are usually red.
- Slowly angle the transducer back and forth across the valve plane in order to locate any eccentric areas of turbulence. Demonstrate the size and location of any regurgitation or turbulent flow.
- Color can also be used to locate the peak flow velocity across the valve allowing for easy placement of the CW Doppler cursor.

N O T E : Regurgitation or any pathology should be demonstrated in more than one view.

Continuous-Wave Doppler Survey

- CW is best for determining peak flow velocities. Place the cursor so it bisects the opening of the valve that is to be sampled. If the peak velocity across a valve exceeds its normal velocity, the peak should then be measured. Three profiles are measured and averaged. Do not measure post PVC beats. If the patient is in atrial fibrillation, average at least five or six beats.
- The peak velocity of tricuspid regurgitation is also measured to help with the evaluation of pulmonary hypertension.

N O T E : If unable to find a peak velocity on any valve, tricuspid or aortic regurgitation, a nonimaging, stand-alone CW probe should be used. Due to the smaller footprint of the transducer and the lower frequency, the peak velocity can be easily found.

Pulsed-Wave Doppler Survey

- Pulsed Doppler demonstrates exactly where a flow disturbance occurs and is then used to map out the direction and size of the disturbance. Place the cursor or Doppler "gate" slightly above the valve opening. Slowly move below the valve, then across the valve plane in both directions. If regurgitation is detected, follow the flow into the chamber as far back as it goes, mapping the length and also the width of the turbulent area.

N O T E :   If any additional flow disturbances (e.g., ASD, VSD) are visualized, they too should be evaluated with color, CW, and PW Doppler.

Standard Doppler Positions

View	Structure
Parasternal long axis	Interventricular septum
Parasternal short axis:	
–Aortic valve level	Tricuspid valve, pulmonic valve, right ventricular outflow tract (RVOT), pulmonary artery, ductal flow
–Mitral to left ventricle	Interventricular septum
Right ventricular inflow	Tricuspid valve
Right ventricular outflow	Pulmonic valve, RVOT
Right parasternal	Aortic valve flow
Apical four-chamber	Mitral valve, tricuspid valve
Apical five-chamber	Aortic valve, left ventricular outflow tract (LVOT)
Apical two-chamber	Mitral valve
Apical long axis	Mitral valve, aortic valve, LVOT
Subcostal four-chamber	Interatrial and interventricular septums, IVC
Suprasternal	Ascending, arch and descending aorta, pulmonary flow

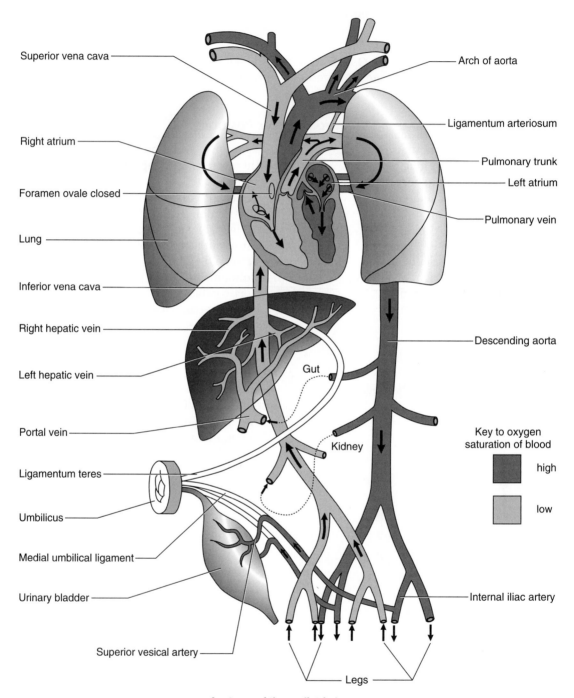

Superior vena cava

Right atrium

Foramen ovale closed

Lung

Inferior vena cava

Right hepatic vein

Left hepatic vein

Portal vein

Ligamentum teres

Umbilicus

Medial umbilical ligament

Urinary bladder

Superior vesical artery

Arch of aorta

Ligamentum arteriosum

Pulmonary trunk

Left atrium

Pulmonary vein

Descending aorta

Gut

Kidney

Key to oxygen
saturation of blood

high

low

Internal iliac artery

Legs

Anatomy of the pediatric heart

Pediatric Echocardiography Scanning Protocol

CHAPTER
22

Maureen E. McDonald

ANATOMY AND PHYSIOLOGY

- See Adult Echocardiography Scanning Protocol, Chapter 21.

SONOGRAPHIC APPEARANCE

- The pericardium is the brightest structure and appears almost white.
- The valves tend to be the next brightest, appearing light gray to almost white depending upon how perpendicular the valve is to the ultrasound beam.
- The myocardium has a homogeneous texture and appears gray.
- The area within the chambers, vessels, and any fluid appear anechoic.

PATIENT PREP

- An infant or young child may need to be sedated if he or she is uncooperative with the exam. Special arrangements should be made to have a physician administer chloral hydrate prior to the exam.
- EKG leads should be attached to the right shoulder, left shoulder, and left hip regions.

PATIENT POSITION

- Neonates and infants may remain supine.
- Children (classified as anyone under the age of seventeen) should be in the left lateral decubitus position.

TRANSDUCER

- 7.5 MHz used for preemies.
- 5 to 7.5 MHz used for neonates to infants.
- 5 to 3.5 MHz for toddlers (depending upon the body surface area).
- 3.5 to 2.5 MHz used for children and teenagers (depending upon body habitus).

BREATHING TECHNIQUES

- Normal respiration.

TRANSDUCER ORIENTATION

- Images are obtained from the following four windows: Parasternal, Apical, Subcostal, and Suprasternal.

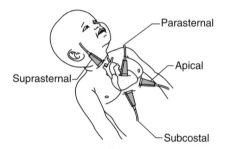

- Scanning is performed in the anatomically corrected position; therefore, the sector is inverted for the subcostal and apical views. The study thus provides an anatomical reference for the surgeon.

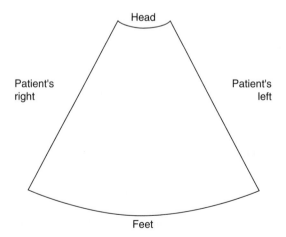

- The EKG rate is increased to 100% for neonates due to the higher infant heart rate. This allows for easier interpretation of the Doppler and EKG.

HEART SURVEY

1. Begin by placing the transducer midline on the abdomen, below the xiphoid process. Flip the sector, so the point appears at the bottom of the screen. Looking at the monitor, the image should be oriented so the structures on the patient's left appear to the right of the screen. Point directly anterior to posterior, visualizing the liver and cross sections of the IVC (found on the patient's right) and aorta (to the patient's left). This establishes normal situs of the abdominal structures.

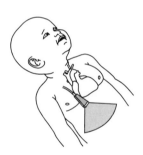

2. Slowly angle superiorly, demonstrating the entry of the hepatic veins into the inferior vena cava (IVC) and eventually the IVC into the right atrium (RA). Continue to angle superiorly until the four chambers of the heart are observed. Verify the orientation of the heart, its chambers, and valves. The apex should appear to the right of the screen. Look for the four pulmonary veins to enter the left atrium (LA). Use color Doppler and pulsed-wave (PW) Doppler to assess the flow across the mitral and tricuspid valves. Color Doppler the interatrial septum and interventricular septums to assess for the presence of a shunt. Pulse any turbulence observed. Use continuous-wave (CW) Doppler to evaluate any high velocities (e.g., ventricular septal defect, tricuspid regurgitation).

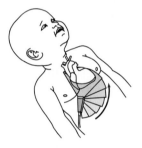

3. Continue to angle the transducer more superiorly, opening the left ventricular outflow tract (LVOT) and the aorta. Color and PW Doppler these, looking for the presence of regurgitation or turbulence.

4. Tilting the transducer even more superiorly will open the right ventricular outflow region, pulmonic valve (PV), and pulmonary artery (PA). Color and PW Doppler the PV for turbulence and assess for the presence of a patent ductus arteriosus (PDA).

5. Slowly tilt inferiorly to return to the four-chamber view, then rotate the transducer clockwise 90 degrees. This is the orientation for the subcostal short axis views. Begin by directing the transducer toward the right shoulder, demonstrating the entry of the superior and inferior vena cavas into the right atrium. Color Doppler the IVC and SVC. PW to establish normal flow profiles.

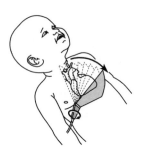

6. Slowly begin to angle the transducer toward the left shoulder, first demonstrating the interatrial septum, then the PA, PV, and aortic valve (AV). Color Doppler and PW any turbulence observed. Continue to sweep leftward through the mitral and tricuspid valves, assessing thickness and motion, to the cross section of the left (LV) and right (RV) ventricles. Slowly sweep beyond the papillary muscles to the apical region, all the while assessing thickness and contractility. Repeat using color Doppler, looking for any shunts.

7. Move the transducer to the left flank, directing the beam towards the right shoulder. This will dissect the heart from apex to base and the apical four-chamber view is visualized. The left side of the heart should appear to the right of the screen. The LA, LV, RA, and RV are visualized as well as the mitral (MV) and tricuspid (TV). Assess the chamber sizes and valves. Color and PW Doppler both the valves using CW Doppler for any high velocities.

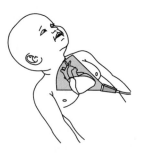

8. Angle the transducer slightly anterior to open the LVOT and aorta. This is the apical five-chamber view. Color and PW Doppler the aortic valve and LVOT.

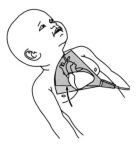

9. Rotate the transducer clockwise to open the outflow tract even more. This produces the apical long axis. In addition, the AV, LA, LV, and MV are visualized. Again, color the LVOT region and PW Doppler up the IVS looking for a step-up in velocity or any turbulence.

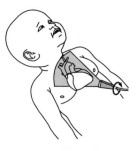

10. Flip the sector to its original position, with the point at the top of the screen. Move the transducer to the left of the sternum to the region known as parasternal. The image should be oriented so a long axis of the left ventricle appears to the left of the screen and the aorta to the right. The anterior portion of the aortic root and the interventricular septum (IVS) should run continuous and the posterior part of the aortic root and the anterior mitral valve leaflet are continuous. Evaluate the size of the LA, MV, LV, posterior LV wall, IVS, and the RV for anatomic relationships, size, thickness, and motion. Use color Doppler to evaluate the valves and IVS. CW Doppler any high velocities.

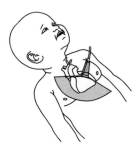

11. Slowly angle the transducer inferior and medial to open the right ventricular inflow view. This will visualize the RA, RV, and TV, which are the most anterior structures of the heart. Assess the tricuspid valve with color Doppler and CW Doppler for any high velocities. Slowly return to the parasternal long axis view, using color Doppler to evaluate the IVS. CW Doppler any high velocities.

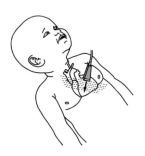

12. Angle the transducer towards the left shoulder to open the right ventricular outflow region. This includes the RV outflow tract, PV, and main PA. Color Doppler and PW Doppler any turbulence. Again return to the long axis view.

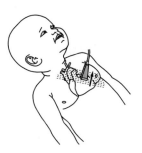

13. Rotate the transducer clockwise 90 degrees to obtain the short axis parasternal views. Begin by directing the beam towards the right shoulder demonstrating the aortic valve, LA, RA, PV, and PA. Assess the number of cusps of the aortic valve. Slowly angle slightly above the level of the leaflets to evaluate for the presence of the right and left coronary arteries. Color Doppler the interatrial septum, tricuspid, and pulmonic valves. Angle slightly anterior and leftward to open the right and left pulmonary arteries and PW each. Color Doppler for the presence of a PDA and PW and CW Doppler if present.

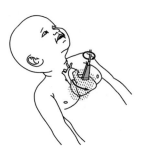

14. Slowly begin sweeping the transducer to the left, moving through the level of the mitral valve to the left ventricle and as far towards the apex as possible, all the while assessing thickness and contractility. Repeat the sweep, this time using color Doppler, looking for any turbulence across the septum. CW Doppler any high velocities.

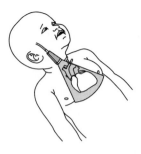

15. Move the transducer near the sternoclavicular notch in the suprasternal region. Direct the beam inferior, looking for a long axis of the aortic arch. Identify the branching vessels and establish aortic orientation. Look for any areas of narrowing, using color Doppler to identify turbulent areas. PW Doppler the ascending, arch, and descending aorta, and CW Doppler any increased velocities. Evaluate the LA posterior to the right pulmonary artery and look for the presence of pulmonary veins.

16. Rotate the transducer clockwise 90 degrees, opening the branching PA's. Color and PW Doppler each branch. A cross section of the aorta is also visualized.

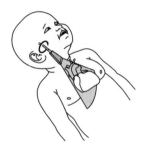

REQUIRED IMAGES

NOTE: The following views are all recorded on videotape, allowing for real-time assessment of cardiac structures. At least 8-10 beats of each view is recorded with additional images for color, PW, and CW Doppler.

1. Subcostal view demonstrating the orientation of the aorta and IVC.

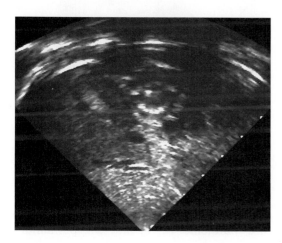 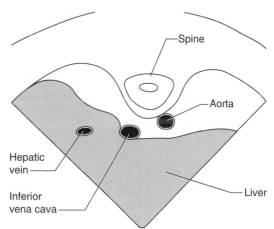

2. Subcostal four-chamber view.

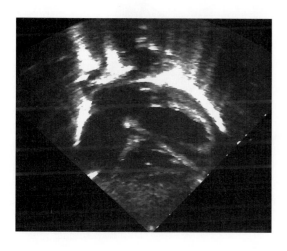 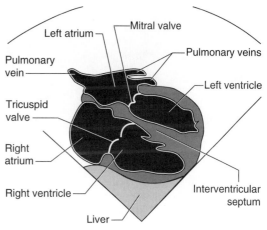

3. Subcostal five-chamber view showing the aorta and the left ventricular outflow tract.

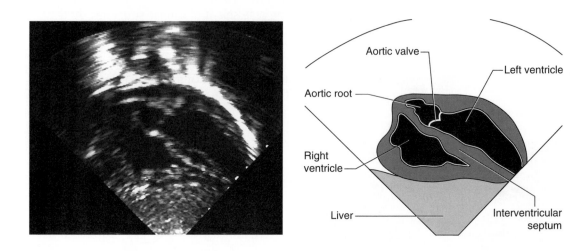

4. Subcostal long axis angled anteriorly to demonstrate the RV outflow tract, pulmonic valve, and the pulmonary artery.

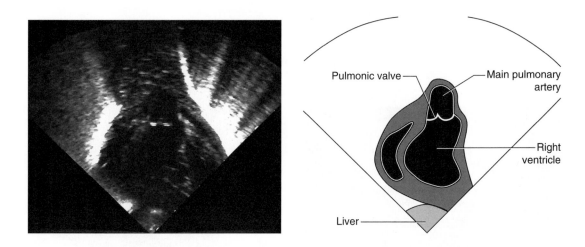

5. Short axis subcostal showing the IVC and SVC entering the right atrium.

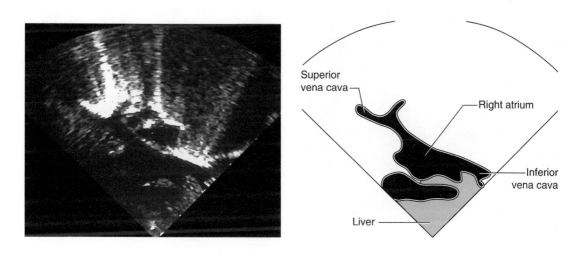

6. Short axis subcostal demonstrating the aortic valve, pulmonary artery, and interatrial septum.

N O T E :   A small angulation may be needed to fully visualize the interatrial septum.

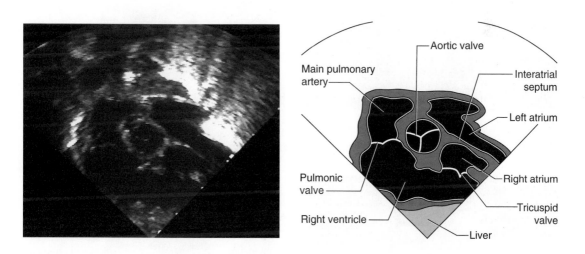

7. Short axis subcostal of the mitral valve.

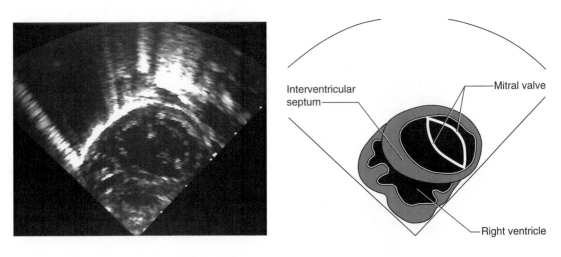

8. Short axis subcostal of the left and right ventricles.

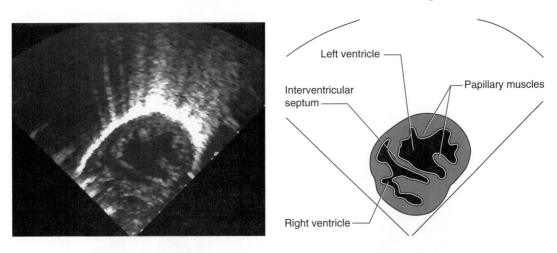

9. Apical four-chamber view.

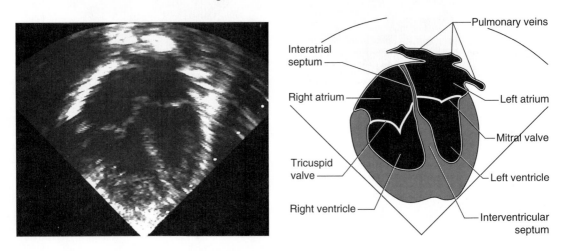

10. Apical long axis documenting the left ventricular outflow tract.

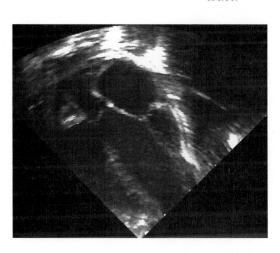

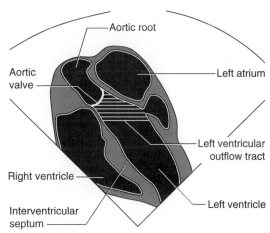

11. Parasternal long axis.

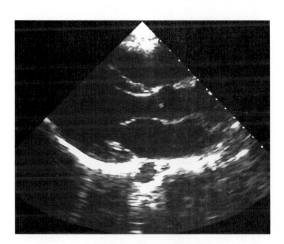

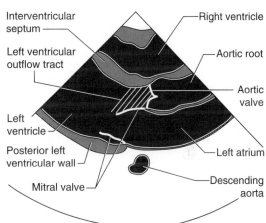

12. Right ventricular inflow view.

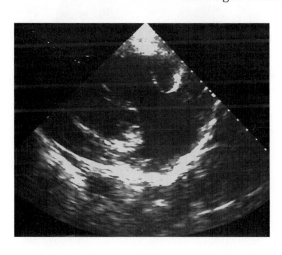

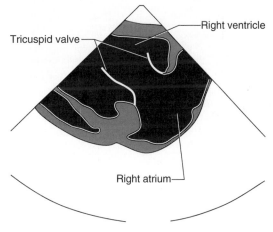

13. Right ventricular outflow view.

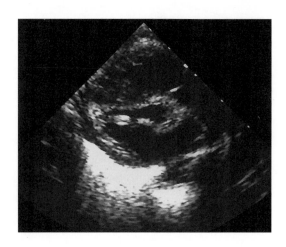

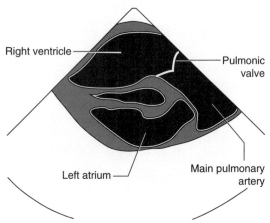

14. Parasternal short axis at the level of the aortic valve to document the orientation of the great vessels.

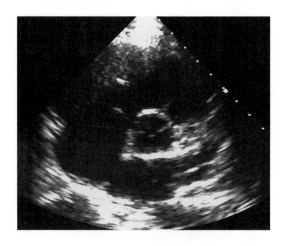

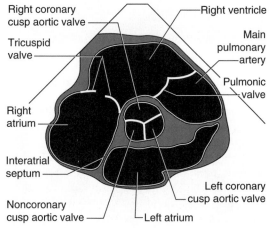

15. Parasternal short axis documenting the left coronary artery.

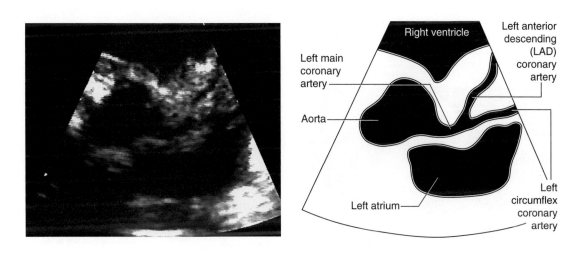

N O T E :   Angle slightly above the aortic valve leaflets and zoom in on the region to simplify coronary evaluation.

16. Parasternal short axis documenting the right coronary artery.

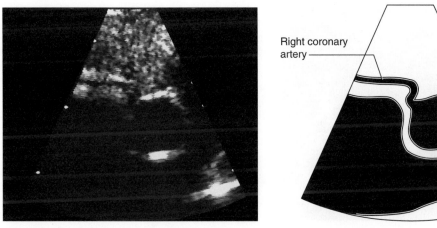
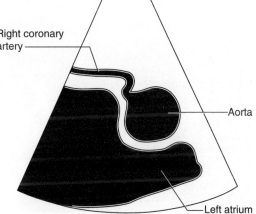

17. Parasternal short axis to document the right and left pulmonary branches and the presence/absence of a patent ductus arteriosus.

N O T E :   If a ductus is present, demonstrate its connection to the aorta.

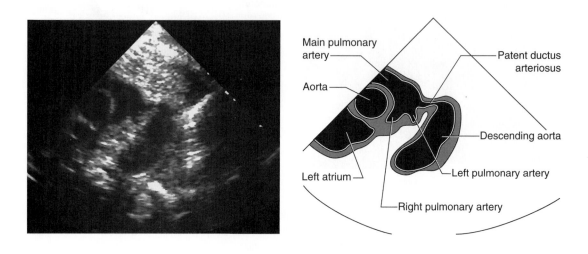

Main pulmonary artery
Aorta
Patent ductus arteriosus
Descending aorta
Left atrium
Left pulmonary artery
Right pulmonary artery

18. Parasternal short axis at the level of the mitral valve to document thickness and motion of the leaflets.

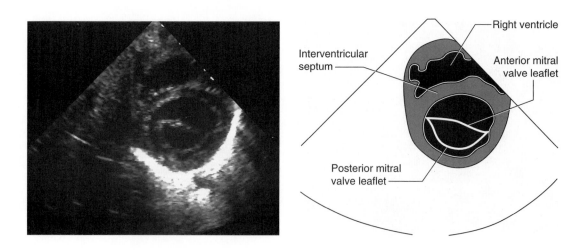

Interventricular septum
Right ventricle
Anterior mitral valve leaflet
Posterior mitral valve leaflet

19. Parasternal short axis at the level of the papillary muscles.

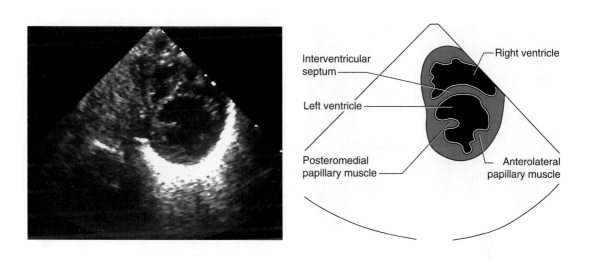

20. Suprasternal notch documenting the aortic arch and its branches.

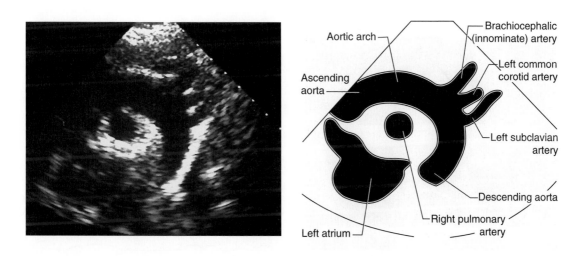

21. Suprasternal notch documenting the branch pulmonary arteries and short axis of the aorta.

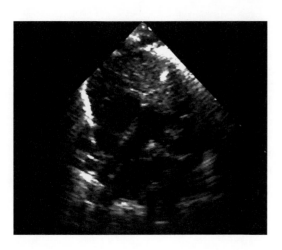
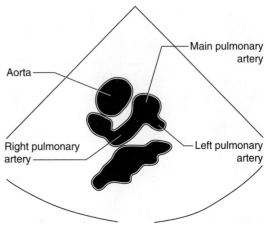

REQUIRED M-MODE IMAGES

- An M-mode should be performed from either the parasternal long or parasternal short axis by placing the cursor through the following three levels:

1. Aortic valve level.

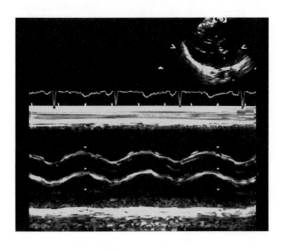
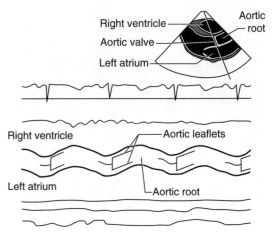

2. Mitral valve level.

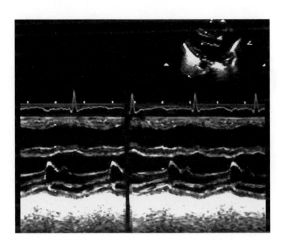
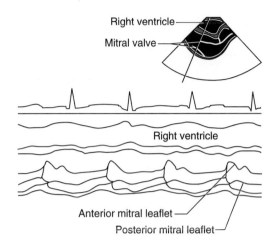

3. Left ventricular level.

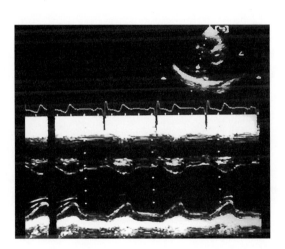
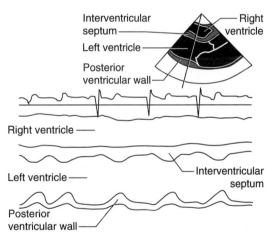

- Attention is given to sizes of the chambers, motion of the valves, ventricular contractility, and structural continuity.

N O T E :   Sweep speed of the M-Mode is increased to 100% to accommodate the increased heart rate of neonates.

COLOR PLATES

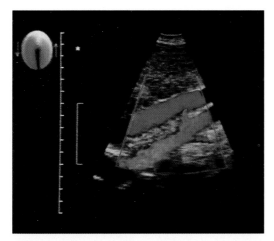

Plate 1. Color Doppler image demonstrating renal artery origins. (Courtesy of Diasonics, Inc., Milpitas, California.)

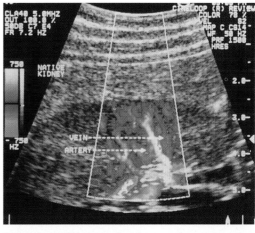

Plate 2. Color Doppler image demonstrating renal perfusion. (Courtesy of ATL, Bothell, Washington.)

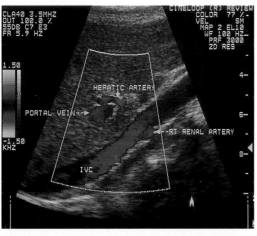

Plate 3. Color Doppler image demonstrating flow in the region of the porta hepatis. (Courtesy of ATL, Bothell, Washington.)

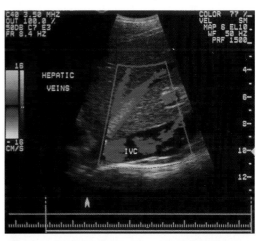

Plate 4. Example of color flow Doppler in hepatic veins. (Courtesy of ATL, Bothell, Washington.)

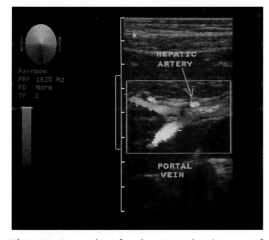

Plate 5. Example of color Doppler image of flow in the portal vein.

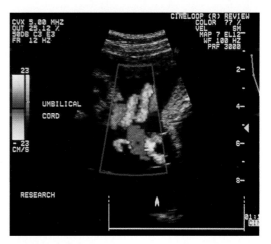

Plate 6. Color Doppler image of a three-vessel umbilical cord.

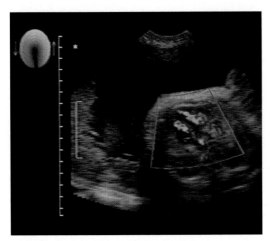

Plate 7. Color Doppler image of a fetal four-chamber heart. (Courtesy of Diasonics, Inc., Milpitas, California. Diasonics does not have the Food and Drug Administration approval to market their probes for this fetal Doppler application. However, the final decision as to how a medical device will be used is the prerogative of the medical practitioner. Please check FDA approval for all manufacturers' probes used in any examination.)

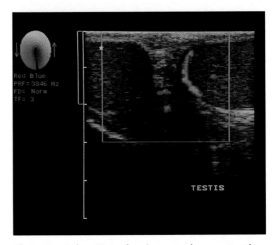

Plate 8. Color Doppler image demonstrating arterial flow in a testicular artery. (Courtesy of Diasonics, Inc., Milpitas, California.)

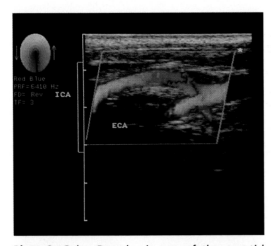

Plate 9. Color Doppler image of the carotid artery bifurcation. (Courtesy of Diasonics, Inc., Milpitas, California.)

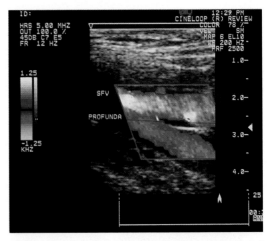

Plate 10. Color flow Doppler image at the level of the SFV and profunda vein insertions. (Courtesy of ATL, Bothell, Washington.)

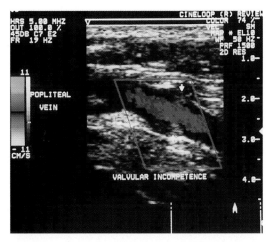

Plate 11. Color Doppler image demonstrating valvular incompetence. (Courtesy of ATL, Bothell, Washington.)

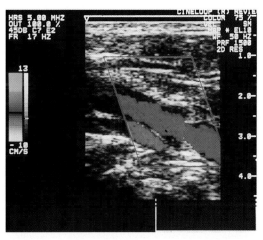

Plate 12. Color Doppler image of popliteal vein and artery. (Courtesy of ATL, Bothell, Washington.)

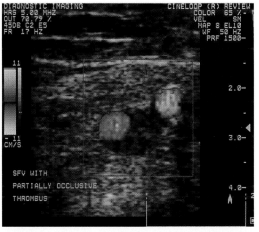

Plate 13. Color Doppler image demonstrating thrombus in the SFV. (Courtesy of ATL, Bothell, Washington.)

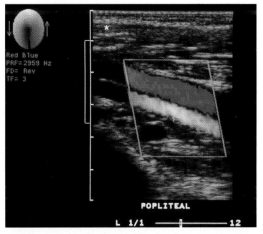

Plate 14. Color Doppler image of the popliteal artery. (Courtesy of Diasonics, Inc., Milpitas, California.)

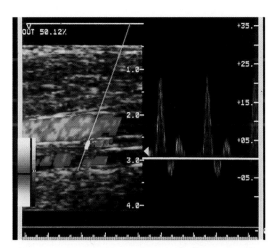

Plate 15. Spectral analysis of the posterior artery, demonstrating normal triphasic flow. (Courtesy of ATL, Bothell, Washington.)

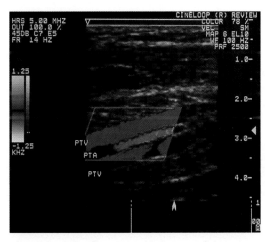

Plate 16. Color flow Doppler image of the posterior tibial artery and vein. (Courtesy of ATL, Bothell, Washington.)

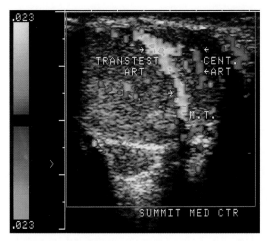

Plate 17. Color flow image of a normal variant.

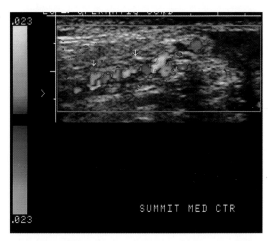

Plate 18. Color flow image of spermatic cord.

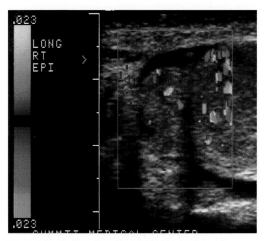

Plate 19. Color flow image of epididymis.

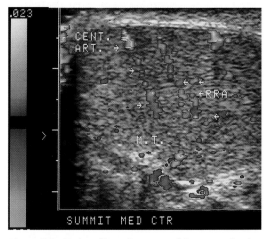

Plate 20. Color flow image of intratesticular arteries.

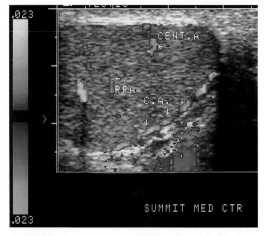

Plate 21. Color flow image of intratesticular arteries.

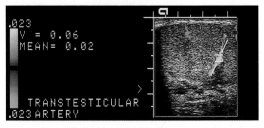

Plate 22. Color flow image and waveform of intratesticular arteries.

Abbreviation Glossary

AIUM: American Institute of Ultrasound in Medicine

ALARA: As low as reasonably acceptable

ANT: Anterior

ART: Artery

AV: Atrioventricular

AV: Atrioventricular valves

BIF: Bifurcation

CBD: Common bile duct

cc: Cubic centimeter

CD: Common duct

CERX: Cervix

CFA: Common femoral artery

CFV: Common femoral vein

CHD: Common hepatic duct

cm: Centimeter

COR: Coronal

CR: Crown rump

C-SPINE: Cervical spine

CW: Continuous wave Doppler

DECUB: Decubitus

DP: Dorsalis pedis artery

EKG: Electrocardiogram

ER: Endorectal

EV: Endovaginal

Fd: Doppler shift frequency

Fo: Operating frequency

GB: Gallbladder

GS: Gestational sac

Hz: Hertz

IN: Inches

INF: Inferior

IVC: Inferior vena cava

IVS: Interventricular septum

kHz: Kilohertz

KID: Kidney

LA: Left atrium

LAD: Left anterior descending

LAT: Lateral

LLD: Left lateral decubitus

LPO: Left posterior oblique

L-SPINE: Lumbar spine

LT: Left

LV: Left ventricular

LVOT: Left ventricular outflow tract

MED: Medical

MHz: Megahertz

ML: Midline

mm: Millimeter

MV: Mitral valve

NIP: Nipple

OBL: Oblique

OV: Ovary

PA: Pulmonary artery

PDA: Patent ductus arteriosus

PFV: Profunda femoris vein

POP: Popliteal artery

POST: Posterior

PRF: Time and depth limitations

PROX: Proximal

PT: Posterior tibial artery

PV: Pulmonic valve

PW: Pulsed wave Doppler

RA: Right atrium

RCA: Right coronary artery

RI: Resistive indices

RLD: Right lateral decubitus

RPO: Right posterior oblique

RT: Right

RV: Right ventricle

SA: Sinoatrial node

SAG: Sagittal

SEM V: Seminal vesicles

SFA: Superficial femoral artery

SFV: Superficial femoral vein

SMA: Superior mesenteric artery

SUP: Superior

SVC: Superior vena cava

TGC: Time-gain compensation

TRV: Transverse

T-SPINE: Thoracic spine

TV: Tricuspid valve

UT: Uterus

VAG: Vagina

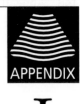

Guidelines for Performance of the Abdominal and Retroperitoneal Ultrasound Examination*

The following are proposed guidelines for ultrasound evaluation of the upper abdomen. The document consists of two parts:

Part I: Equipment and Documentation Guidelines
Part II: Guidelines for a General Examination of the Abdomen and Retroperitoneum

These guidelines have been developed to provide assistance to practitioners performing ultrasound studies in the abdomen and retroperitoneum. In some cases, additional and/or specialized examinations may be necessary. While it is not possible to detect every abnormality, adherence to the following guidelines will maximize the probability of detecting most of the abnormalities that occur in the abdomen and retroperitoneum.

PART I

≡ GUIDELINES FOR EQUIPMENT AND DOCUMENTATION

Equipment

Abdominal and retroperitoneal studies should be conducted with a real-time scanner, preferably using sector or curved linear transducers. Static B-scan images may be obtained as a supplement to the real-time images when indicated. The transducer or scanner should be adjusted to operate at the highest clinically appropriate frequency, realizing that there is a trade-off between resolution and beam penetration. With

*From American Institute of Ultrasound in Medicine. Additional copies of guidelines can be ordered from the AIUM at the cost of $6.00 for AIUM members and $20.00 for nonmembers. Mail orders to AIUM Publications Department, 11200 Rockville Pike, Suite 205, Rockville, MD 20852-3139.

447

modern equipment, these frequencies are usually between 2.25 and 5.0 MHz.

Documentation

Adequate documentation is essential for high-quality patient care. This should be a permanent record of the ultrasound examination and its interpretation. Images of all appropriate areas, both normal and abnormal, should be recorded in appropriate imaging or storage format. Variations from normal size should be accompanied by measurements. Images are to be appropriately labeled with the examination date, patient identification, and image orientation. A report of the ultrasound findings should be included in the patient's medical record, regardless of where the study is performed. Retention of the ultrasound examination should be consistent both with clinical needs and with relevant legal and local health care facility requirements.

PART II

≡ GUIDELINES FOR THE ABDOMEN AND RETROPERITONEUM ULTRASOUND EXAMINATION

The following guidelines describe the examination to be performed for each organ and anatomical region in the abdomen and retroperitoneum. A complete examination would include all of the following. A limited examination would include only one or more of these areas, but not all of them.

Liver

The liver survey should include both long axis (coronal or sagittal) and transverse views. If possible, views comparing the echogenicity of the liver to the right kidney should be performed. The major vessels (aorta/inferior vena cava) in the region of the liver should be imaged, including the position of the inferior vena cava where it passes through the liver.

The regions of the ligamentum teres on the left and of the dome of the right lobe with the right hemidiaphragm and right pleural space should be imaged. The main lobar fissure should be demonstrated.

Survey of right and left lobes should include visualization of the hepatic veins. The right and left branches of the portal vein should be identified. The intrahepatic bile ducts should be evaluated for possible dilatation.

Gallbladder and Biliary Tract

The gallbladder evaluation should include long axis (coronal or sagittal) and transverse views obtained in the supine position. Left lateral decubitus (left side down), erect, or prone positions may also be necessary to allow a complete evaluation of the gallbladder and its surrounding area.

The intrahepatic ducts can be evaluated, as described under the liver, by obtaining a view of the liver demonstrating the right and left hepatic branches of the portal vein. The extrahepatic ducts can be evaluated in supine, left lateral decubitus, and/or semierect positions. The size of the intrahepatic and extrahepatic ducts should be assessed. With these views the relationship among the bile ducts, hepatic artery, and portal vein can be shown. When possible, the common bile duct in the pancreatic head should be visualized.

Pancreas

The pancreatic head, uncinate process, and body should be identified in transverse, and when possible, long axis (coronal or sagittal) projections. If possible, the pancreatic tail should also be imaged, and the pancreatic duct demonstrated. The peripancreatic region should be assessed for adenopathy.

Spleen

Representative views of the spleen in long axis, either sagittal or coronal, and in transverse projection should be performed. An attempt should be made to demonstrate the left pleural space. When possible, the echogenicity of the upper pole of the left kidney should be compared to that of the spleen.

Kidneys

Representative long axis (coronal or sagittal) view of each kidney should be obtained, visualizing the cortex and the renal pelvis. Transverse views of both the left and right kidney should include the upper pole, middle section at the renal pelvis, and the lower pole. When possible, comparison of renal echogenicity with the adjacent liver and spleen should be performed. The perirenal regions should be assessed for possible abnormality.

Aorta and Inferior Vena Cava

The aorta and inferior vena cava should be imaged in long axis (either sagittal or coronal) and transverse planes. Scans of both vessels should be attempted from the diaphragm to the bifurcation (usually at the level of the umbilicus). If possible, images should also include the adjacent common iliac vessels.

Abnormalities should be assessed. The surrounding soft tissues should be evaluated for adenopathy.

Guidelines for Performance of the Scrotal Ultrasound Examination*

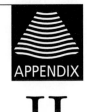

APPENDIX

II

The following are proposed guidelines for ultrasound evaluation of the scrotum. The document consists of two parts:

Part I: Equipment and Documentation Guidelines
Part II: Guidelines for a General Examination of the Scrotum

These guidelines have been developed to provide assistance to practitioners performing ultrasound studies in the scrotum. In some cases, additional and/or specialized examinations may be necessary. While it is not possible to detect every abnormality, adherence to the following guidelines will maximize the probability of detecting most of the abnormalities that occur in the scrotum.

PART I

≡ GUIDELINES FOR EQUIPMENT AND DOCUMENTATION

Equipment

Scrotal studies should be conducted with a real-time scanner, preferably using sector or curved linear transducers. Static B-scan images may be obtained as a supplement to the real-time images when indicated. The transducer or scanner should be adjusted to operate at the highest clinically appropriate frequency, realizing that there is a trade-off between resolution and beam penetration. With modern equipment, these frequencies are usually between 2.25 and 5.0 MHz or greater.

C O M M E N T : Resolution should be of sufficient quality to routinely differentiate small cystic from solid lesions.

*From American Institute of Ultrasound in Medicine. Additional copies of guidelines can be ordered from the AIUM at the cost of $6.00 for AIUM members and $20.00 for nonmembers. Mail orders to AIUM Publications Department, 11200 Rockville Pike, Suite 205, Rockville, MD 20852-3139.

Documentation

Adequate documentation is essential for high-quality patient care. This should be a permanent record of the ultrasound examination and its interpretation. Images of all appropriate areas, both normal and abnormal, should be recorded in any image format. Variations from normal size should be accompanied by measurements. Images are to be appropriately labeled with the examination date, patient identification, and image orientation. A report of the ultrasound findings should be included in the patient's medical record, regardless of where the study is performed. Retention of the ultrasound examination should be consistent both with clinical need and with relevant legal and local health care facility requirements.

PART II

≡ GUIDELINES FOR THE SCROTAL ULTRASOUND EXAMINATION

The testes should be studied in at least two projections, long axis and transverse. Views of each testicle should include the superior, mid, and inferior portions as well as its medial and lateral borders. The adjacent epididymis should be evaluated. The size and echogenicity of each testicle and epididymis should be compared to its opposite side.

Any abnormality should be documented and all extratesticular structures evaluated. Additional techniques such as Valsalva maneuver or upright positioning can be utilized as needed.

Guidelines for Performance of the Antepartum Obstetrical Ultrasound Examination*

These guidelines have been developed for use by practitioners performing obstetrical ultrasound studies. A limited examination may be performed in clinical emergencies or if used as a follow-up to a complete examination. In some cases, an additional and/or specialized examination may be necessary. While it is not possible to detect all structural congenital anomalies with diagnostic ultrasound, adherence to the following guidelines will maximize the possibility of detecting many fetal abnormalities.

Equipment

These studies should be conducted with real-time scanners, using an abdominal and/or vaginal approach. A transducer of appropriate frequency (3 MHz or higher abdominally, 5 MHz or higher vaginally) should be used. A static scanner (3 to 5 MHz) may be used but should not be the sole method of examination. The lowest possible ultrasonic exposure settings should be used to gain the necessary diagnostic information.

C O M M E N T : Real-time is necessary to reliably confirm the presence of fetal life through observation of cardiac activity, respiration, and active movement. Real-time studies simplify evaluation of fetal anatomy as well as the task of obtaining fetal measurements. The choice of frequency is a trade-off between beam penetration and resolution. With modern equipment, 3- to 5-MHz abdominal transducers allow sufficient penetration in nearly all patients, while providing adequate resolution. During early pregnancy, a 5-MHz abdominal or a 5- to 7-MHz vaginal transducer may provide adequate penetration and produce superior resolution.

---

*From American Institute of Ultrasound in Medicine. Additional copies of guidelines can be ordered from the AIUM at the cost of $6.00 for AIUM members and $20.00 for nonmembers. Mail orders to AIUM Publications Department, 11200 Rockville Pike, Suite 205, Rockville, MD 20852-3139.

Documentation

Adequate documentation of the study is essential for high-quality patient care. This should include a permanent record of the ultrasound images, incorporating whenever possible the measurement parameters and anatomical findings proposed in the following sections of this document. Images should be appropriately labeled with the examination date, patient identification, and if appropriate, image orientation. A written report of the ultrasound findings should be included in the patient's medical record regardless of where the study is performed.

≡ GUIDELINES FOR FIRST TRIMESTER SONOGRAPHY

Overall Comment: Scanning in the first trimester may be performed either abdominally or vaginally. If an abdominal scan is performed and fails to provide definitive information concerning any of the following guidelines, a vaginal scan should be performed whenever possible.

1. The location of the gestational sac should be documented. The embryo should be identified and the crown-rump length recorded.

C O M M E N T :   The crown-rump length is an accurate indicator of fetal age. Comparison should be made to standard tables. If the embryo is not identified, characteristics of the gestational sac including mean diameter of the anechoic space to determine fetal age and analysis of the hyperechoic rim should be noted. During the late first trimester, biparietal diameter and other fetal measurements may also be used to establish fetal age.

2. Presence or absence of fetal life should be reported.

C O M M E N T :   Real-time observation is critical in this diagnosis. It should be noted that fetal cardiac activity may not be visible prior to 7 weeks abdominally and frequently at least 1 week earlier vaginally as determined by crown-rump length. Thus, confirmation of fetal life may require follow-up evaluation.

3. Fetal number should be documented.

C O M M E N T :   Multiple pregnancies should be reported only in those instances where multiple embryos are seen. Due to variability in fusion between the amnion and chorion, the appearance of more than one sac-like structure in early pregnancy is often noted and may be confused with multiple gestation or amniotic band.

4. Evaluation of the uterus (including cervix) and adnexal structures should be performed.

C O M M E N T :   This will allow recognition of incidental findings of potential clinical significance. The presence, location, and size of myomas and adnexal masses should be recorded.

≡ GUIDELINES FOR SECOND AND THIRD TRIMESTER SONOGRAPHY

1. Fetal life, number, and presentation should be documented.

C O M M E N T :   Abnormal heart rate and/or rhythm should be reported. Multiple pregnancies require the reporting of additional information: placental number, sac number, comparison of fetal size, and when visualized, fetal genitalia, and presence or absence of an interposed membrane.

2. An estimate of the amount of amniotic fluid (increased, decreased, normal) should be reported.

C O M M E N T :   While this evaluation is subjective, there is little difficulty in recognizing extremes of amniotic fluid volume. Physiological variation with stage of pregnancy must be taken into account.

3. The placental location, appearance, and its relationship to the internal cervical os should be recorded.

C O M M E N T :   It is recognized that placental position early in pregnancy may not correlate well with its location at the time of delivery.

4. Assessment of gestational age should be accomplished using combination of biparietal diameter (or head circumference) and femur length. Fetal growth and weight (as opposed to age) should be assessed in the third trimester and requires the addition of abdominal diameters or circumferences. If previous studies have been performed, an estimate of the appropriateness of interval change should be given.

C O M M E N T :   Third trimester measurements may not accurately reflect gestational age. Initial determination of gestational age should therefore be performed prior to the third trimester whenever possible. If one or more previous studies have been performed, the gestational age at the time of the current examination should be based on the earliest examination that permits measurement of crown-rump length, biparietal diameter, head circumference, and/or femur length by the equation: current fetal age equals initial embryo/fetal age plus number of weeks from first study. The current measurements should be compared with norms for the gestational age based on standard tables. If previous studies have been performed, interval change in the measurements should be assessed.

4A. Biparietal diameter at a standard reference level (which should include the cavum septi pellucidi and the thalamus) should be measured and recorded.

C O M M E N T :   If the fetal head is dolichocephalic or brachycephalic, the biparietal diameter alone may be misleading. On occasion, the computation of the cephalic index, a ratio of the biparietal diameter to fronto-occipital diameter, is needed to make this determination. In such situations, the head circumference or corrected biparietal diameter is required.

4B. Head circumference is measured at the same level as the biparietal diameter.

4C. Femur length should be measured routinely and recorded after the 14th week of gestation.

C O M M E N T :   As with biparietal diameter, considerable biological variation is present late in pregnancy.

4D. Abdominal circumference should be determined at the level of the junction of the umbilical vein and portal sinus.

C O M M E N T :   Abdominal circumference measurement may allow detection of growth retardation and macrosomia—conditions of the late second and third trimester. Comparison of the abdominal circumference with the head circumference should be made. If the abdominal measurement is below or above that expected for a stated gestation, it is recommended that circumferences of the head and body be measured and the head circumference/abdominal circumference ratio be reported. The use of circumferences is also suggested in those instances where the shape of either the head or body is different from that normally encountered.

5. Evaluation of the uterus and adnexal structures should be performed.

C O M M E N T :   This will allow recognition of incidental findings of potential clinical significance. The presence, location, and size of myomas and adnexal masses should be recorded.

6. The study should include, but not necessarily be limited to, the following fetal anatomy: cerebral ventricles, four-chamber view of the heart (including its position within the thorax), spine, stomach, urinary bladder, umbilical cord insertion site on the anterior abdominal wall, and renal region.

C O M M E N T :   It is recognized that not all malformations of the above-mentioned organ systems (such as the spine) can be detected using ultrasonography. Nevertheless, a careful anatomical survey may allow diagnosis of certain birth defects that would otherwise go unrecognized. Suspected abnormalities may require a specialized evaluation.

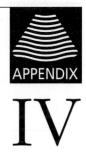

Guidelines for Performance of the Ultrasound Examination of the Female Pelvis*

The following are proposed guidelines for ultrasound evaluation of the female pelvis. The document consists of two parts:

Part I: Equipment and Documentation Guidelines
Part II: Guidelines for the General Examination of the Female Pelvis

These guidelines have been developed to provide assistance to practitioners performing ultrasound studies of the female pelvis. In some cases, additional and/or specialized examinations may be necessary. While it is not possible to detect every abnormality, adherence to the following guidelines will maximize the probability of detecting most of the abnormalities that occur.

PART I

≡ GUIDELINES FOR EQUIPMENT AND DOCUMENTATION

Equipment

Ultrasound examination of the female pelvis should be conducted with a real-time scanner, preferably using sector or curved linear transducers. Static B-scan images may be obtained as a supplement to the real-time images when indicated. The transducer or scanner should be adjusted to operate at the highest clinically appropriate frequency, realizing that there is a trade-off between resolution and beam penetration. With modern equipment, studies performed from the anterior abdominal wall can usually use frequencies of 3.5

---

*From American Institute of Ultrasound in Medicine. Additional copies of guidelines can be ordered from the AIUM at the cost of $6.00 for AIUM members and $20.00 for nonmembers. Mail orders to AIUM Publications Department, 11200 Rockville Pike, Suite 205, Rockville, MD 20852-3139.

MHz or higher, while scans performed from the vagina should use frequencies of 5 MHz or higher.

Care of the Equipment

Vaginal probes should be covered by a protective sheath prior to insertion. Following the examination, the sheath should be disposed and the probe cleaned in an antimicrobial solution. The type of solution and amount of time for cleaning depends on manufacturer and infectious disease recommendations.

Documentation

Adequate documentation is essential for high-quality patient care. There should be a permanent record of the ultrasound examination and its interpretation. Images of all appropriate areas, both normal and abnormal, should be recorded in an imaging or storage format. Variations from normal size should be accompanied by measurements. Images are to be appropriately labeled with the examination date, patient identification, and image orientation. A report of the ultrasound findings should be included in the patient's medical record. Retention of the permanent record of the ultrasound examination should be consistent both with clinical need and with the relevant legal and local health care facility requirements.

PART II

≡ GUIDELINES FOR PERFORMANCE OF THE ULTRASOUND EXAMINATION OF THE FEMALE PELVIS

The following guidelines describe the examination to be performed for each organ and anatomic region in the female pelvis. Identifying all relevant structures should be identified by the abdominal or vaginal approach; in some cases, both will be necessary.

General Pelvic Preparation

For a pelvic sonogram performed from the abdominal wall, the patient's urinary bladder should be filled. For a vaginal sonogram, the urinary bladder is usually empty. The vaginal transducer may be introduced by the patient, the sonographer, or the sonologist. It is recommended that a woman should be present in the examining room at all times during a vaginal sonogram, either as an examiner or a chaperone.

Uterus

The vagina and uterus provide an anatomic landmark that can be utilized as a reference point for the remaining normal and abnormal pelvic structures. In evaluating the uterus, the following should be documented: a) the uterine size, shape, and orientation; b) the endometrium; c) the myometrium; and d) the cervix. The vagina should be imaged as a landmark for the cervix and lower uterine segment.

Uterine size can be obtained. Uterine length is evaluated in long axis from the fundus to the cervix (the external os, if it can be identified). The depth of the uterus (anteroposterior dimension) is measured in the same long axis view from its anterior to posterior walls, perpendicular to the length. The width is measured from the transaxial or coronal view. Cervical diameters can be similarly obtained.

Abnormalities of the uterus should be documented. The endometrium should be analyzed for thickness, echogenicity, and its position within the uterus. The myometrium and cervix should be evaluated for contour changes, echogenicity, and masses.

Adnexa (Ovaries and Fallopian Tubes)

When evaluating the adnexa, an attempt should be made to identify the ovaries first since they can serve as the major point of reference for adnexal structures. Frequently the ovaries are situated anterior to the internal iliac (hypogastric) vessels, which serve as a landmark for their identification. The following ovarian findings should be documented: a) size, shape, contour, and echogenicity and b) position relative to the uterus. The ovarian size can be determined by measuring the length in long axis, usually along the axis of the hypogastric (internal iliac) vessels, with the anteroposterior dimension measured perpendicular to the length. The ovarian width is measured in the transaxial or coronal view. A volume can be calculated.

The normal fallopian tubes are not commonly identified. This region should be surveyed for abnormalities, particularly dilated tubular structures.

If an adnexal mass is noted, its relationship to the ovaries and uterus should be documented. Its size and echopattern (cystic, solid, or mixed) should be determined.

Cul-de-Sac

The cul-de-sac and bowel posterior to the uterus may not be clearly defined. This area should be evaluated for the presence of free fluid or mass. If a mass is detected, its size, position, shape, echopattern (cystic, solid, or complex), and its relationship to the ovaries and uterus should be documented. Differentiation of normal loops of bowel from a mass may be difficult if only an abdominal examination is performed. If a suspected mass is imaged that might represent fluid and feces within normal rectosigmoid colon and a vaginal scan is not performed, an ultrasound water enema study or a repeat examination after a cleansing enema may be indicated.

APPENDIX

V

Guidelines for Performance of the Ultrasound Examination of the Prostate (and Surrounding Structures)*

The following are proposed guidelines for the ultrasound evaluation of the prostate and surrounding structures. The document consists of two parts:

Part I: Equipment and Documentation
Part II: Ultrasound Examination of the Prostate and Surrounding Structures

These guidelines have been developed to provide assistance to practitioners performing an ultrasound study of the prostate. In some cases, an additional and/or specialized examination may be necessary. While it is not possible to detect every abnormality, adherence to the following will maximize the detection of most abnormalities.

PART I

≡ EQUIPMENT AND DOCUMENTATION

Equipment

A prostate study should be conducted with a real-time transrectal (also termed endorectal) transducer using the highest clinically appropriate frequency, realizing that there is a trade-off between resolution and beam penetration. With modern equipment, these frequencies are usually 5 MHz or higher.

*From American Institute of Ultrasound in Medicine. Additional copies of guidelines can be ordered from AIUM at the cost of $6.00 for AIUM members and $20.00 for nonmembers. Mail orders to AIUM Publications Department, 11200 Rockville Pike, Suite 205, Rockville, MD 20852-3139.

Documentation

Adequate documentation is essential for high-quality patient care. There should be a permanent record of the ultrasound examination and its interpretation. Images of all appropriate areas, both normal and abnormal, should be accompanied by measurements. Images are to be appropriately labeled with the examination date, patient identification, and image orientation. A report of the ultrasound findings should be included in the patient's medical record. Retention of the permanent record of the ultrasound examination should be consistent both with clinical need and with the relevant legal and local health care facility requirements.

Care of the Equipment

Transrectal probes should be covered by a disposable sheath prior to insertion. Following the examination, the sheath should be disposed, and the probe soaked in an antimicrobial solution. The type of solution and amount of time for soaking depends on manufacturer and infectious disease recommendations. Following the examination, if there is a gross tear in the sheath, the fluid channels in the probe should be thoroughly flushed with the antimicrobial solution. Tubing and stop cocks should be disposed after each examination.

PART II

≡ ULTRASOUND EXAMINATION OF THE PROSTATE AND SURROUNDING STRUCTURES

The following guidelines describe the examination to be performed for the prostate and surrounding structures.

Prostate

The prostate should be imaged in its entirety in at least two orthogonal planes, sagittal and axial or sagittal and coronal, from the apex to the base of the gland. In particular, the peripheral zone should be thoroughly imaged. The gland should be evaluated for size, echogenicity, symmetry, and continuity of margins. The periprostatic fat and vessels should be evaluated for asymmetry and disruption in echogenicity.

Seminal Vesicles and Vas Deferens

The seminal vesicles should be examined in two planes from their insertion into the prostate via the ejaculatory ducts to their cranial and lateral extents. They should be evaluated for size, shape, position, symmetry, and echogenicity. Both vas deferens should be evaluated.

Perirectal Space

Evaluation of the perirectal space, in particular the region that abuts on the prostate and perirectal tissues, should be performed. If rectal pathology is clinically suspected, the rectal wall and lumen should be studied.

Index

Note: Page numbers in *italic* refer to illustrations: those followed by t refer to tables.

ISBN 0-7216-6879-8